Brain Tumors

Edited by Amit Agrawal

Published in London, United Kingdom

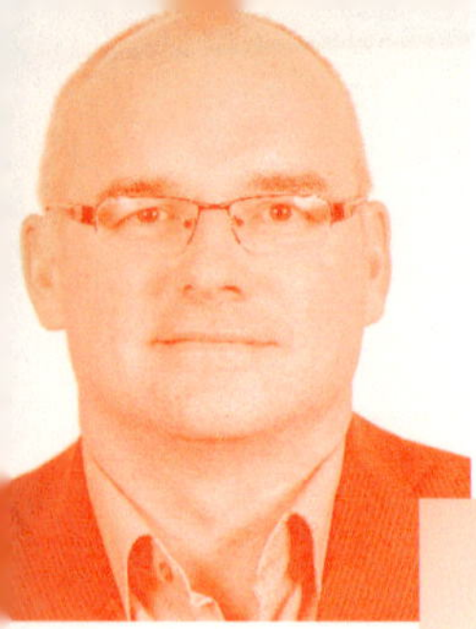
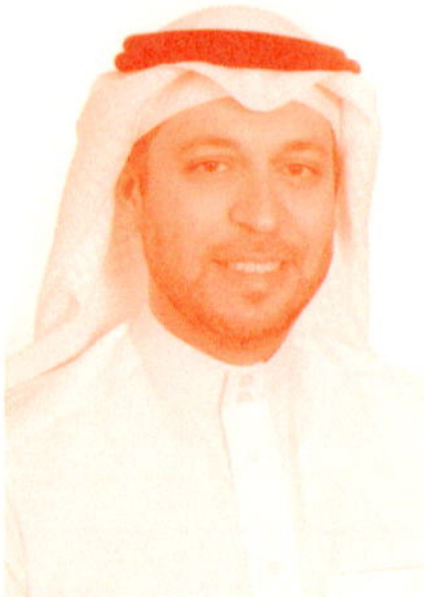
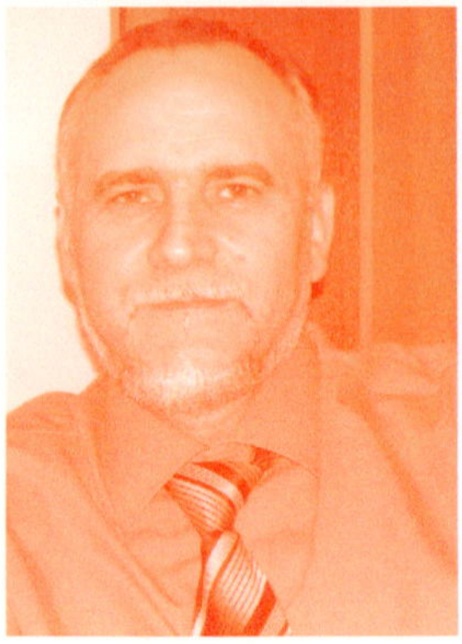
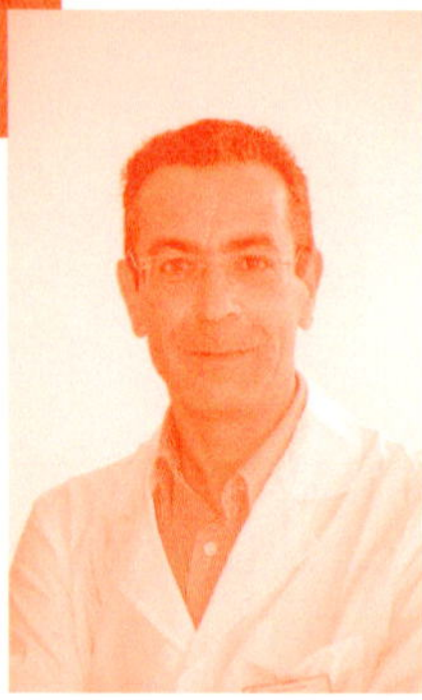
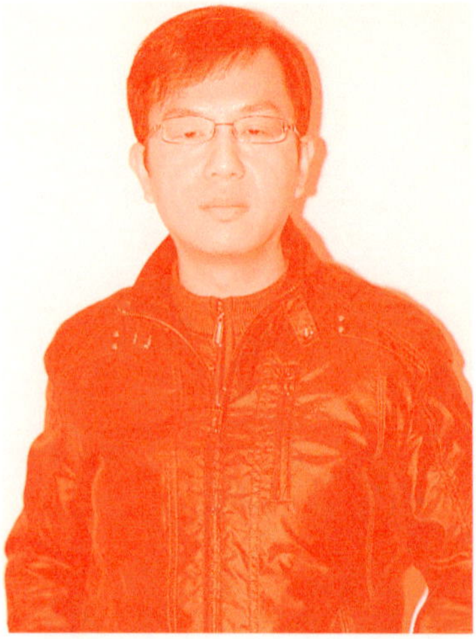
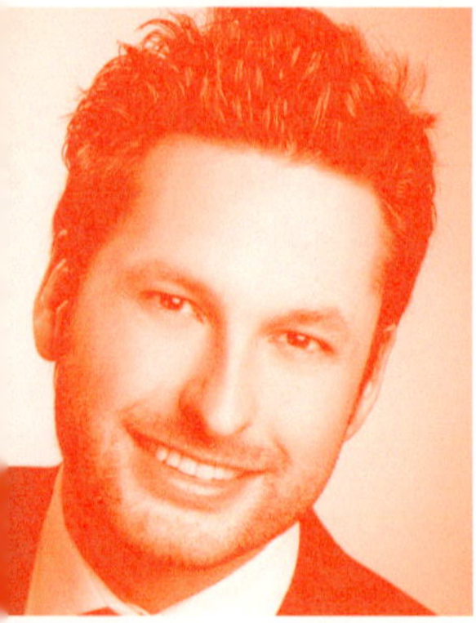
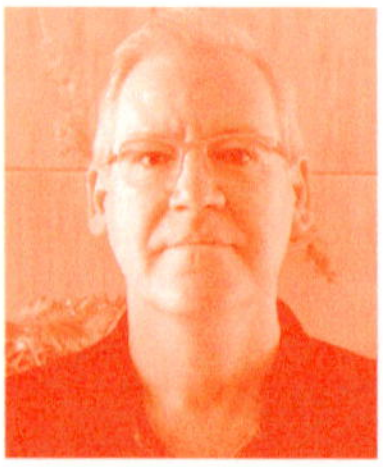

IntechOpen

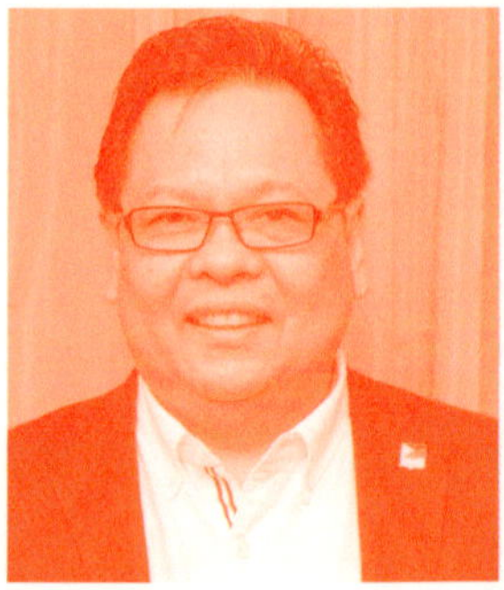
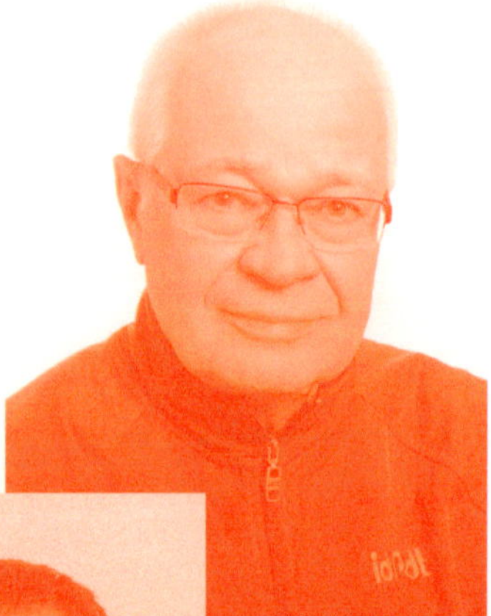
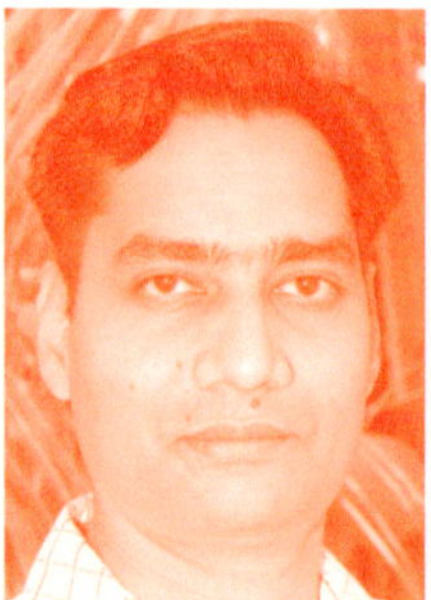
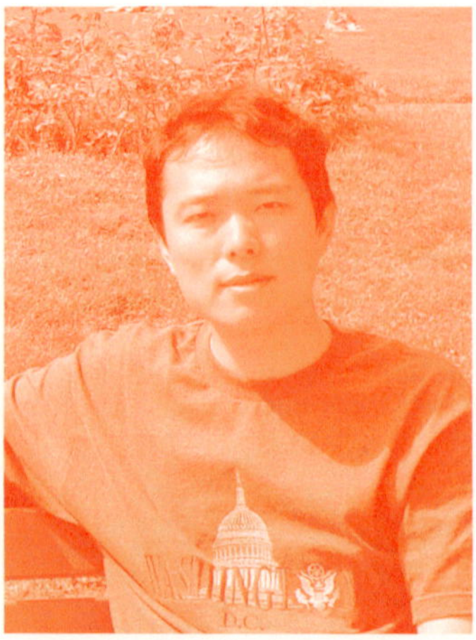
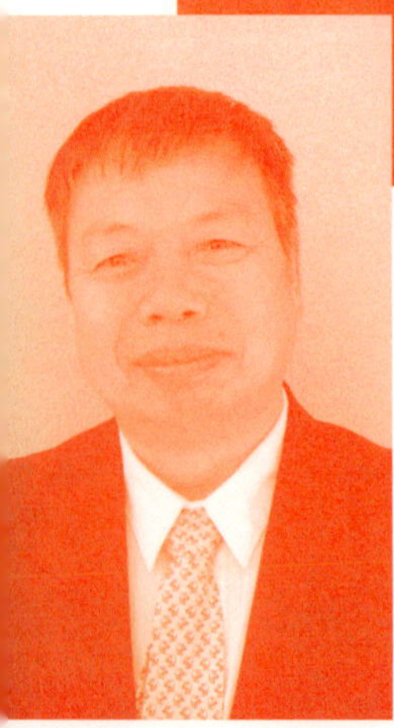
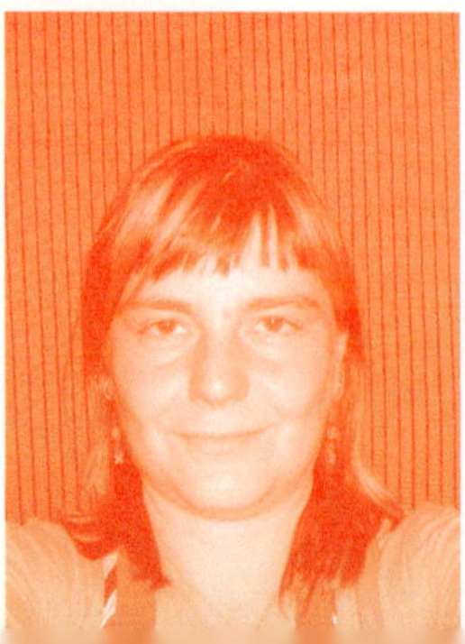

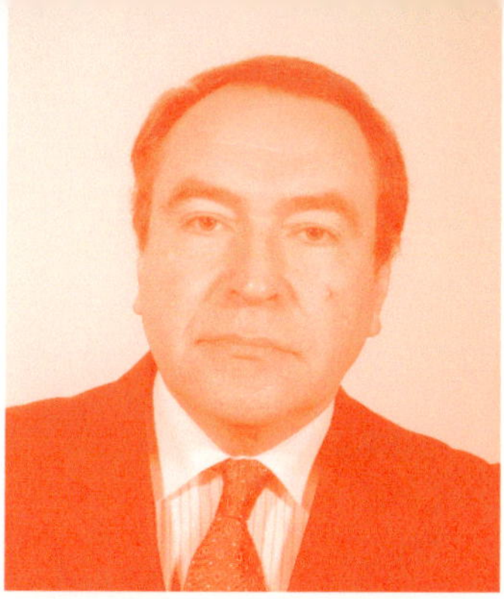
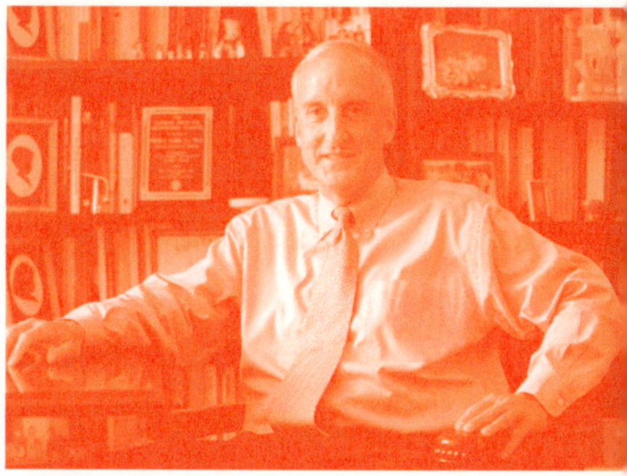
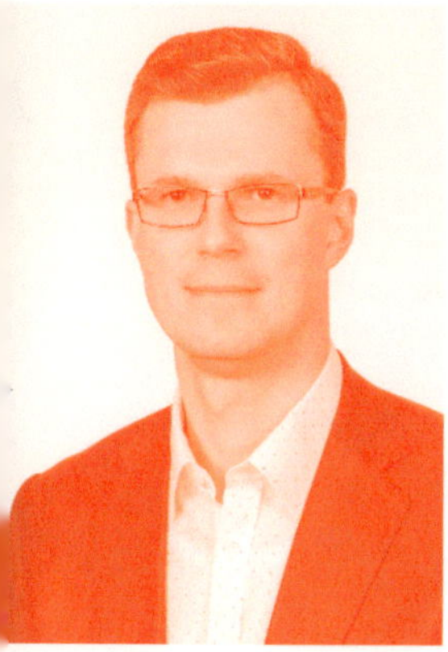
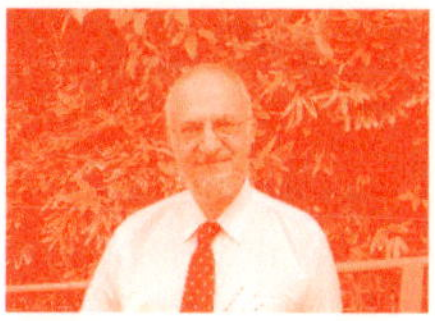
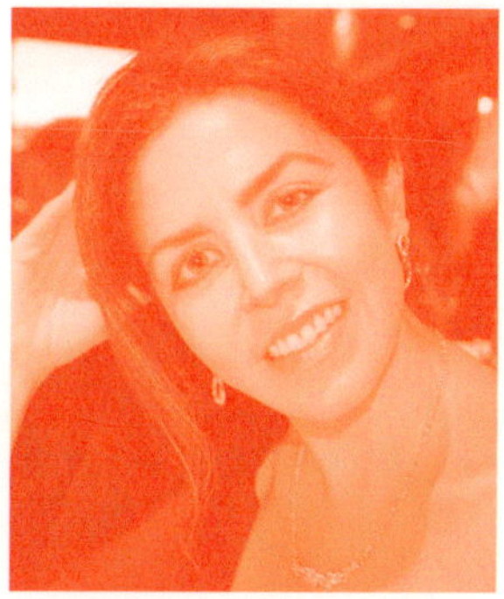

Supporting open minds since 2005

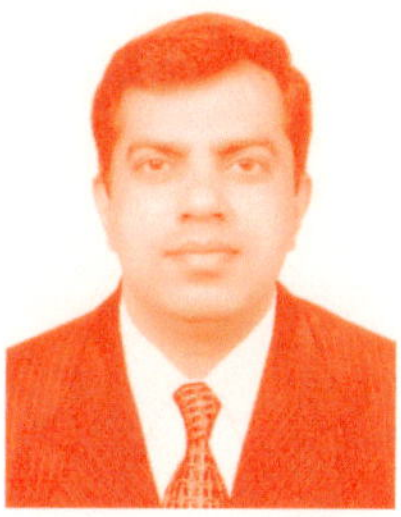
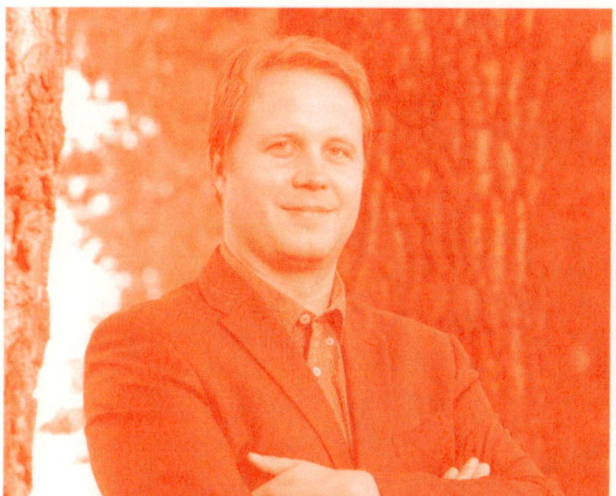
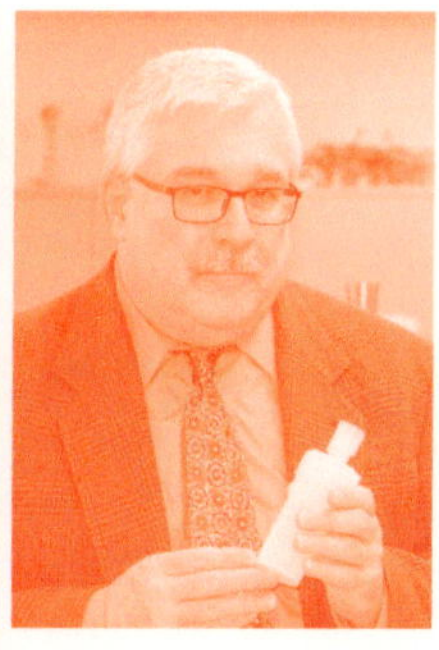
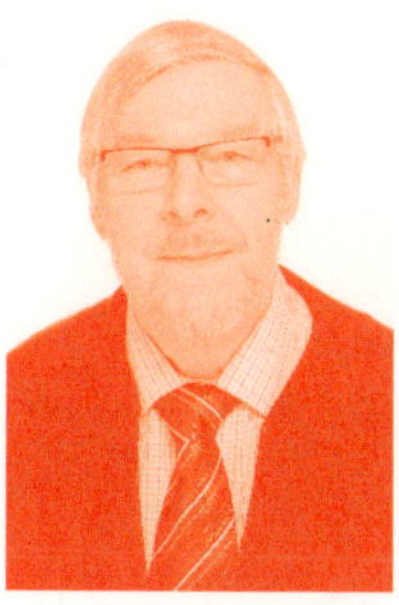
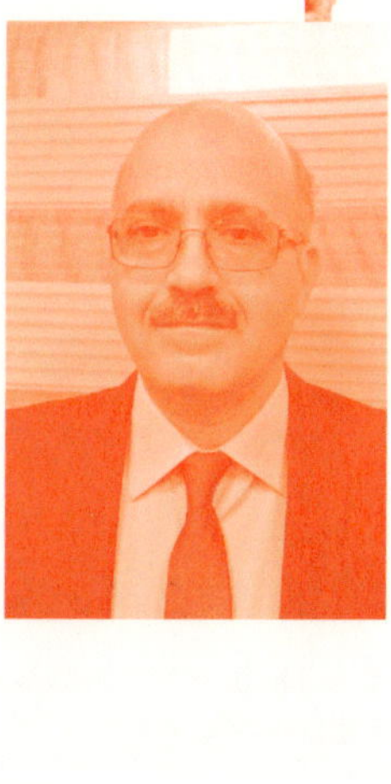
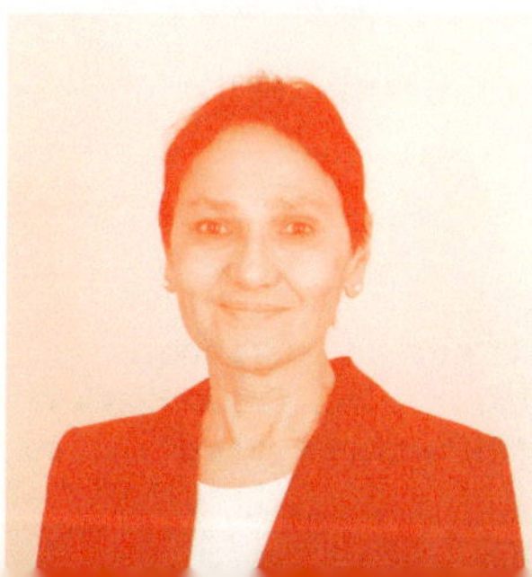
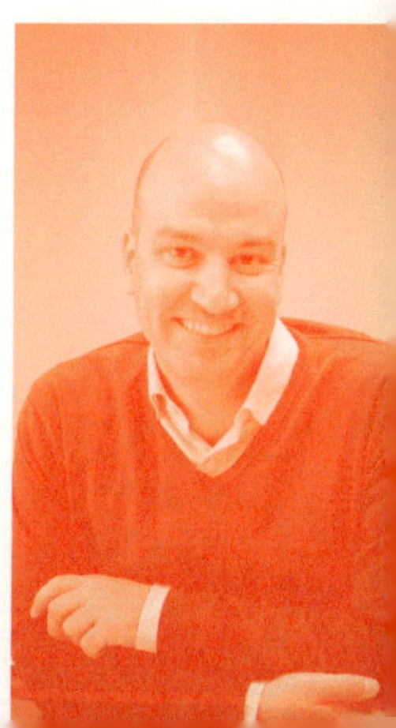

Brain Tumors
http://dx.doi.org/10.5772/intechopen.94814
Edited by Amit Agrawal

Contributors
John A. Ozolek, Tak Lap Poon, Ka Wing See, José Luis Navarro-Olvera, Armando Armas-Salazar, José Damián Carrillo-Ruiz, Jesús Q. Beltrán, Gustavo Parra-Romero, Gustavo Aguado-Carrillo, Manimekalai Pichaivel, Gayathri Anbumani, Murugananthan Gopal, Panneerselvam Theivendren, Sukanya Bhunia, Arabinda Chaudhuri, Catherine T. Flores, Mathew Sebastian, Bayli DiVita Dean, Andres F. Cardona, Juan Esteban Garcia-Robledo, Camila Ordóñez-Reyes, Alejandro Ruiz-Patiño, Álvaro Muñoz, Oscar Arrieta, Enrique Jiménez, Fernando Hakim, Diego Gómez, Juan Fernando Ramón, Julio Plata-Bello, Helga Fariña-Jeronimo, Yaiza Pérez-Martín

First published in London, United Kingdom, 2022 by IntechOpen
IntechOpen is the global imprint of INTECHOPEN LIMITED, registered in England and Wales, registration number: 11086078, 5 Princes Gate Court, London, SW7 2QJ, United Kingdom
Printed in Croatia

British Library Cataloguing-in-Publication Data
A catalogue record for this book is available from the British Library

Additional hard and PDF copies can be obtained from orders@intechopen.com

Brain Tumors
Edited by Amit Agrawal
p. cm.
Print ISBN 978-1-83969-803-3
Online ISBN 978-1-83969-804-0
eBook (PDF) ISBN 978-1-83969-805-7

For EU product safety concerns:
IN TECH d.o.o., Prolaz Marije Krucifikse Kozulić 3, 51000 Rijeka, Croatia, info@intechopen.com or visit our website at intechopen.com.

Meet the editor

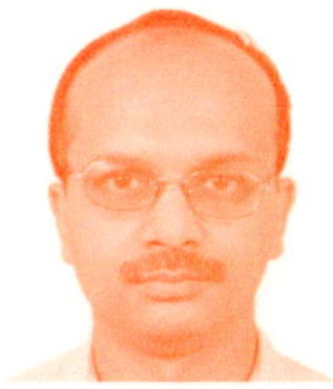

Dr. Agrawal completed his neurosurgery training at the National Institute of Mental Health and Neurosciences, Bangalore, India, in 2003. He is a self-motivated, enthusiastic, and results-oriented professional with more than eighteen years of experience in research and development, as well as teaching and mentoring in the field of neurosurgery. He is proficient in managing and leading teams for running successful process operations and has experience in developing procedures and service standards of excellence. He has attended and participated in many international and national symposiums and conferences and delivered lectures on vivid topics. Dr. Agrawal has published more than 750 scientific articles in various national and international journals. His expertise is in identifying training needs, designing training modules, and executing the same while working with limited resources. He has excellent communication, presentation, and interpersonal skills with proven abilities in teaching and training various academic and professional courses. Presently, he is working at the All India Institute of Medical Sciences, Bhopal, Madhya Pradesh, India.

Contents

Preface

Central nervous system (CNS) groups of tumours have no pathognomonic presentation, however, they do present with clinical features such as increased intracranial pressure, focal neurological deficits, or seizures (generalized or partial). Recent advances in genetic testing have improved our understanding of brain tumours and have been helpful in deciding management and follow-up strategies. It is anticipated that life expectancy will increase and thus it will be important to further define management protocols and identify potential targets for future clinical trials to improve outcomes as well as the quality of life in patients with brain tumours. Recent advances in genetic testing are continuously improving our understanding of meningiomas and have been helpful in deciding management and follow up strategies. It is further anticipated that an increase in life expectancy shall further increase the incidence of symptomatic meningiomas and thus it will be important to further define the management protocols and identify potential targets for future clinical trials to improve outcomes, as well as the quality of life in these patients. This book is a collection of high-quality research work on brain tumours, including meningiomas, and their treatment.

Amit Agrawal
Professor,
Department of Neurosurgery,
All India Institute of Medical Sciences,
Bhopal, India

Chapter 1

An Overview of Brain Tumor

Manimekalai Pichaivel, Gayathri Anbumani, Panneerselvam Theivendren and Muruganantham Gopal

Abstract

Brain tumor is an abnormal growth of mass of cells in (or) around the brain. Brain tumors can be malignant (cancerous) or being non-cancerous. It is the most common malignant primary intracranial tumors of central nervous system. Brain tumor can affect brain function if they grow large enough to press on surrounding nerves, blood vessels and tissues. Only one third of tumors formed in the brain are formed as cancerous cells. Brain tumors release molecular information to the circulation. Liquid biopsies collect and analyse tumor component in the body fluid and there is an increasing interest in investigation of liquid biopsies as substitute from tumor markers. Tumor-derived biomarkers include nucleic acids, proteins and tumor-derived extracellular vesicles that accumulate in blood (or) cerebrospinal fluid. Circulating biomarkers like O-6-methylguanine DNA methyl transferase, epidermal growth factor, isocitrate dehydrogenase, circulating tumor cells, circulating cell free micro RNAs, circulating extracellular vesicles plays and important role in causing a cancer. Brain tumor can be treated by surgery, radiation therapy (or) targeted therapy. Radiation therapy is often given afterwards. As a consequence, the most recent review reviewed the present state of research with the hopes of discovering a new brain tumor inhibitor that may be used to treat advanced malignancies.

Keywords: brain tumor, bio-markers, circulating bio-marker, O-6-methylguanine DNA methyl transferase

1. Introduction

A brain tumor is one of the most malignant tumors in humans. It accounts for approximately 1.35% of all malignant neoplasm and 29.5% of cancer-related death [1]. Brain and CNS tumors include tumors of the brain, cranial nerves, spinal nerves, spinal cord, and the meninges. The tumor can be broadly classified as malignant and non-malignant (or benign) tumors. The world health organization (WHO) classification specifies a grading system ranging from grade, whereas, grade III/IV are malignant or high grade [2]. A brain tumor is a diverse group of neoplasm with different types of primary brain tumor (or) metastatic cancer. The most common malignant brain tumors are glioblastoma that originates from glial cells [3]. Metastatic brain tumors (MBTs) account for the majority of an intra-axial brain tumors in adult patients. It is estimated that up to one-third of patients diagnosed with a primary malignancy will develop central nervous system metastatic lesions during their disease course [4]. Pediatric central nervous system (CNS) tumors are the second most common childhood malignancy and the most common solid tumor in children [5]. Early diagnosis and treatment of brain tumors are imperative to prevent permanent damage to the brain (or) death of the patient. At the level of medical data analysis, the features election and classification process are the ones intensively used to identify the patient data whether it is normal (or) abnormal [6]. Once the tumor is detected under the microscope. It is often too late for effective treatment prognosis in patients is correlated with the stage of disease at the time of detection and therefore, it is important to find markers that allow the early detection of the tumor. The treatment options for patients with brain metastases include corticosteroids, surgery, chemotherapy, whole-brain radiation therapy, and stereotactic radiosurgery [7]. A patient with a brain tumor suffers from a significant problem called neurocognitive dysfunction. To diagnose the neurocognitive dysfunction in the brain tumor needs new strategies for the early initiation of appropriate neurocognitive rehabilitation. Raman spectroscopy technique is used for the differentiation of brain tumors. This leads to accurate identification of two essential factors such as brain tumor boundary and the complete resection of the tumor which is important for removal of glioma tumor in brain surgery [8].

2. Pathophysiology

In the 19th century, Stephen Paget postulated the "seed and soil" hypothesis, which considers that metastatic growth depends on cancer cells (the seed) interactions with and affinity for specific distant organ tissues (the soil). Paget's assertion that a nutritional microenvironment is imperative for metastatic cells to grow in distant tissues is supported by conceptual frameworks of contemporary cancer research [9]. A more advanced understanding of the complex and multifactorial mechanisms of metastasis formation consists of three premises: first, the existence of tumor heterogeneity, including morphologically- and phenotypically-distinct profiles of cancer cells with different proliferative, angiogenic, invasive, and metastatic characteristics; second, a metastatic process that is selective for tumor cells that accomplish all the key steps of the metastatic cascade; and third, the metastatic potential of a tumor, which depends on multiple, reciprocal interactions between the primary tumor and the tumor microenvironment, as well as homeostatic mechanisms [10]. This reciprocal cross-talk determines tumor progression and the potential for metastatic growth. As in the periphery, a brain tumor's microenvironment plays a critical role in metastatic colonization of the brain; but the outgrowth of tumor cells to the brain depend on specific behaviors of the tumor cells and conditions in the brain tumor microenvironment. In the literature, at least three microenvironments have been considered involved in brain metastasis formation: the perivascular niche, the brain parenchyma, and the cerebrospinal fluid also termed the leptomeningeal niche [11]. As the brain tumor grows it creates pressure on and changes the function of surrounding cells and it leads to symptoms. Most cases of Brain Tumor travel by hematogenous spread and occur most often at the gray-white matter junction [4]. The markers involved in the brain tumor are as follows:

A. Circulating tumor cells

B. O-6 methylguanine-DNA mutations

C. Epidermal growth factor receptor

D. Isocitrate dehydrogenase

E. Circulating free DNA

F. Circulating proteins

G. Tumor protein39.

H. Tumor protein 53.

A. Circulating tumor cells

Circulating tumor cells (CTCs) are cells that are shed from primary or metastatic tumors in the body fluids, including blond, cerebrospinal fluid, and urine. CTCs determine the ability of epithelial tumor cells to metastasize [12]. These different types of potential biomarkers in the blood can be present in cell-free forms, attached to lipid or protein structures, or delivered by circulating extracellular vesicles or platelets [13]. CTCs are also used in the monitoring of glioblastoma patients. The level of CTCs detected after chemotherapy is significantly lower compared to their level before the treatment, which may provide invaluable insight in differentiating tumor progression from radiation necrosis [14, 15].

B. O-6 methylguanine-DNA methyltransferase mutations (MGMT)

The gene encoding O-6-methylguanine DNA methyltransferase (MGMT) is found on chromosome 10q26 [4]. By methylating DNA base pairs, alkylating chemotherapeutic drugs such as temozolomide impair DNA replication. Active MGMT reverses the effect of temozolomide, enabling normal DNA replication to occur within a tumor [16]. O-6-methyl transferase DNA methyltransferase contributes to DNA repair by reversing DNA alkylation and eliminating the guanine-alkyl group, therefore preventing apoptosis. MGMT has recently been established as a biomarker for tumor diagnosis [17]. Methylation promotes the gene code for MGMT in glioblastoma and is the genetic fingerprint with the greatest influence on clinical practice. The presence of O-6-methylguanine-DNA methyltransferase (MGMT) suggests that the current standard of treatment, adjuvant chemoradiotherapy with the alkylating drug temozolomide, is more effective [18–20].

C. Epidermal growth factor receptor

Most signaling pathways and physiological responses, including migration, proliferation, survival, and tumor development, are activated by the epidermal growth factor receptor (EGFR). EGF, TGF-, heparin-binding epidermal growth factor-like factor (HB-EGF), amphiregulin (AR), betacellulin (BTC), neuregulins (NRGs), also known as neuregulin; neu differentiation factors; glial growth factors; acetylcholine receptor inducing activity; and epiregulin are all members of the EGF superfamily (EPR) [21, 22].

D. Isocitrate dehydrogenase

Isocitrate dehydrogenase (IDH) is a protein enzyme that encodes genes on chromosome 2, the main function of IDH in the Krebs cycle is to catalyze oxidative decarboxylation [4]. IDH has been grouped into two classes (IDH 1 and IDH 2). Mutation of isocitrate dehydrogenase 1 (IDH-1) in glioblastoma was first noted by following an integrated genomic analysis of human glioblastoma samples [16]. The IDH-1 protein protects the cytoplasm against oxidative damage. In 12% of glioblastoma samples, a heterozygous point mutation at R132 was discovered. Glioblastomas that were known to have developed from lower-grade tumors had a considerably greater prevalence of IDH-1 mutation (83%) [23]. Grade II/III astrocytomas, oligoastrocytomas, and oligodendrogliomas all have isocitrate dehydrogenase, which can be utilized to distinguish primary from secondary glioblastomas [24, 25].

E. Circulating free DNA

Cell-free DNA (cfDNA) as a double-stranded, DNA fragments released for the breakdown of cancer tissue by bloodstream that is approximately 150 to 200 base pairs in length, corresponding to nucleosome-associated DNA, can be released by cells under physiological and pathological conditions as well. It is suggested that cfDNA could be derived from apoptotic or necrotic cells, rapidly dividing cells, or CTCs [4]. Blood cfDNA is mostly derived from genomic DNA released during inflammation or cell death in people without cancer. Due to phagocyte clearance, the concentration of cfDNA in the blood is low in physiological settings. Circulating protein markers may be used to track the efficacy of therapy in patients with brain tumors. Current MR imaging techniques cannot effectively detect the unique biological tumor characteristics and complicated tissue changes produced by various cancer treatments [26, 27].

The incidence of detectable ctDNA varies significantly across patients with various tumor types. The concentration of cancer cell-generated ctDNA in plasma in glioblastoma is low when compared to other cancer types, which might be due to the existence of the blood–brain barrier. In glioblastoma, ctDNA analysis presents a number of difficulties. Aside from the common issues of short half-lives (1.5 h) of ctDNA fragments, distinguishing mutant from wild-type alleles, and developing mutation thresholds, the primary issue is the low amount of ctDNA in the samples [28].

F. Circulating proteins

Several tumor-derived circulating nucleic acids (e.g., ctDNA, cmtDNA, mRNA, non-coding RNAs including miRNAs, long non-coding RNAs) that can be detected from blood or other types of body fluids like urine, cerebrospinal fluid (CSF), saliva, pleural fluid, and ascites. In brain tumor patients, the secretion of the proteins may lead to an increase in the level of circulating proteins (CPs) in the blood and urine and/or CSF [4]. Angiogenesis-related protein markers were discovered in malignancies. The amount of vascular endothelial growth factor was shown to be substantially greater in brain tumor patients than in healthy persons, and even higher in patients with brain metastases [29]. There are two types of prognostic CP indicators: tumor-associated markers and related markers with endogenous systemic stress responses. Overall survival was adversely associated with the tumor-related plasma markers YKL-40, the extracellular domain of EGFR, and osteopontin [30, 31].

G. Tumor protein 39 (TP39)

Tumor protein 39A (TP39A) belongs to the Transmembrane protein 39 families (TMEM39), consisting of TMEM39A and TMEM39B. The two TMEM39 isoforms are produced via alternative splicing. The

TMEM39A-encoding gene may be a susceptibility causes the brain tumor [4]. Transmembrane proteins across the plasma membrane from one side to the other. The movement of materials across biological membranes is regulated by several transmembrane proteins. Multiple sclerosis susceptibility may be linked to the TMEM39A-encoding gene. TMEM39A has also been linked to systemic lupus erythematosus [32, 33].

H. Tumor protein 53 (TP53)

TP53 is a typical tumor suppressor gene located in 17p13.1. This encodes the nuclear protein p53. To regulate the expression of its target genes the p53 protein responds to diverse cellular stresses, thereby inducing cell cycle arrest, apoptosis, senescence, DNA repair, or metabolic changes. Several human malignancies, including Li-Fraumeni syndrome and numerous hereditary gliomas, are linked to mutated TP53 genes and overexpressed aberrant p53 protein, which has a longer half-life than wild type p53 [4]. If p53 mutations are important in the start of malignant transformation of glial cells, i.e., if they play the function of "mutator" mutations, families with hereditary mutations of one of the p53 alleles would be expected to develop CNS malignancies. Furthermore, the histological kind of glioma that was found should match the usual histology of gliomas with a p53 mutation [34].

The well-known tumor suppressor protein p53 is encoded by the TP53 gene. It is known as the genome's guardian, and it has a variety of tasks in preventing tumor development. Secondary brain cancers (90 percent) have considerably more TP53 point mutations than initial brain tumor (30%), and in rare cases, primary lesions had none at all [35, 36].

3. Epidemology

Population-based studies are generally considered more accurate and less biased than the more limited clinical (or) autopsy-based series [37]. The exact incidence of brain metastases is unknown. The epidemiological study is done by using the hospital records, tumor registers, and death certificates. Finally from this study, the incidence of brain metastases seems equal to the incidence of gliomas [38]. The survival rate by histology is summarized in **Figure 1**.

A. Meningiomas

Meningiomas are the most common brain tumors in adults accounts about 36% of all brain tumors in the central brain tumor registry of the united states (CBTRUS). In 2015 CBTRUS estimates that there will be approximately 24,000 new meningiomas diagnosed in the united states [37]. The incidence of meningioma steadily increases with age being twice as common in women as in men and 20% more common in blacks than in whites. A majority of meningiomas are benign (grade I), with 5–20% atypical (grade II) and 1–3% malignant in type (grade III) [38, 39].

Although benign meningiomas are a minor cause of death, skull-based tumors can cause considerable morbidity. Atypical and malignant meningiomas, on the other hand, are linked to high rates of recurrence and substantial morbidity and death [40, 41]. Meningioma is shown in **Figure 2**. Because telomerase activity is detected in all anaplastic/malignant (WHO grade III)

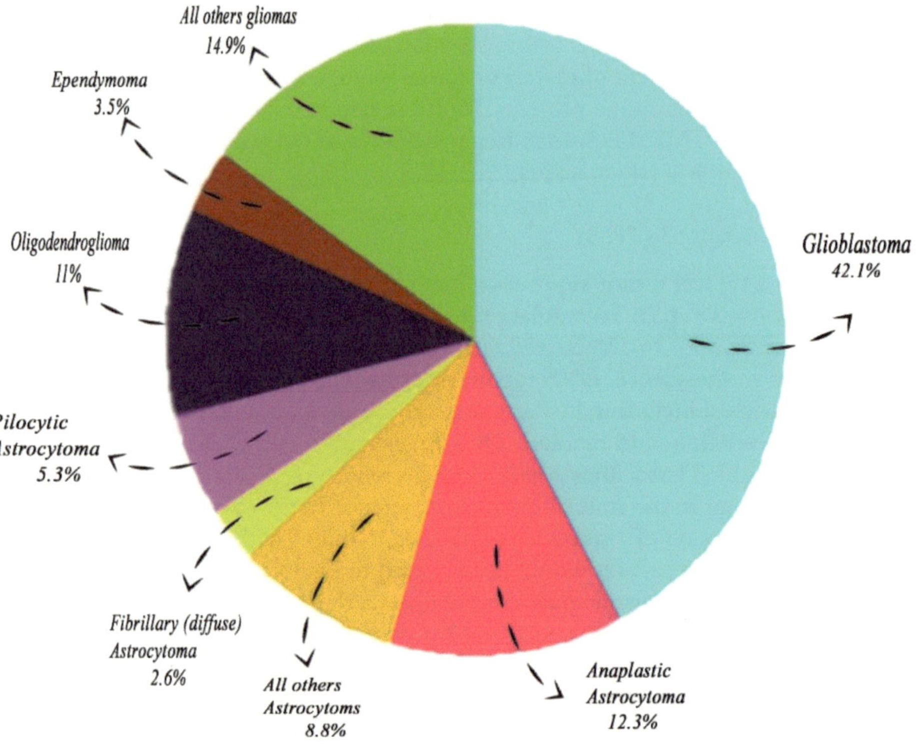

Figure 1.
CNS tumor epidemiology -the incidence of brain tssumor in different regions of brain.

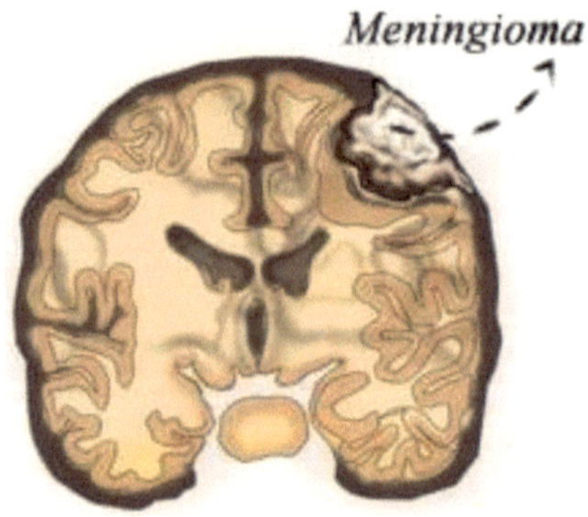

Figure 2.
Brain meningioma.

and the majority of atypical (WHO grade II) meningiomas, there is a link between telomerase activity and tumor grading in meningiomas [42, 43].

B. Glioma

Glioma is the second most common brain tumor in adults. In 2015 the CBTRUS estimates approximately 20,000 newly diagnosed gliomas in the united states. Approximately one-half of gliomas is glioblastoma, the commonest malignant primary brain tumor in adults. Glioma occurs almost in all four lobes in the brain: frontal (23.6%), temporal (17.4%), parietal (10.6%), occipital (2.8%), a small percentage in the brain stem, cerebellum and spinal cord [20].

Glioma is shown in **Figure 3.** Secondary glioblastomas are considered to develop as a result of progression from pre-existing astrocytomas, thus this finding is fascinating [44].

C. Pituitary tumor

The third most common brain tumor in adults is the pituitary tumor and it accounts for 15%. A majority of brain tumors are benign adenomas [45]. Even people who do not produce hormones might have symptoms as a result of the intracranial mass effect. Hormones that control normal pituitary function, as well as growth factors implicated in normal fetal pituitary development, appear to stimulate tumor growth [46, 47]. Pituitary tumor is shown in **Figure 4**.

D. Pediatric brain tumor

CNS tumors in children are the second most frequent malignancy in children and the most common solid tumor in children. According to CBTRUS, about 2000 children in the United States are diagnosed with a brain tumor before the age of 14. The most frequent solid tumor in babies and toddlers is a brain tumor. More than 8% of children and adolescent cancers are caused by genetic predisposition syndromes, and this percentage is anticipated to climb as research continues [3].

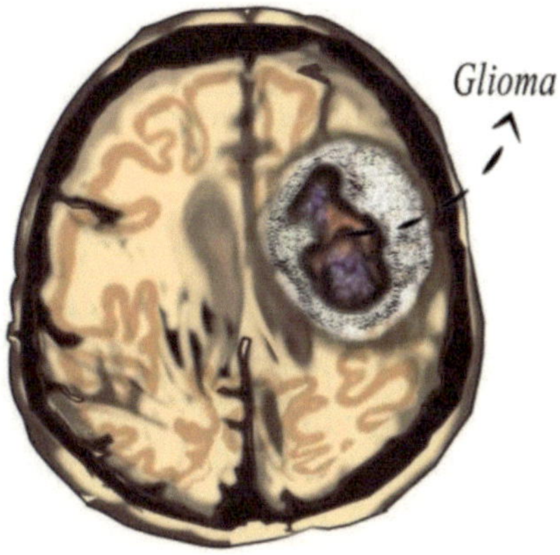

Figure 3.
Glioma.

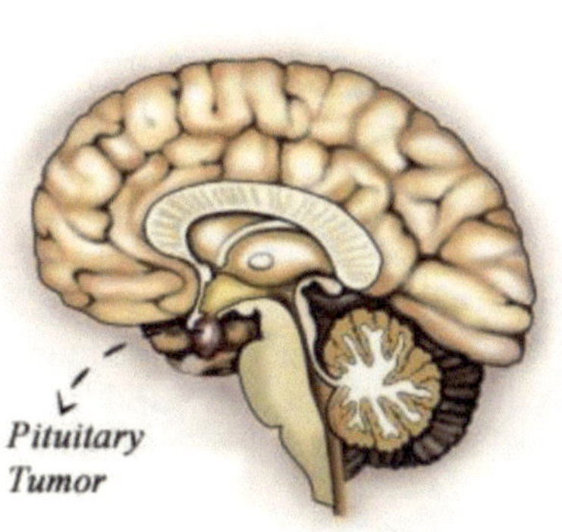

Figure 4.
Pituitary tumor.

Non–posterior fossa embryonal tumors, also known as CNS-primitive neuroectodermal tumors (PNETs), are a kind of uncommon juvenile brain tumor that accounts for less than 3% of all cases and has a dismal prognosis [46]. All CNS embryonal tumors are very malignant and are classified as WHO grade IV tumors by the World Health Organization. Many tumors classified as supratentorial embryonal tumors histologically cluster with other tumor types, such as high-grade gliomas and ependymomas, according to molecular studies; this has major therapeutic implications in terms of the amount of radiotherapy required for tumor control and the choice of adjuvant chemotherapy or biologic therapy [47, 48].

4. Signs and symptoms

A. Headache

Headache occurs commonly in all brain tumor patients. The headache is said to develop in the temporal and the spatial, relation to the neoplasm and resolves 7 days of surgical removal or treatment with corticosteroids [48].

Headache in pituitary brain tumor

The presence of headache has been shown to be more highly associated with family history than the tumor size [47].

Headache in pediatric brain tumor

Headache appears to be the most common presenting symptom (41% of patients in some studies). It tends to occur with other symptoms such as vomiting, unsteadiness, behavioral problems, and cranial nerve palsies, and most commonly nocturnally (or) in the early morning [49].

Mechanism of headache in brain tumor

The mechanism of headache in brain tumors may include the traction on vascular structure, cranial or central sensitization through neurogenic inflammation as well as the component of central sensitization through trigeminovascular afferents on the meninges and the cranial nerves [50].

B. Nausea and vomiting

Nausea and vomiting occur when the chemo trigger zone in the area postrema, located on the floor of the fourth ventricle is stimulated. Raised intracranial pressure leads to vomiting. It can also occur in the absence of elevated intracranial pressure in brain stem tumors involving the nucleus solitarius [51].

Mechanism of vomiting

Nausea and vomiting are highly conserved responses and the survival advantages in survival vertebrates. Vomiting is primitive, low-threshold, brain stem response that allows the human to purge the gastrointestinal tract of orally consumed noxious substances. Vomiting is multidimensional having a higher cognitive brain center, emotions, and interoceptive domains is more common disabling, and more difficult to control than vomiting [52].

C. Altered mental status

Mental and cognitive abnormalities may be specific, or nonspecific. Specific findings include aphasia, agnosia, abulia, alexia, or apraxia. In about 16–34%

of patients, the symptoms for brain tumor patients include irritability, change in personality, emotional liability, forgetfulness, lack of enthusiasm or spontaneity, and slowed response progressing apathy and lathery [53].

D. Papilledema

Papilledema is an indicator of increased intracranial pressure it is now rarely seen in patients at the time of presentation of the tumor. Like headache, papilledema is seen mostly seen in young adults and children, this is probably because older adults have tumor expansion due to tumor atrophy [53].

Mechanism of papilledema

The mechanism of papilledema is due to axoplasmic flow stasis. High intracranial pressure produces raise in cerebrospinal fluid pressure surrounding the optic nerve, which disturbs the normal gradient between intraocular pressure retro lamellar pressure leading to high pressure within the nerves and this leads to papilledema [54].

E. Seizures

Seizure is the most frequent symptom in patients with brain tumors. The incidence of brain tumors varies 30–100% depending on the tumor type and location with a slow-growing tumor that is being epileptogenic [53]. Brain tumor patients with epilepsy will have a high risk of seizure-related morbidities, mortality as well as experience a low quality of life [55].

Mechanism of seizure

The mechanism of seizure in brain tumor patients involves changes in aminoacid neurotransmission is the most important mechanism underlying tumor-related seizures and changes in extracellular ions also play an important role. Hypoxia, acidosis, metabolic, immunological, and inflammatory changes may also be involved in seizure occurrence [56].

5. Diagnosis

Diagnostic tests to detect these changes using biomarkers show significant potential for early detection [57]. Development of neurologic deficits and new-onset seizures are commonly followed by neurologic workup that includes magnetic resonance imaging (MRI). Computer tomography (CT) with contrast enhancement is less sensitive in detecting the typical features of glioblastoma [58].

A. WCFS-IBMDNT

Many recent studies have attempted to define the characteristics of brain tumors to diagnose the illnesses. However, with a large dataset, the correlations across brain tumor characteristics limit the illness diagnosis performance. Furthermore, when using standard approaches for categorization, misclassification outcomes might arise. The WCFS-IBMDNL approach employs the IBMDNN classifier after selecting a subset of characteristics for efficient brain tumor diagnosis with low time complexity. The most significant diagnostic approach used to diagnose brain tumors is Weighted Co-relation Feature Selection Based Iterative Bayesian Multivariate Deep Neural Learning (WCFS-IBMDNT). The WCFS-IBMDNT approach was created to enhance brain tumor diagnosis by requiring the least amount of time [59]. The major importance of WCFS-IBMDNT are as follows:

1. The WCFS-IBMDNT technique was designed to enhance the prediction of brain tumors based on classification. Weighed correlation-based feature selection is the traditional method and performs WC-FS for highlighting the characterization of brain tumors by the subset of medicinal hights [59]

2. First it is proposed to enhance the performance of brain tumor prediction via a classification technique. The proposed WCFS-IBMDNL technique is designed with the implementation of WC-FS and IBMDNN classifier [59].

3. The feature selection procedure for providing effective brain tumor detection diagnostic is carried out using WC-FS. The Pearson correlation coefficient is used in WCFS-IBMDNL, which is a first. The Pearson correlation coefficient is used to determine the relationship between two medical variables to choose a group of medical parameters that are most important to the categorization of brain tumors [59].

4. The IBMDNN classifier is used in the proposed WCFSIBMDNL method to improve brain tumor diagnostic classification performance. BMLR is also utilized in the IBMDNN classifier to analyze medical characteristics to categorize patients as normal or abnormal. The least absolute error is calculated after the categorization. Finally, to reduce the error rate, the IRLS technique is utilized. This contributes to a higher illness detection rate while lowering the FAR [59].

B. Magnetic resonance imaging (MRI)

MRI is the most important technique for the diagnosis of brain tumors. MRI is used in the biomedical to detect and visualize finer details in the internal structure of the body. This technique is used to detect the differences in the tissues. MRI is fundamentally better than CT scanning [60]. This study proposes the computer-assisted computed organization feature extraction with abnormal MRI images of brain tumors to develop the accuracy of classification results according to the original feature classification. The initial input database images are fed for pre-processing and the images are transferred as 3×3 blocks. Then for each image of 3×3 blocks, 22 number of texture feature was extracted. Then the extracted feature was used to classify the brain tumor as normal as unusual [61].

The most prevalent metabolites of the brain, such as N-acetyl aspartate (NAA), choline (Cho), creatine (Cr), lipid, and lactate, may be quantified using MR spectroscopy (MRS) [57]. Choline is considered to correspond with cell turnover, therefore variations in Cho might be linked to the stage of radio-necrosis. Cho rises in the first few months following radiation therapy, according to two studies, but it declines as radionecrosis develops, according to Rock et al. Rapid Cho, on the other hand, is a common characteristic of tumor recurrence due to high cell turnover [62].

C. CT Scanning (computer tomography)

Computer tomography has a high accuracy than magnetic resonance imaging MRI. CT uses ionizing radiation for the diagnosis of brain tumors. This is used for the diagnosis of primary glaucoma and lymphoma of the Central Nervous System (CNS) was performed [59]. A CT scan may reveal hypodensity in the white matter, as well as a mass effect on surrounding structures. In vascular metastases, localized bleeding may be observed [63].

D. Fused MRI and CT Analysis

Tumor identification is done using a combination of computed tomography CT and MRI scans. Multiple modalities such as CT and MRI are utilized to create the merged pictures (MRI). CT pictures, which are utilized to determine the difference in tissue density, and MRI images, which give a good contrast between distinct bodily tissues, play a vital role in medical image processing [64]. CT pictures show differences in tissue density based on the tissues' capacity to respond to X-rays, whereas MRI images show the contrast between soft tissues. When compared to the source pictures, the fused image retains the complementary and redundant information from both source images, including tumor size and position, allowing for better tumor detection [65].

E. Positron emission tomography [PET]

The brain's major energy source is aerobic glucose metabolism. The most commonly used PET radiotracer, F18-FDG, is actively transported across the BBB and accumulates in areas where aerobic glucose metabolism is enhanced. FDG accumulation is proportional to glucose metabolism in the cell, and higher accumulation correlates to higher cellular metabolism. The brain's typical strong metabolic activity causes high uptake in the normal brain parenchyma, resulting in poor tumor-to-brain contrast. Another possible stumbling block is the nonspecific nature of FDG absorption, which may be seen in inflammatory and infectious processes [66].

PET radiolabelled amino acids increase proportionately to cellular proliferation due to enhanced transport. Tumors increase transporter activity, metabolic enzyme activity, and demand, resulting in increased radiotracer accumulation proportionate to protein synthesis and food demand [67].

F. Single-photon emission computed tomography [SPECT]

SPECT is a low-cost imaging technique that is readily available and may be used in conjunction with CT and MRI to evaluate tumors and RN. In the post-treatment context, a variety of SPECT radiotracers are available for brain tumor imaging. Thallium201 is very accurate for post-treatment evaluation of tumor burden because it concentrates on living tumors; nevertheless, Thallium201 has nonspecific absorption in non-neoplastic processes such as granulomatous or fungal etiologies [66].

Thallium201 absorption is unaffected by the BBB and is primarily determined by the pace of cell growth, making it highly selective for brain tumors. Thallium201-SPECT had a sensitivity of 71.7 percent and a specificity of 80.9 percent for supratentorial brain tumors, according to a retrospective analysis of 90 patients. Because tumor growth rates are substantially greater than normal brain parenchyma, thalllium201 accumulates in brain malignancies without considerable absorption in the normal brain parenchyma, producing good tumor-to-background contrast [68, 69].

6. Types of brain tumor

The brain plays an important role in the body by controlling voluntary and involuntary processes. It is highly necessary to maintain a healthy brain to live longer. But some factors like environmental and genetic factors tumors in the brain can be developed [70]. These tumor causes the damage in healthy tissues and increases the pressure in the brain. Thus, some tissues may get pushed against the skull.

The tumors are classified according to the place they occur and the type of cell as follows:

1. The type and grade

2. Primary or secondary tumor

3. Malignant or benign tumor

4. Tumor location [71].

According to WHO (World Health Organization) brain tumors are classified as:

1. Astrocytoma

2. Glioblastoma

3. Oligodendroglioma [71].

1. Astrocytoma

   Astrocytoma tumors arise from the supportive glial cells of the brain. About 7% of the primary brain tumor are astrocytoma. A star-shaped tumor that begins in the brain is called astrocytoma. In adults, the astrocytoma most often arises in the cerebrum, wherein in children it occurs in the brain stem [63].

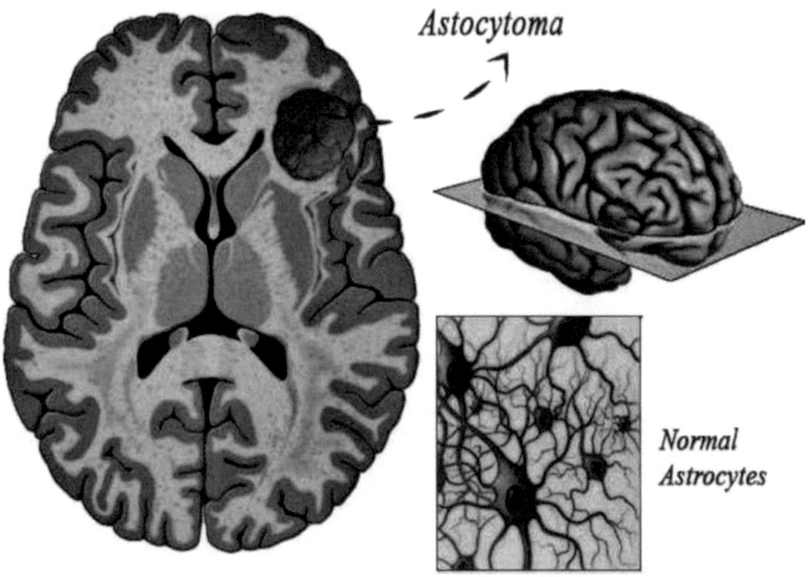

Figure 5.
Astrocytoma.

Astrocytoma is shown in **Figure 5.** The basal ganglia and thalamus are the two most likely locations where the long-term prognosis is poorer than for hemisphere injuries [72]. Post-operative radiation is a treatment option for low-grade gliomas. However, one disadvantage of radiation is that it causes neurocognitive damage and does not result in considerable improvement. As a result, radiation is often reserved for individuals with tumors that are at high risk of malignant transformation [73].

2. Glioblastoma

Glioblastomas (GBMs) is the most common and primary aggressive brain tumor. Glioblastoma is shown the **Figure 6**. Glioblastoma accounts for 45.6% of primary malignant brain tumors. Typical molecular changes in glioblastoma include mutation in gene-regulating receptor tyrosine kinase (RTK) / phosphoinositide 3-kinase (PI3K), p53, and retinoblastoma protein (RB) signaling [71]. Secondary glioblastoma is a kind of glioblastoma that develops in younger people when a previous malignancy, such as grade II astrocytoma or anaplastic astrocytoma, somatically mutates into a glioblastoma [74].

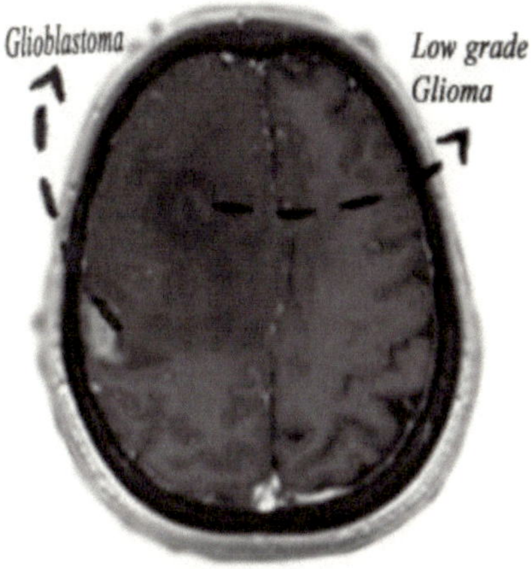

Figure 6.
Glioblastoma.

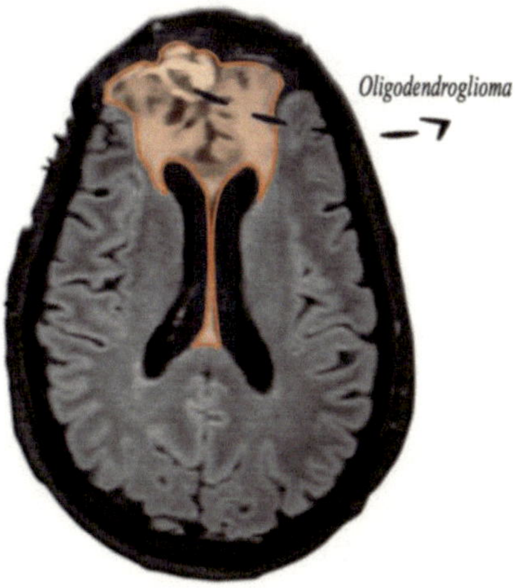

Figure 7.
Oligodendroglioma.

3. Oligodendroglioma

   Oligodendroglioma is a rare form of brain tumor. The brain is made up of many supporting cells that are called glial cells. Any tumor of these glial cells is called glioma. A tumor that arises from the glial cells (oligodendrocyte cells) is called oligodendroglioma [72]. Oligodendrogliomas vary from other glial tumors in their molecular genetic makeup. On chromosome 1p and chromosome 19q, LOH is seen often in oligodendrogliomas of all grades [75]. Oligodendroglioma is shown in **Figure 7.**

7. Pediatric brain tumor

The pediatric brain tumor is the second most childhood malignant brain tumor and the most common solid tumor in children. The genetic syndromes that cause brain tumors are due to NF-1, tuberous sclerosis, Li-Fraumeni syndrome, and other less common inherited conditions, such as Gorlin syndrome or Turcot syndrome [76].

1. low-grade glioma

   Low-grade gliomas (LGGs) is the most common pediatric central nervous system (CNS) tumor and it comprises for 30–40% of all CNS tumor. LGGs are infiltrative and incurable primary brain tumors with a typical slow evolution. Treatment of this low-grade glioma includes chemotherapy, radiation therapy, and targeted therapy [77].

2. High-grade glioma

   High grade comprises up to 12% of pediatric CNS tumors and it includes anaplastic astrocytoma (WHO grade III) and glioblastoma (WHO grade IV). The symptoms depend on tumor location. The treatment method includes chemotherapy regimens that have been studied in the patients with high-grade gliomas, including temozolomide, lomustine, and thalidomide but have unfortunately not resulted in significant improvement in survival rates [78].

3. Medulloblastoma

   Medulloblastoma is the most common CNS embryonal tumor. It represents about 10% of all pediatric brain tumors [79]. Medulloblastoma is the most common malignant brain tumor in children accounting for approximately 25% of pediatric brain tumors, with many reports indicating an increase in medulloblastoma in recent years [80].

4. Ependymoma

   Ependymomas are tumors of the central nervous system that derive from the ependymal cells that line the ventricles of the brain and the central canal of the spinal cord [81]. Ependymoma can occur throughout the neuroaxis-supratentorial, posterior fossa, and spinal cord; however, 90% of pediatric ependymomas occur intracranially with 2/3 in the posterior fossa and 1/3 supratentorially [82].

8. Molecular genetics of brain tumor

The molecular genetics of brain tumors is due to the mutation in enzymatic activity. The mutation rate that commonly occurs in various gene to cause brain tumor are:

1. Astrocytoma a grade II, III type of brain tumor is due to IDH mutation, P53 mutation, ATRX mutation.

2. Glioblastoma a grade IV type is due to amplification of EGFR, PDGFRA amplification mutation of EGFRvIII, deletion of PTEN homozygous, CDKN2A homozygous deletion, BRAF V600E mutation, (epithelioid GBM) TP53 mutation.

3. Oligodendroglioma a grade II, III is due to IDH mutation, 1p/19q codeletion, CIC/FUBP1 mutation, TERTp mutation [83].

A. Mutation IDH1/2

IDH catalyzes the oxidative decarboxylation of isocitrate to generate (-KG) and CO2, however, mutant IDH1/2 preferentially binds -KG rather than isocitrate outside of the citric acid cycle, resulting in the formation and accumulation of the oncometabolite 2-hydroxyglutarate (2HG) [84].

HIF1 (Hypoxia Inducible Factor) levels and alterations in the HIF1 downstream pathway are modulated by -KG–dependent prolyl hydroxylases, resulting in an increase in reactive oxygen species levels and potentially contributing to the risk of cancer [85].

B. TP53 mutation

TP53 is a tumor suppressor gene that encodes the nuclear protein p53 and is found on the 17p13.1 chromosome [86]. Several human malignancies, including Li-Fraumeni syndrome and numerous hereditary gliomas, are linked to mutated TP53 genes and over-expressed aberrant p53 protein, which has a longer half-life than wild type p53 [87].

C. ATRX is an X-linked gene of α- Thalassemia and mental retardation syndrome

ATRX is a 280-kDa nuclear protein that has been implicated in a variety of biological activities including DNA recombination, repair, and transcription control. It is found on chromosome 21.1 and encodes a 280-kDa nuclear protein [88]. When ATRX and DAXX connect, the resulting complex acts as a histone chaperone, allowing histone variation H3.3 to be deposited into heterochromatic repeats such as pericentric, telomeric, and ribosomal DNA repeat regions [89].

D. EGFR amplification and EGFRvIII truncation mutation

EGFR, also known as Erb1 or HER1, is an ErbB family receptor tyrosine kinase that is found on chromosome 7q12. EGFR over-expression is linked to EGFR amplification. The EGFRvIII mutation is a frame deletion of 801 bytes from exons 2 to 7 of the EGFR gene, which is linked to EGFR amplification, antibody response, and poor prognosis [90, 91].

E. BRAF mutation

Pilocytic astrocytoma is defined by BRAF V600E mutations and BRAF fusions with KIAA1549 or FAM131B. A tandem duplication at 7q34 was verified, and a novel fusion gene was discovered in pilocytic astrocytoma, which was previously uncharacterized by a fusion between the KIAA1549 and BRAF genes [92].

9. Treatment method of brain tumor

A. Immunotherapy

When it comes to treating brain tumors, immunotherapy is a potential treatment option. Chemotherapy, radiation treatment, and surgery have all been used to treat it in the past. An immune-based cancer therapy uses the body's immune system to destroy cancer cells [93]. If the cells are no longer required or pose a hazard, apoptosis, or programmed cell death, will occur to halt cell growth [94]. Cancer progresses and develops through eight processes, which are as follows:

1. Stained proliferation

2. Evasion of growth suppressor

3. Cell death resistance

4. Replicative immortality

5. Angiogenesis

6. Metastasis

7. Reprogrammed metabolism

8. Evasion of immune destruction [95].

The evasion of immune destruction has been studied for decades. Because EphA2 is abundantly expressed in glioblastoma but only at low levels in normal brain tissue, CAR T cell treatment targeting the glioblastoma antigen EphA2 is an appealing strategy to enhance outcomes [93].

Since brain tumor immunotherapy has been extensively studied [94–96], we will focus in this work on the most recent and late-stage clinical trial treatments, as well as the engineering problems these immunotherapies confront in the brain tumor environment [96].

i. Vaccines

Traditional vaccinations against viral illnesses (for example, influenza) employ attenuated or live viruses in combination with a danger signal (as an adjuvant) to activate DCs. DCS then takes up the viral antigen, digests it, moves to lymph nodes through lymphatic channels, and activates T-cells via the presentation of various peptide antigens/antigenic epitopes on MHC molecules [93].

a. Peptide vaccines

Immunization using peptide vaccine when released at the tumor site, peptide vaccinations stimulate T-cell responses by releasing antigen-specific peptides. APCs take up peptides, which are often associated with carrier proteins and adjuvants, and display them on the cell surface by way of MHC [97]. The treatment method by peptide vaccine is explained in **Figure 8**.

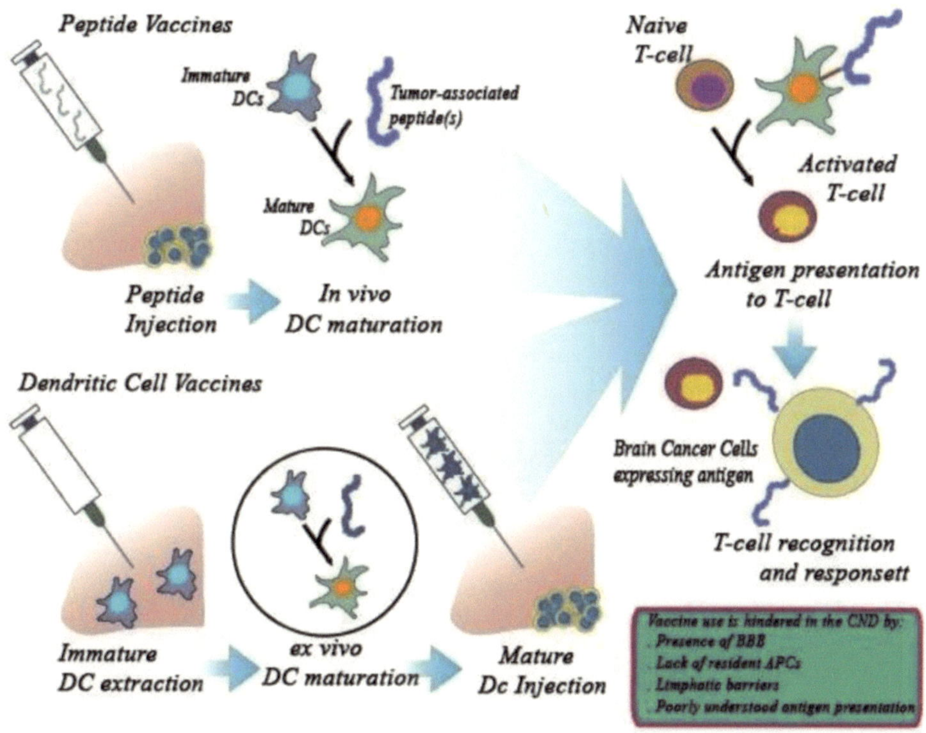

Figure 8.
Dendritic vaccine therapy and treatment method by peptide vaccine.

APCs take up peptides, which are often associated with carrier proteins and adjuvants, and display them on the cell surface by way of MHC. Molecules of human leukocyte antigens (HLA) MHC I (HLA) [98].

b. Dendric cell vaccines

If you are looking for an alternative to peptide vaccines in situ, you may also use direct activation of DCs ex vivo to create a cancer vaccine. Autologous dendritic cells derived from peripheral blood monocytes primed with tumor-related antigens have been utilized in cancer immunotherapy instead of injecting a peptide that is given to an APC [99]. If there are inflammatory signals, immature CD4+ T cells can deliver antigen to T-cells that recognize it in an MHC-restricted way as a result of immature DC maturation. T-cells activated with CD8 + antigens and MHC I complexes may now identify tumor cells and seek to lyse them [100]. Dendritic vaccine therapy is explained in **Figure 8.**

ii. Adaptive cell therapy (ACT)

T-cells, x-cells, and other tumor infiltrating lymphocytes (TILs) can be activated directly via Adoptive Cell Therapy (ACT) instead of DC activation [101].

Adaptive cell therapy is shown in **Figure 9**. It is most usual to utilize cytokine-induced killer (CIK) and CAR T-cells in the ACT process.

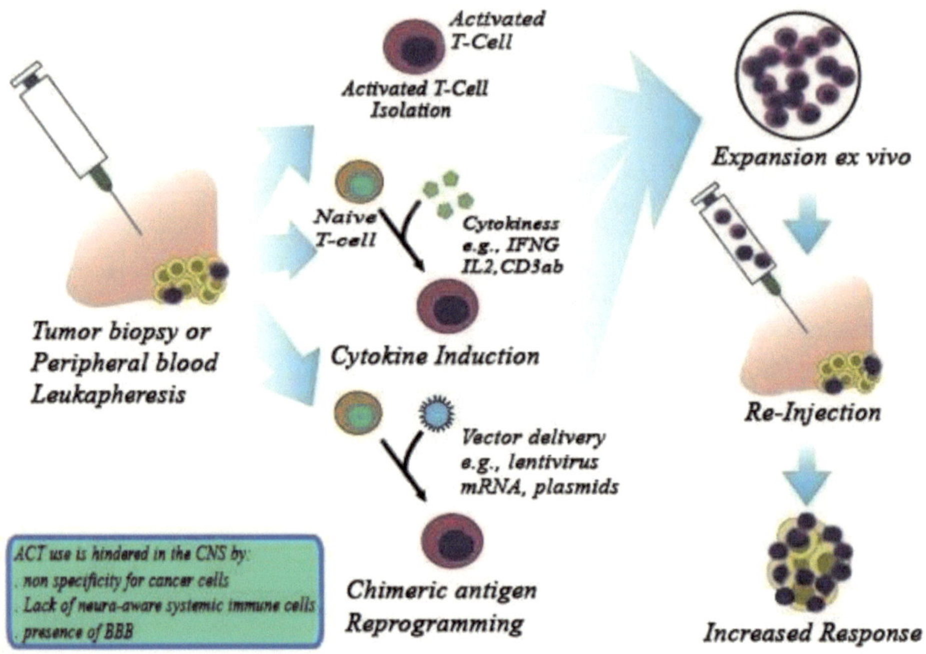

Figure 9.
Adaptive cell therapy.

IFN, IL2, and CD3 monoclonal antibodies are used to induce peripheral blood lymphocytes into CIK cells in vitro. Cells that have been modified to express a single or many costimulatory tumor antigens are called CAR T-cells [102].

iii. Monoclonal antibodies

Using monoclonal antibodies is a passive method of immunotherapy that does not need the body's immune system. **Figure 10** shows the monoclonal antibodies treatment method [93]. Antibodies that target abnormally expressed surface receptors in malignancies or receptors implicated in carcinogenesis are generally selected. However, Nimotuzumab, another monoclonal antibody widely used in brain tumors, is an anti-EGFR inhibitor that has only slightly improved overall survival when administered in children with high-grade gliomas [103].

To some extent, monoclonal antibody treatment in the brain has suboptimal survival benefits because monoclonal antibodies are unable to penetrate the BBB without causing considerable barrier disruption and because patient-specific antigen mutations affect antibody binding efficiency [104].

iv. Virotherapy

Non-pathogenic viruses are used in oncolytic virotherapy to selectively infiltrate or express proteins in brain tumor cells that can directly destroy cancer cells or else activate an immune response. Many virotherapy techniques have been investigated, but their broad use in the brain remains a problem [105]. The virotherapy method for brain tumor treatment is shown in **Figure 11**.

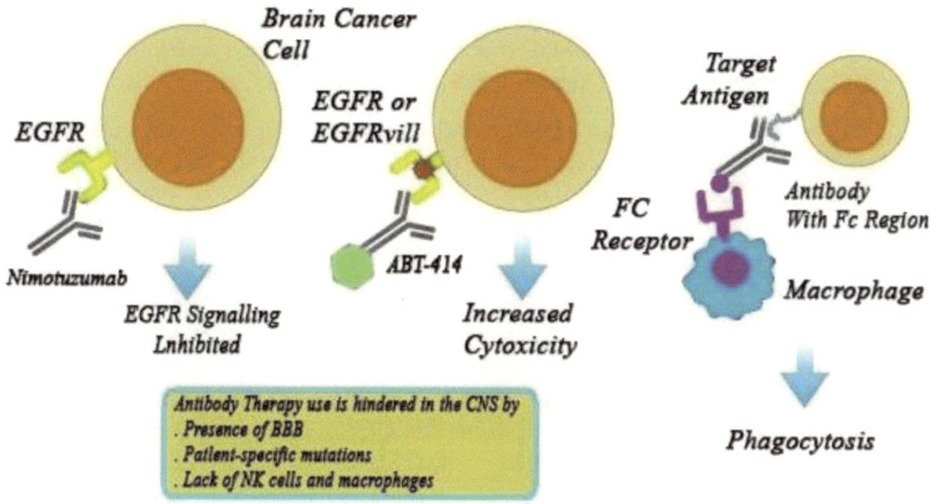

Figure 10.
Monoclonal antibodies treatment method.

Furthermore, the targeting of non-neuronal lineage cells may make a method like PVSRIPO appealing; nevertheless, other component cells in the CNS may be misidentified for cancer cells, resulting in negative side effects. The BBB can also limit viral migration to the tumor site, which is important in virotherapy for brain cancers [106].

B. Radiation therapy

Patients with primary brain tumors benefit from radiation therapy because it helps them maintain local control or prolong their progression-free life. In the treatment of primary brain tumors, radiation therapy (RT) plays a crucial role, with the majority of patients experiencing local control or prolonged progression-free survival. On the other hand, RT can have a negative

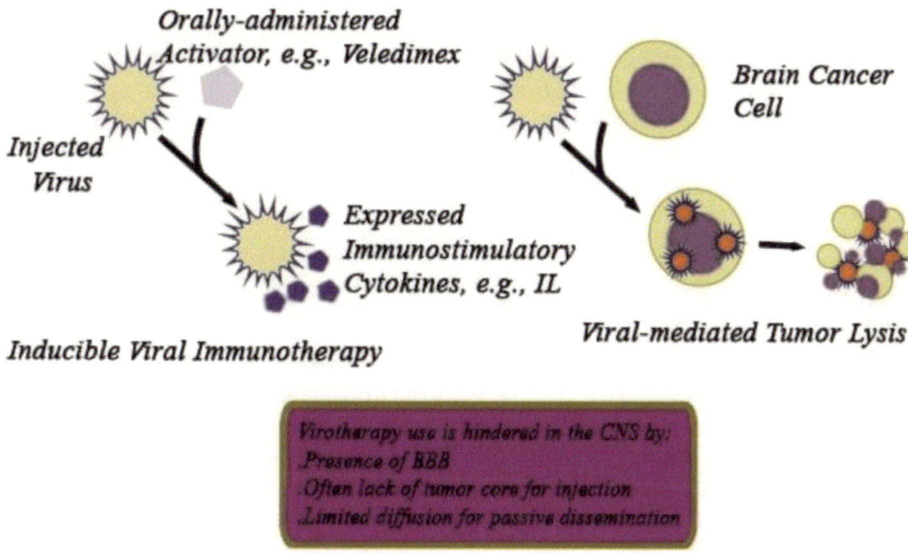

Figure 11.
Virotherapy method for brain tumor treatment.

influence on cognitive performance, which can have a detrimental effect on the quality of life. When one or more cognitive processes, such as attention, memory, language, and executive function are impaired [107, 108].

Primary brain tumors, both benign and malignant, are commonly treated with radiation therapy (RT). Post-treatment neurocognitive deterioration has been documented with RT in verbal and visuospatial memory most commonly (i.e., difficulty encoding, retaining, and retrieving visual information) [109, 110].

C. Surgery

The majority of therapy is surgical resection. Patients with persistent hydrocephalus despite tumor excision require a third ventriculostomy or CSF diversion to cure the condition. A cardiac examination should be performed on neonates suspected of having tuberous sclerosis before an intraventricular tumor is surgically removed [111].

D. Chemotherapy

The discovery of chromosomal markers that indicate greater chemosensitivity in patients with low-grade astrocytoma and other histopathologies has sparked renewed interest in using chemotherapy in the treatment of low-grade astrocytoma patients with other histopathologies. Temozolomide is the most widely used chemotherapy regimen in adult low-grade astrocytoma patients, followed by procarbazine, CCNU, and vincristine (PCV) if temozolomide fails [112].

The Southwest Oncology Group conducted an early randomized trial to see if treating low-grade astrocytoma patients with single-agent CCNU after radiation was beneficial. In this research, adding CCNU to the therapy schedule had no further benefits. Furthermore, individuals in the CCNU arm experienced a high rate of hematologic adverse effects after chemotherapy [113].

The effectiveness of temozolomide, an oral alkylating drug, in treating patients with low-grade astrocytoma is now a staple of adjuvant treatment, although it is also being investigated in several trials [114]. Response rates range from 31 to 61 percent when minor replies are considered. Despite the short duration of follow-up, the median time to advancement ranged from 31 months to >36 months. It was concluded by Brada and co-workers (2003, in a phase 2 study) that the drug temozolomide has single-agent action against low-grade astrocytoma and may also assist control seizures in this patient group and that it is safe and effective in this patient population [115].

10. Recent research in brain tumor

In 2020, A new improved WOA is used to propose a comprehensive method for brain tumor detection based on optimal feature extraction and feature selection. On a set of benchmark cases, IWOA's experimental results are compared to those of other common optimizers, and the results are verified [116].

Z.U. Rehman, M.S. Zia, G.R. Bojja, and F. Jinchao explained Two recent and useful trends for brain tumor localization: (1) using the texton-map to create the image in texture form (2) extracting the features from the superpixels The three contributions were used in this paper. First, superpixel segmentation is performed on texton-map images, which reduces the computational cost of image segmentation in small regions, improves spatial smoothness of superpixels, and improves low-level feature accuracy. Second, we covered the concept of data balancing, which aids in the development of vision-based classifiers. Third, we created a quick comparison of four different classifiers and examined their performance in terms of model training accuracy. Initially, our image denoising method is shown to effectively remove false-positive regions [117].

Ratan et al. developed watershed segmentation and used edge detection, contrast, and greyscale on 2D and 3D images to detect brain tumors. Somasundaram and Kalaiselvi used ten data sets with normal and abnormal subjects to detect brain tumors. Muscles, scalp, skull, and fats the unwanted brain areas are removed first in their proposed framework, followed by fuzzy segmentation. Finally, for tumor region detection, and intensity-based extended maxima transform is used [18]. proposes a systematic model that starts with a diagnosis of the brain tumor and then extracts the brain tumor region. A classifier called Naive Bayes is used to diagnose the tumor from brain MR images. After a diagnosis, the brain tumor region is extracted using K-mean clustering and boundary detection techniques. It had an accuracy rate of over 80%. To detect the brain tumor region, researchers propose a segmentation method based on color and edge detection. Edge detection is done with the Prewitt, Canny, Sobel, and Laplacian of Gaussian operators, while color-based segmentation is done with the K-mean clustering technique [118].

Alexander Winkler-Schwartz and his colleagues have created a comprehensive research framework for studying oncological neurosurgery's technical performance and resection extent. This platform works by incorporating a low-cost alginate-based artificial brain tumor into an ex-vivo calf brain in a controlled operative environment. To our knowledge, this is the first time an artificial tumor has been created using the biomechanical properties of human specimens obtained through resection. Given that its components are relatively inexpensive and combined in small quantities, the overall cost of the artificial tumor is well under 2 cents/mL. To put this into perspective, 1 kg of alginate and 5800 mL of calcium sulphate, respectively, can yield 40,000 and 5800 mL of final tumor. Gadobutrol (Bayer AG) or its analogues, arguably the most expensive compound in the mix, can often be obtained for a low price from clinical units' expired stockpiles. Even if one were to pay the full cost for an average 30-mL vial, this would yield 27,000 mL of tumor. A 10e100-mL pipette and a laboratory-grade scale are required, but they are both one-time purchases. The recordings from the surgical microscope and ceiling-mounted camera, as well as the movements generated by the instrument-mounted fiducial markers, can be used to evaluate operative "performance" [119].

Medical imaging is still the gold standard for detecting, diagnosing, and examining gliomas and other diseases. Magnetic resonance imaging (MRI), diffusion tensor imaging (DTI), functional MRI, computed tomography, and positron emission tomography is the most commonly used imaging techniques in clinical practice [120].

11. Discussion

The brain is responsible to control all activities of the human body. It is well-known that a disease occurred in the brain may affect human life negatively. A brain tumor is one of the critical diseases that originate from the abnormal growth of cells in the brain. Automatic brain tumor classification plays an important role in the early stage of tumor detection and this system allows patients to be diagnosed in time and chance of survival. Also, this system may help radiologists in decision-making and treatment plans. In this paper, we proposed a new scheme to classify three types of brain tumors, namely, Meningioma, Glioma, and Pituitary tumors from MRI images. First, pre-processed is applied to images [70].

Recent laboratory advances in primary brain tumors have shown that specific molecular signatures can predict the biological behavior of tumors. Current brain tumor classification systems based on histology and morphology may soon be supplemented by a system based on molecular markers of tumor differentiation and progression [74].

12. Conclusion

The quantitative, domain-specific data acquired through these studies will improve our understanding of brain toxicity and cognitive decline associated with radiation dosage to non-targeted tissue and can provide the basis for evidence-based cognition-sparing brain radiotherapy. Interestingly, this study introduces an association between certain WM diffusion changes and radiation-induced memory decline, which may indicate that there are other ROIs not studied in this paper that should be investigated as potentially vulnerable areas contributing to post-RT cognitive decline. Further research is needed to investigate the dynamic trajectories of tissue response to radiation to better understand how MRI changes can be used to predict important neurocognitive trajectories post-treatment [60].

Treatments and better outcomes for primary brain tumors have long lagged behind those of other tumors. However, a new era in neuro-oncology has emerged, with major advances in both cancer and CNS immunology, and progress in genomics [55].

Abbrevations

ATRX	Alpha- Thalassemia X- linked mental Retardation
BBB	Blood Brain Barrier
CAR T cells	Chimeric Antigen Receptor
CDKN2A	Cyclin-Dependent Kinase inhibitor 2A
CD4+	Cluster of Differentiation 4
CD3	Cluster of differentiation 3
IFN	Interferon
IL-2	Interleukin-2
MIB-1	Monoclonal antibody-1
qRT- PCR	Quantitative Real-Time Polymerase Chain Reaction
NK	Natural Killer
MHC	Major histocompatibility complex

Author details

Manimekalai Pichaivel[1*], Gayathri Anbumani[1], Panneerselvam Theivendren[2] and Muruganantham Gopal[3]

1 Department of Pharmacology, Swamy Vivekananda College of Pharmacy, Namakkal, Tamilnadu, India

2 Department of R&D, Swamy Vivekananda College of Pharmacy, Namakkal, Tamilnadu, India

3 Department of Pharmacognosy, Swamy Vivekananda College of Pharmacy, Namakkal, Tamilnadu, India

*Address all correspondence to: mekalaivel@gmail.com

References

[1] Lapointe S, Perry A, Butowski NA. Primary brain tumours in adults. The Lancet. 2018;**392**(10145):432-446

[2] Clifton W, Reimer R. Metastatic brain tumors. In: Comprehensive Overview of Modern Surgical Approaches to Intrinsic Brain Tumors. Elsevier: Academic Press; 2019. pp. 159-167. DOI: 10.1016/b978-0-12-811783-5.00008-2

[3] Udaka YT, Packer RJ. Pediatric brain tumors. Neurologic clinics. 2018;**36**(3): 533-536. DOI: 10.1016/j.ncl.2018.04.009

[4] Jelski W, Mroczko B. Molecular and circulating biomarkers of brain tumors. International Journal of Molecular Sciences. 2021;**22**(13):7039

[5] Hendrix P, Hans E, Griessenauer CJ, Simgen A, Oertel J, Karbach J. Neurocognitive status in patients with newly-diagnosed brain tumors in good neurological condition: the impact of tumor type, volume, and location. Clinical Neurology and Neurosurgery. 2017;**156**:55-62

[6] Mehta S, Shah A, Jung H. Diagnosis and treatment options for sequelae following radiation treatment of brain tumors. Clinical Neurology and Neurosurgery. 2017;**163**:1-8

[7] Kumar A, Ramachandran M, Gandomi AH, Patan R, Lukasik S, Soundarapandian RK. A deep neural network based classifier for brain tumor diagnosis. Applied Soft Computing. 2019;**82**:105528

[8] Zhou Y, Liu CH, Wu B, Zhang C, Yu X, Cheng G, et al. Invited article: Molecular biomarkers characterization for human brain glioma grading using visible resonance Raman spectroscopy. APL Photonics. 2018;**3**(12):120802

[9] Seiler A, Sood AK, Jenewein J, Fagundes CP. Can stress promote the pathophysiology of brain metastases? A critical review of biobehavioral mechanisms. Brain, Behavior, and Immunity. 2020;**87**:860-880

[10] Esquenazi Y, Lo VP, Lee K. Critical care management of cerebral edema in brain tumors. Journal of Intensive Care Medicine. 2017;**32**(1):15-24

[11] Staedtke V, a Dzaye OD, Holdhoff M. Actionable molecular biomarkers in primary brain tumors. Trends in Cancer. 2016;**2**(7):338-349

[12] Birkó Z, Nagy B, Klekner Á, Virga J. Novel molecular markers in glioblastoma—Benefits of liquid biopsy. International Journal of Molecular Sciences. 2020;**21**(20):7522

[13] Plaks V, Koopman CD, Werb Z. Circulating tumor cells. Science. 2013; **341**(6151):1186-1188

[14] Yu M, Stott S, Toner M, Maheswaran S, Haber DA. Circulating tumor cells: Approaches to isolation and characterization. Journal of Cell Biology. 2011;**192**(3):373-382

[15] Pantel K, Speicher MR. The biology of circulating tumor cells. Oncogene. 2016;**35**(10):1216-1224

[16] Shan S, Hui G, Hou F, Shi H, Zhou G, Yan H, et al. Expression of metastasis- associated protein 3 in human brain glioma related to tumor prognosis. Neurological Sciences. 2015; **36**(10):1799-1804

[17] Watanabe T, Katayama Y, Komine C, Yoshino A, Ogino A, Ohta T, et al. O6-methylguanine-DNA methyltransferase methylation and TP53 mutation in malignant astrocytomas and their relationships with clinical course. International Journal of Cancer. 2005;**113**(4):581-587

[18] Lamb KL, Liu Y, Ishiguro K, Kwon Y, Paquet N, Sartorelli AC, et al.

Tumor-associated mutations in O6-methylguanine DNA-methyltransferase (MGMT) reduce DNA repair functionality. Molecular Carcinogenesis. 2014;**53**(3):201-210

[19] Yip S, Iafrate AJ, Louis DN. Molecular diagnostic testing in malignant gliomas: a practical update on predictive markers. Journal of Neuropathology & Experimental Neurology. 2008;**67**(1):1-5

[20] Davis ME. Epidemiology and overview of gliomas. Seminars in Oncology Nursing. 2018;**34**(5):420-429

[21] Szopa W, Burley TA, Kramer-Marek G, Kaspera W. Diagnostic and therapeutic biomarkers in glioblastoma: Current status and future perspectives. BioMed Research International. 2017; **2017**:1-13

[22] William D, Mokri P, Lamp N, Linnebacher M, Classen CF, Erbersdobler A, et al. Amplification of the EGFR gene can be maintained and modulated by variation of EGF concentrations in in vitro models of glioblastoma multiforme. PLoS One. 2017;**12**(9):e0185208

[23] Thon N, Kreth S, Kreth FW. Personalized treatment strategies in glioblastoma: MGMT promoter methylation status. Oncotargets and Therapy. 2013;**6**:1363

[24] Chen JR, Yao Y, Xu HZ, Qin ZY. Isocitrate dehydrogenase (IDH) 1/2 mutations as prognostic markers in patients with glioblastomas. Medicine. 2016;**95**(9):1-13

[25] Sarkar A, Chiocca EA. Glioblastoma and malignant astrocytoma. In: Brain Tumors. WB Saunders. Elsevier specific brain tumor. 2012;**21**:384-407. DOI: 10.1016/b978-0-443-06967-3.00021-1

[26] Aili Y, Maimaitiming N, Mahemuti Y, Qin H, Wang Y, Wang Z. Liquid biopsy in central nervous system tumors: The potential roles of circulating miRNA and exosomes. American Journal of Cancer Research. 2020;**10**(12):4134

[27] Wang J, Bettegowda C. Applications of DNA-based liquid biopsy for central nervous system neoplasms. The Journal of Molecular Diagnostics. 2017;**19**(1):24-34

[28] Bettegowda C, Sausen M, Leary RJ, Kinde I, Wang Y, Agrawal N, et al. Detection of circulating tumor DNA in early-and late-stage human malignancies. Science Translational Medicine. 2014;**6**(224):224ra24

[29] Birkó Z, Nagy B, Klekner Á, Virga J. Novel molecular markers in glioblastoma—Benefits of liquid biopsy. International Journal of Molecular Sciences. 2020;**21**(20):7522

[30] Keup C, Mach P, Aktas B, Tewes M, Kolberg HC, Hauch S, et al. RNA profiles of circulating tumor cells and extracellular vesicles for therapy stratification of metastatic breast cancer patients. Clinical Chemistry. 2018; **64**(7):1054-1062

[31] Cortez MA, Bueso-Ramos C, Ferdin J, Lopez-Berestein G, Sood AK, Calin GA. MicroRNAs in body fluids—the mix of hormones and biomarkers. Nature Reviews. Clinical Oncology. 2011;**8**(8):467-477

[32] Park J, Lee H, Tran Q, Mun K, Kim D, Hong Y, et al. Recognition of transmembrane protein 39A as a tumor-specific marker in brain tumor. Toxicological Research. 2017;**33**(1): 63-69

[33] Bustany P, Chatel M, Derlon JM, Darcel F, Sgouropoulos P, Soussaline F, et al. Brain tumor protein synthesis and histological grades: a study by positron emission tomography (PET) with C11-L-methionine. Journal of Neuro-Oncology. 1986;**3**(4):397-404

[34] Bögler O, Su Huang HJ, Kleihues P, Cavenee WK. The p53 gene and its role in human brain tumors. Glia. 1995;**15**(3): 308-327

[35] Alvarado-Ortiz E, de la Cruz-López KG, Becerril-Rico J, Sarabia-Sánchez MA, Ortiz-Sánchez E, García-Carrancá A. Mutant p53 gain-of-function: Role in cancer development, progression, and therapeutic approaches. Frontiers in Cell and Development Biology. 2021;**8**:1868

[36] Park SH, Won J, Kim SI, Lee Y, Park CK, Kim SK, et al. Molecular testing of brain tumor. Journal of Pathology and Translational Medicine. 2017;**51**(3):205

[37] Gavrilovic IT, Posner JB. Brain metastases: Epidemiology and pathophysiology. Journal of Neuro-Oncology. 2005;**75**(1):5-14

[38] Fox BD, Cheung VJ, Patel AJ, Suki D, Rao G. Epidemiology of metastatic brain tumors. Neurosurgery Clinics of North America. 2011;**22**(1):1-6

[39] Falchetti M, Larocca L, Pallini R. Telomerase in brain tumors. Child's Nervous System. 2002;**18**(3–4):112-117

[40] Lah TT, Novak M, Breznik B. Brain malignancies: Cancer cell trafficking in and out of the niches. Elsevier. Seminars in Cancer Biology. 2019.

[41] Charles NA, Holland EC, Gilbertson R, Glass R, Kettenmann H. The brain tumor microenvironment. Glia. 2012;**60**(3):502-514

[42] Noreen N, Palaniappan S, Qayyum A, Ahmad I, Imran M, Shoaib M. A deep learning model based on concatenation approach for the diagnosis of brain tumor. IEEE Access. 2020;**5**(8):55135-55144

[43] McNeill KA. Epidemiology of brain tumors. Neurologic Clinics. 2016;**34**(4): 981-998

[44] Platten M, Reardon DA. Concepts for immunotherapies in gliomas. Seminars in Neurology. 2018;**38**(01): 062-072

[45] Gittleman H, Ostrom QT, Farah PD, Ondracek A, Chen Y, Wolinsky Y, et al. Descriptive epidemiology of pituitary tumors in the United States, 2004–2009. Journal of Neurosurgery. 2014;**121**(3): 527-535

[46] Ostrom QT, de Blank PM, Kruchko C, Petersen CM, Liao P, Finlay JL, et al. Alex's Lemonade Stand Foundation infant and childhood primary brain and central nervous system tumors diagnosed in the United States in 2007–2011. Neuro-Oncology. 2015;**16**(suppl. 10):x1-x36

[47] Nelson S, Taylor LP. Headaches in brain tumor patients: primary or secondary? Headache: The Journal of Head and Face Pain. 2014;**54**(4):776-785

[48] Malbari F, Lindsay H. Genetics of common pediatric brain tumors. Pediatric Neurology. 2020;**104**:3-12

[49] Lecler A, Charbonneau F, Psimaras D, Metten MA, Gueguen A, Xuan KH, et al. Remote brain microhaemorrhages may predict haematoma in glioma patients treated with radiation therapy. European Radiology. 2018;**28**(10):4324-4333

[50] Taylor LP. Mechanism of brain tumor headache. Headache: The Journal of Head and Face Pain. 2014;**54**(4):772-775

[51] Preuß M, Preiss S, Syrbe S, Nestler U, Fischer L, Merkenschlager A, et al. Signs and symptoms of pediatric brain tumors and diagnostic value of preoperative EEG. Child's Nervous System. 2015;**31**(11):2051-2054

[52] Wickham RJ. Revisiting the physiology of nausea and vomiting—challenging the paradigm. Supportive Care in Cancer. 2020;**28**(1):13-21

[53] Alentorn A, Hoang-Xuan K, Mikkelsen T. Presenting signs and symptoms in brain tumors. Handbook of Clinical Neurology. 2016;**134**:19-26

[54] Rigi M, Almarzouqi SJ, Morgan ML, Lee AG. Papilledema: Epidemiology, etiology, and clinical management. Eye and Brain. 2015;**7**:47

[55] Vargo M. Brain tumor rehabilitation. American Journal of Physical Medicine & Rehabilitation. 2011;**90**(5):S50-S62

[56] Chen DY, Chen CC, Crawford JR, Wang SG. Tumor-related epilepsy: epidemiology, pathogenesis and management. Journal of Neuro-Oncology. 2018;**139**(1):13-21

[57] Laddha RR, Ladhake SA. A review on brain tumor detection using segmentation and threshold operations. International Journal of Computer Science and Information Technologies. 2014;**5**(1):607-611

[58] Karpathiou G, Dumollard JM, Dridi M, Dal Col P, Barral FG, Boutonnat J, et al. Chordomas: a review with emphasis on their pathophysiology, pathology, molecular biology, and genetics. Pathology, Research and Practice. 2020;**216**:153089

[59] Kumar A, Ramachandran M, Gandomi AH, Patan R, Lukasik S, Soundarapandian RK. A deep neural network based classifier for brain tumor diagnosis. Applied Soft Computing. 2019;**82**:105528

[60] Tiwari A, Srivastava S, Pant M. Brain tumor segmentation and classification from magnetic resonance images: Review of selected methods from 2014 to 2019. Pattern Recognition Letters. 2020;**131**:244-260

[61] Ginat DT, Swearingen B, Curry W, Cahill D, Madsen J, Schaefer PW. 3 Tesla intraoperative MRI for brain tumor surgery. Journal of Magnetic Resonance Imaging. 2014;**39**(6): 1357-1365

[62] Ellenbogen GR, Scott MR. Choroid plexus tumors. In: Kaye HA, Laws RE, editors. Brain Tumors. Elsevier. 2011;**25**: 450-462. DOI: 10.1016/b978-0-443-06967-3.00025-9

[63] Wirsching HG, Galanis E, Weller M. Glioblastoma. In: Handbook of Clinical Neurology. Elsevier. 2016;**134**(3): 381-397. DOI: 10.1016/b978-0-12-802997-8.00023-2

[64] Noreen N, Palaniappan S, Qayyum A, Ahmad I, Imran M, Shoaib M. A deep learning model based on concatenation approach for the diagnosis of brain tumor. IEEE Access. 2020;**8**:55135-55144

[65] Işın A, Direkoğlu C, Şah M. Review of MRI-based brain tumor image segmentation using deep learning methods. Procedia Computer Science. 2016;**102**:317-324

[66] Zhang J, Traylor KS, Mountz JM. PET and SPECT imaging of brain tumors. Seminars in Ultrasound, CT and MRI. 2020;**41**(6):530-540

[67] Suchorska B, Tonn JC, Jansen NL. PET imaging for brain tumor diagnostics. Current Opinion in Neurology. 2014;**27**(6):683-688

[68] Matsunaga S, Shuto T, Takase H, Ohtake M, Tomura N, Tanaka T, et al. Semiquantitative analysis using thallium-201 SPECT for differential diagnosis between tumor recurrence and radiation necrosis after gamma knife surgery for malignant brain tumors. International Journal of Radiation Oncology, Biology, Physics. 2013;**85**(1):47-52

[69] Balasooriya NM, Nawarathna RD. A sophisticated convolutional neural network model for brain tumor

classification. Ministry of Higher Education & Scientific Research Al-Nahrain University College of Engineering. In: 2017 IEEE International Conference on Industrial and Information Systems (ICIIS). Vol. 89. IEEE; 2017. pp. 1-5. DOI: 10.1109/ICIINFS.2017.8300364

[70] Kaplan K, Kaya Y, Kuncan M, Ertunç HM. Brain tumor classification using modified local binary patterns (LBP) feature extraction methods. Medical Hypotheses. 2020;**139**:109696

[71] Sarkar A, Chiocca EA. Glioblastoma and malignant astrocytoma. In: Brain Tumors. WB Saunders. Elsevier specific brain tumor. 2012;**21**:384-407. DOI: 10.1016/b978-0-443-06967-3.00021-1

[72] Sanai N, Chang S, Berger MS. Low-grade gliomas in adults: A review. Journal of Neurosurgery. 2011;**115**(5): 948-965

[73] Ivan ME, Mohammadi AM, De Deugd N, Reyes J, Rodriguez G, Shah A, et al. Laser ablation of newly diagnosed malignant gliomas: a meta-analysis. Neurosurgery. 2016;**79**(suppl. 1):S17-S23

[74] Doolittle ND. State of the science in brain tumor classification. Seminars in Oncology Nursing. 2004;**20**(4):224-230

[75] Shah SS, Dellarole A, Peterson EC, Bregy A, Komotar R, Harvey PD, et al. Long-term psychiatric outcomes in pediatric brain tumor survivors. Child's Nervous System. 2015;**31**(5):653-663

[76] Reon BJ, Anaya J, Zhang Y, Mandell J, Purow B, Abounader R, et al. Expression of lncRNAs in low-grade gliomas and glioblastoma multiforme: An in silico analysis. PLoS Medicine. 2016;**13**(12):e1002192

[77] Kumthekar P, Raizer J, Singh S. Low-grade glioma. Current Understanding and Treatment of Gliomas. 2015;**163**:75-87

[78] Wang Y, Jiang T. Understanding high grade glioma: Molecular mechanism, therapy and comprehensive management. Cancer Letters. 2013; **331**(2):139-146

[79] Kim JY, Koralnik IJ, LeFave M, Segal RA, Pfister LA, Pomeroy SL. Medulloblastomas and primitive neuroectodermal tumors rarely contain polyomavirus DNA sequences. Neuro-Oncology. 2002;**4**(3):165-170

[80] León MM. Meduloblastoma pediátrico, revisión y puesta al día. Radiología. 2011;**53**(2):134-145

[81] Gerstner ER, Pajtler KW. Ependymoma. Seminars in Neurology. 2018;**38**(01):104-111

[82] Reni M, Gatta G, Mazza E, Vecht C. Ependymoma. Critical Reviews in Oncology/Hematology. 2007;**63**(1):81-89

[83] Park SH, Won J, Kim SI, Lee Y, Park CK, Kim SK, et al. Molecular testing of brain tumor. Journal of Pathology and Translational Medicine. 2017;**51**(3):205

[84] Kelley MJ, Shi J, Ballew B, Hyland PL, Li WQ, Rotunno M, et al. Characterization of T gene sequence variants and germline duplications in familial and sporadic chordoma. Human Genetics. 2014;**133**(10):1289-1297

[85] Borger DR, Tanabe KK, Fan KC, Lopez HU, Fantin VR, Straley KS, et al. Frequent mutation of isocitrate dehydrogenase (IDH) 1 and IDH2 in cholangiocarcinoma identified through broad-based tumor genotyping. The Oncologist. 2012;**17**(1):72

[86] Vaidya M, Sugaya K. DNA associated with circulating exosomes as a biomarker for glioma. Genes. 2020; **11**(11):1276

[87] Ogi H, Tanaka T, Yoshitake Y, Shinohara M, Nakayama H, Imamura T.

A rare mandibular osteosarcoma case of Li-Franmeni syndrome with a germline p53R273H mutation. Journal of Oral and Maxillofacial Surgery, Medicine, and Pathology. 2020;**32**(2):132-135

[88] Liu XY, Gerges N, Korshunov A, Sabha N, Khuong-Quang DA, Fontebasso AM, et al. Frequent ATRX mutations and loss of expression in adult diffuse astrocytic tumors carrying IDH1/IDH2 and TP53 mutations. Acta Neuropathologica. 2012;**124**(5):615-625

[89] Yamamichi A, Ohka F, Aoki K, Suzuki H, Kato A, Hirano M, et al. Immunohistochemical ATRX expression is not a surrogate for 1p19q codeletion. Brain Tumor Pathology. 2018;**35**(2): 106-113

[90] Hobbs J, Nikiforova MN, Fardo DW, Bortoluzzi S, Cieply K, Hamilton RL, et al. Paradoxical relationship between degree of EGFR amplification and outcome in glioblastomas. The American Journal of Surgical Pathology. 2012;**36**(8):1186

[91] Stichel D, Ebrahimi A, Reuss D, Schrimpf D, Ono T, Shirahata M, et al. Distribution of EGFR amplification, combined chromosome 7 gain and chromosome 10 loss, and TERT promoter mutation in brain tumors and their potential for the reclassification of IDH wt astrocytoma to glioblastoma. Acta Neuropathologica. 2018;**136**(5):793-803

[92] Wang J, Yao Z, Jonsson P, Allen AN, Qin AC, Uddin S, et al. A secondary mutation in BRAF confers resistance to RAF inhibition in a BRAF V600E-mutant brain tumor. Cancer Discovery. 2018;**8**(9):1130-1141

[93] Platten M, Reardon DA. Concepts for immunotherapies in gliomas. Seminars in Neurology. 2018;**38**(01): 062-072

[94] Lyon JG, Mokarram N, Saxena T, Carroll SL, Bellamkonda RV. Engineering challenges for brain tumor immunotherapy. Advanced Drug Delivery Reviews. 2017;**114**:19-32

[95] Ho YJ, Li JP, Fan CH, Liu HL, Yeh CK. Ultrasound in tumor immunotherapy: Current status and future developments. Journal of Controlled Release. 2020;**323**:12-23

[96] Wang SS, Bandopadhayay P, Jenkins MR. Towards immunotherapy for pediatric brain tumors. Trends in Immunology. 2019;**40**(8):748-761

[97] Wei X, Chen F, Xin K, Wang Q, Yu L, Liu B, et al. Cancer-testis antigen peptide vaccine for cancer immunotherapy: Progress and prospects. Translational Oncology. 2019;**12**(5):733-738

[98] Yoshimura K, Minami T, Nozawa M, Kimura T, Egawa S, Fujimoto H, et al. A phase 2 randomized controlled trial of personalized peptide vaccine immunotherapy with low-dose dexamethasone versus dexamethasone alone in chemotherapy-naive castration-resistant prostate cancer. European Urology. 2016;**70**(1):35-41

[99] Chandramohan V, Mitchell DA, Johnson LA, Sampson JH, Bigner DD. Antibody, T-cell and dendritic cell immunotherapy for malignant brain tumors. Future Oncology. 2013;**9**(7): 977-990

[100] Everson RG, Jin RM, Wang X, Safaee M, Scharnweber R, Lisiero DN, et al. Cytokine responsiveness of CD8+ T cells is a reproducible biomarker for the clinical efficacy of dendritic cell vaccination in glioblastoma patients. Journal for Immunotherapy of Cancer. 2014;**2**(1):1-1

[101] Deepa AR, Emmanuel WS. An efficient detection of brain tumor using fused feature adaptive ficrefly backpropagation neural network.

Multimedia Tools and Applications. 2019;**78**(9):11799-11814

[102] Keidar M, Yan D, Beilis II, Trink B, Sherman JH. Plasmas for treating cancer: Opportunities for adaptive and self-adaptive approaches. Trends in Biotechnology. 2018;**36**(6):586-593

[103] Han L, Liu C, Qi H, Zhou J, Wen J, Wu D, et al. Systemic delivery of monoclonal antibodies to the central nervous system for brain tumor therapy. Advanced Materials. 2019;**31**(19): 1805697

[104] Ait-Belkacem R, Berenguer C, Villard C, Ouafik LH, Figarella-Branger D, Beck A, et al. Monitoring therapeutic monoclonal antibodies in brain tumor. MAbs. 2014;**6**(6):1385-1393

[105] Friedman GK, Bernstock JD, Chen D, Nan L, Moore BP, Kelly VM, et al. Enhanced sensitivity of patient-derived pediatric high-grade brain tumor xenografts to oncolytic HSV-1 virotherapy correlates with nectin-1 expression. Scientific Reports. 2018; **8**(1):1-0

[106] Thaci B, Ahmed AU, Ulasov IV, Tobias AL, Han Y, Aboody KS, et al. Pharmacokinetic study of neural stem cell-based cell carrier for oncolytic virotherapy: targeted delivery of the therapeutic payload in an orthotopic brain tumor model. Cancer Gene Therapy. 2012;**19**(6):431-442

[107] Tringale KR, Nguyen TT, Karunamuni R, Seibert T, Huynh-Le MP, Connor M, et al. Quantitative imaging biomarkers of damage to critical memory regions are associated with post–radiation therapy memory performance in brain tumor patients. International Journal of Radiation Oncology, Biology, Physics. 2019; **105**(4):773-783

[108] Haldbo-Classen L, Amidi A, Wu LM, Lukacova S, Oettingen GV, Gottrup H, et al. Long-term cognitive dysfunction after radiation therapy for primary brain tumors. Acta Oncologica. 2019;**58**(5):745-752

[109] Bouchet A, Potez M, Coquery N, Rome C, Lemasson B, Bräuer-Krisch E, et al. Permeability of brain tumor vessels induced by uniform or spatially microfractionated synchrotron radiation therapies. International Journal of Radiation Oncology, Biology, Physics. 2017;**98**(5):1174-1182

[110] Durand T, Bernier MO, Léger I, Taillia H, Noël G, Psimaras D, et al. Cognitive outcome after radiotherapy in brain tumor. Current Opinion in Oncology. 2015;**27**(6):510-515

[111] Ferraro N, Barbarite E, Albert TR, Berchmans E, Shah AH, Bregy A, et al. The role of 5-aminolevulinic acid in brain tumor surgery: A systematic review. Neurosurgical Review. 2016; **39**(4):545-555

[112] Wang D, Wang C, Wang L, Chen Y. A comprehensive review in improving delivery of small-molecule chemotherapeutic agents overcoming the blood-brain/brain tumor barriers for glioblastoma treatment. Drug Delivery. 2019;**26**(1):551-565

[113] Bhandari A, Bansal A, Singh A, Gupta RK, Sinha N. Comparison of transport of chemotherapeutic drugs in voxelized heterogeneous model of human brain tumor. Microvascular Research. 2019;**124**:76-90

[114] Zhan W, Wang CH. Convection enhanced delivery of chemotherapeutic drugs into brain tumour. Journal of Controlled Release. 2018;**271**:74-87

[115] Chen DY, Chen CC, Crawford JR, Wang SG. Tumor-related epilepsy: epidemiology, pathogenesis and management. Journal of Neuro-Oncology. 2018;**139**(1):13-21

[116] Yin B, Wang C, Abza F. New brain tumor classification method based on an improved version of whale optimization algorithm. Biomedical Signal Processing and Control. 2020;**56**:101728

[117] Rehman ZU, Zia MS, Bojja GR, Yaqub M, Jinchao F, Arshid K. Texture based localization of a brain tumor from MR-images by using a machine learning approach. Medical Hypotheses. 2020; **141**:109705

[118] Khan SR, Sikandar M, Almogren A, Din IU, Guerrieri A, Fortino G. IoMT-based computational approach for detecting brain tumor. Future Generation Computer Systems. 2020; **109**:360-367

[119] Winkler-Schwartz A, Yilmaz R, Tran DH, Gueziri HE, Ying B, Tuznik M, et al. Creating a comprehensive research platform for surgical technique and operative outcome in primary brain tumor neurosurgery. World Neurosurgery. 2020;**144**:e62-e71

[120] Elazab A, Wang C, Gardezi SJ, Bai H, Hu Q, Wang T, et al. GP-GAN: Brain tumor growth prediction using stacked 3D generative adversarial networks from longitudinal MR Images. Neural Networks. 2020;**132**:321-332

Chapter 2

High Grade Meningiomas: Current Therapy Based on Tumor Biology

Juan Esteban Garcia-Robledo, Camila Ordóñez-Reyes, Alejandro Ruiz-Patiño, Álvaro Muñoz, Oscar Arrieta, Enrique Jiménez, Fernando Hakim, Diego Gómez, Juan Fernando Ramón and Andrés F. Cardona

Abstract

Atypical (WHO grade II) and malignant meningiomas (WHO Grade III) are a rare subset of primary intracranial tumors. Due to the high recurrence rate after surgical resection and radiotherapy, there has been a recent interest in exploring other systemic treatment options for these refractory tumors. Recent advances in molecular sequencing of tumors have elucidated new pathways and drug targets currently being studied. This article provides a thorough overview of novel investigational therapeutics, including targeted therapy, immunotherapy, and new technological modalities for atypical and malignant meningiomas. There is encouraging preclinical evidence regarding the efficacy of the emerging treatments discussed in this chapter. Several clinical trials are currently recruiting patients to translate targeted molecular therapy for recurrent and high-grade meningiomas.

Keywords: targeted therapy, molecular biology, progression free survival, overall survival, meningioma, genomics, angiogenesis, immunotherapy, outcomes

1. Introduction

Meningiomas (MN) are a type of central nervous system (CNS) tumors that arise from the leptomeningeal arachnoid covering the encephalon and the spinal cord, more specifically, from the arachnoid cap cells [1]. In adults, MN accounts for approximately 37.6% of all primary brain tumors, and corresponds to the most common intracranial tumor in adults over 35 years [1, 2]. According to Ostrom et al., incidence of MN in the United States (US) is 8.83 per 100,000 per year [3]. Around 90% of all MN cases are diagnosed intracranially, with the rest arising from the spinal arachnoid [4]. The median age at diagnosis for MN is 65 years [4] with the majority of patients being in the range of 55–74 [4]. Cases in the pediatric population are extremely rare, corresponding only to 0.4–4.6% of all pediatric tumors [2]. There is a female predominance in case proportion, with a female:male ratio of 3:1 for all MN, and 9:1 for spinal cord MNs [2, 5]. MNs are characterized for being slow in growth and often not infiltrative, with an insidious development of symptoms. Clinical presentation of MN might vary from patient to patient, with tumor localization being the main determining factor of clinical features. Signs and symptoms might include headaches because of increased intracranial pressure, focal neurological deficits (mainly cranial nerve focalization), and seizures. In the case of MN developing in the frontal lobe, personality changes, altered mental status and mood disturbances might appear [6].

According to the World Health Organization (WHO), MN is classified in three subtypes: common type or WHO grade I, atypical/intermediate type or WHO grade II and the anaplastic/malignant type or WHO grade III. These high-grade tumors might develop *de novo* or as a transformation from a lower grade MN [7]. Approximately 70% of cases are WHO grade I, 28% are WHO grade II and only around 3% are classified as WHO grade III. According to a cohort of 992 patients with MN, the proportion of atypical and anaplastic MN was higher in males than females ($p = 0.003$) [4]. The more aggressive behavior in grade II and III MN is represented by a worse prognosis in terms of overall survival (OS) and recurrence risk after surgical resection (SR). In a cohort of 102 patients with grade II and III MN, 5-year OS (5-yOS) was 97.5% and 67.4% respectively, with a median OS (mOS) of 167 months and 72 months respectively [8]. These results showed a marked increase in survival over the last decades, arguably because of the introduction of better surgical techniques, radiation therapy and some forms of chemotherapy, as previous research showed a 5-yOS of 75% for grade II MN and 32% for grade III MN [9]. Tumor recurrence has been found to be considerably increased in high grade MN, with a 50% and 80% 5-year recurrence for grade II and grade III MN respectively, and only 5–10% for grade I MN [10, 11].

As high-grade MN continue to be a difficult to treat condition, with high recurrence and low response rates, molecular insights into precision medicine have been investigated in the last two decades. With a better understanding of the cellular and molecular pathways underlying MN pathophysiology, recurrence and malignancy, newer therapies have been considered as possible candidates for the treatment of these conditions. Some agents include newer systemic chemotherapeutic agents like trabectedin, inhibitors of the Epidermal Growth Factor Receptor (EGFR) like erlotinib and gefitinib, inhibitors of the Platelet-Derived Growth Factor Receptor (PDGFR), inhibitors of mTOR, especially from the complex 1 (mTORC1) as well as its upstream and downstream elements (AKT/PI3K and MEK). The biological process of angiogenesis is also under research, with ongoing trials with anti-angiogenic agents from the Tyrosine Kinase Inhibitors (TKIs) targeting the Vascular Endothelial Growth Factor (VEGF) pathway, as well as antibody agents like bevacizumab. As it is expected, immunotherapy with checkpoint inhibitors is also under current investigation, with anti-PD1 and anti-PD-L1 monoclonal antibodies being tested in clinical trials. In this chapter we are going to cover the molecular biology of MNs, especially in the cases of grade II and grade III MN. We will also discuss the current knowledge in systemic treatments as well as therapies in clinical trials and possible candidates that are being tested *in vitro*.

2. Molecular biology

Advancements in understanding the pathophysiology and molecular biology of MNs are critical for improving risk evaluation and prognosis. Similarly, to design novel treatments aimed at blocking canonical pathways involved in carcinogenesis and disease evolution. As molecular analyzes of meningiomas continue to evolve, several cytogenetic, genomic, epigenetic, and expression alterations associated with tumor aggressiveness and proclivity for recurrence have been identified as potential biomarkers to enhance risk stratification [12]. Recently, several seminal studies evaluating the genomics of intracranial meningiomas have rapidly changed the understanding of the disease. The importance of NF2 (neurofibromin 2), TRAF7

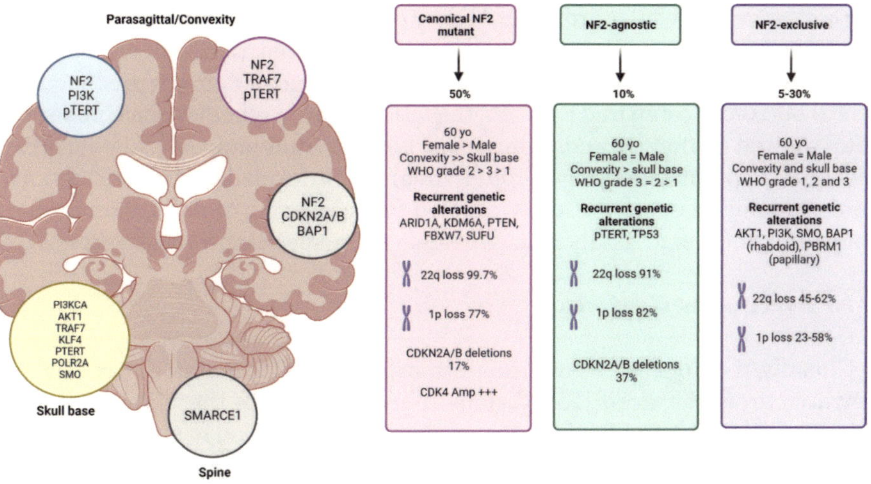

Figure 1.
Main cytogenetic and recurrent genetic alterations in recurrent and high-grade meningiomas according to the WHO classification and anatomical location.

(tumor necrosis factor [TNF] receptor-associated factor 7), KLF4 (Kruppel-like factor-4), AKT1, SMO (smoothened), PIK3CA (phosphatidylinositol-4,5-bisphosphate 3-kinase catalytic subunit alpha), and POLR2 (RNA polymerase II subunit A) demonstrates that there are at least six distinct mutational classes of meningiomas. In addition, six methylation classes of meningioma have been appreciated, enabling improved prognosis prediction compared with traditional WHO grades. Genomic studies have shed light on the nature of recurrent meningioma, distinct intracranial locations and mutational patterns, and a potential embryonic cancer stem cell-like origin [13–16] (**Figure 1**).

2.1 Cytogenetics and genomics

A large number of meningiomas possess a normal karyotype, with an overall low incidence of genomic alterations (including somatic copy number alterations—SCNA, rearrangements, and low mutational burden) [17–19]. However, these disruptions increase following tumor grade, the number of recurrences, and biological aggressiveness. More than half of all identified genomic alterations involve the NF2, which underlies inherited Neurofibromatosis syndrome. Indeed, the most significant SCNA in meningioma is chromosome 22 monosomy, which is present in ~56% of cases and leads to losing the genomic locus containing NF2 (22q12.2) [20, 21]. Among grade I meningiomas, those carrying NF2 alterations are more likely to progress than those with a normal karyotype. In addition, the frequency of NF2 aberrations increases with tumor grade.

Loss of heterozygosity on chromosome 1p is present in 16% of MNs [22]. Characterization of the smallest region of overlapping deletion on this chromosome spans ~3.7 megabases and identified 59 genes, 17 of which have putative tumor-suppressive functions based on gene ontology. The protein methyltransferase and tumor suppressor RIZ1, is located on chromosome 1p, and studies implicate its loss of expression in meningioma progression [23]. Loss of the CDKN2A/CDNK2B locus on chromosome 9q is common in grade II meningiomas that transition to anaplastic lesions [24]. Additionally, a study showed that the levels of p16 and p15, the proteins encoded by CDKN2A and CDKN2B, may hold prognostic significance and/or represent a promising therapeutic target [25]. Recently, Nassiri et al. described four consensus molecular groups of MN by combining DNA somatic copy-number aberrations, DNA somatic point mutations, DNA methylation, and messenger RNA abundance in a unified analysis [26]. These molecular groups predicted clinical outcomes compared with existing classification schemes. Each molecular group showed distinctive and prototypical biology (immunogenic, benign NF2 wild-type, hypermetabolic and proliferative) that informed therapeutic options. Proteogenomic characterization reinforced the robustness of defined molecular groups and uncovered highly abundant and group-specific protein targets [26].

2.2 NF2-related meningiomas

Globally, meningiomas have a low mutation rate (~3.5 mutations per megabase) compared to other cancers [25]. Various efforts to genotype the disease using NGS have identified NF2 mutations as the predominant alteration in spontaneous and Neurofibromatosis syndrome-associated tumors [24], at a frequency of ~40% in low grade and nearly 80% in high-grade tumors [27]. MNs related to alterations in NF2 were more common in the cerebral convexities and posterior skull base than those found in other anatomic locations, and up to 13% were associated with other co-mutations, including single mutations in CREBBP, PIK3CA (R108H), PIK3R1, BRCA1, and SMARCB1 [27]. Unfortunately, within NF2 mutated meningiomas, none of these identified mutations can predict the chance of recurrence, which can vary widely.

TERT promoter mutations have recently been reported in ~6% of all MNs, with ~80% of these also harboring alterations (mutations or deletions) at the NF2 locus [28]. Similar to overall mutational burden, TERT mutations increase with tumor grade. In grade I MN, TERT C228T and C250T mutations are linked with transformation to higher grades [28], prompting many neuro-oncologists to consider standardized testing for TERT promoter mutations. Further studies demonstrate that the presence of C228T and C250T correlates with increased TERT mRNA and functional increases in telomerase activity [29]. In grade II or III tumors, univariate analysis revealed a significant association with decreased PFS (progression-free survival; median 12.5 vs. 26 months, $p = 0.004$) and OS (overall survival; mean 26 vs. 46 months, $p = 0.009$) [30]. In vitro studies demonstrated that TERT mutated meningioma cells show decreased TERT activity in response to YK-4-279, a small molecule inhibitor of ETS transcription factor, suggesting a novel potential strategy for targeting this subgroup of tumors. In addition to individual TERT promoter mutations, recent efforts using targeted sequencing approaches identified an additional TERT promoter in the known hotspot G124A, which like other TERT mutations, seems to correlate with poor prognosis [31].

2.3 Non-NF2 meningioma

Non-NF2 mutated meningiomas, which generally have a benign behavior, are usually chromosomally stable, and often located in the anterior, medial, or skull base regions, possess a distinct mutational landscape [27]. Recent high throughput sequencing studies suggest an average of only 1.56 (SD ± 1.07) genomic alterations (GAs) per non-NF2 mutated tumor [31]. The pro-apoptotic E3 ubiquitin ligase, tumor necrosis factor receptor-associated factor 7 (TRAF7) is mutated ~25% of all meningiomas [31]. Such alterations occur in the C-terminal WD40 protein interaction domain, suggesting they may alter protein-protein interactions with MAPK and NF-kB family members [32]. While TRAF7 mutation is mutually exclusive with NF2 mutations, it is almost always correlated with PI3K and activating E17K mutation in AKT1, with the K409Q alteration of KLF4 [33].

AKT1, also referred to as protein kinase B, is a well-known oncogene. AKT activation relies on the PI3K pathway and is recognized as a critical node in the mTOR pathway. The E17 hotspot is the most characterized of AKT1 mutations and leads to constitutive activation of the protein. Mutations in AKT1 have also been shown to confer resistance to allosteric kinase inhibitors in vitro and are oncogenic in many solid tumors. Specifically, the E17K mutation is found in 7–12% of grade I meningiomas [34], is enriched in the meningothelial subtype [17], and is predictive of decreased PFS in olfactory groove tumors [35]. Altering the same signaling pathway PIK3CA mutations are also found in ~7% of non-NF2 tumors and are mutually exclusive with AKT1 mutation [36]. Targeted sequencing of this gene revealed novel non-synonymous mutations, A3140T and A3140G, which are reported as pathogenic, and C112T, which is also predicted to be pathogenic [31]. Indeed, increased PI3K signaling is related to aggressive behavior, especially within high-grade meningiomas [37], suggesting that therapeutics targeted toward this pathway may be a potential option.

Sequencing of 71 meningiomas genes recently identified two novel missense mutations in FGFR3, T932C, and G1376C, both of which were predicted to be pathogenic [31]. Identifying these mutations in patients with skull base low-grade tumors was associated with a good prognosis, given the absence of recurrence and the requirement of IMRT. KLF4 gene encodes a protein that belongs to the Kruppel family of transcription factors. The encoded zinc finger protein is required to control the G1-to-S transition of the cell cycle following DNA damage by mediating the tumor suppressor gene p53. In addition, KLF4 is involved in the differentiation of epithelial cells and may also function in skin, skeletal, and kidney development [38]. In meningiomas, KLF4 is thought to act as a tumor suppressor gene, expressed in low-grade tumors and downregulated in anaplastic tumors. At the genomic level, KLF4 is mutated in ~12% of grade I meningiomas, virtually all of which are of the secretory sub-type and harbor TRAF7 mutations [39]. All identified KLF4 mutations result in a K409Q substitution within the DNA binding domain, which likely alters several protein functions [40].

SMO (Smoothened, Frizzled Class Receptor) gene encoded a G protein-coupled receptor that interacts with the patched protein, a receptor for hedgehog proteins. Mutations in SMO, which result in L412F or W535L substitutions, lead to functional activation of Hedgehog signaling in meningioma [17, 41]. These mutations are present in ~5.5% of grade I meningiomas and are mutually exclusive with TRAF7, KLF4, and AKT1 mutations [27]. Meningiomas with the L412F mutation are more likely to recur (XX) and are enriched at the midline, perhaps due to the role that Hedgehog signaling plays in hemisphere separation during development [36]. Mutations in the Hedgehog family member SUFU are also found at low frequencies in sporadic meningiomas, and their germinal counterpart is also present in familial meningiomatosis [42]. Additional hedgehog family germline mutations occur in SMARCE1 and SMARCB1, though these carry less risk of recurrence than familial NF2 mutations [43, 44].

POLR2A (RNA Polymerase II Subunit A) catalyzes the transcription of DNA into RNA using the four ribonucleoside triphosphates as substrates. In addition, POLR2A is the largest and catalytic component of RNA polymerase II which synthesizes mRNA precursors and many functional non-coding RNAs. POLR2A encodes RPB1 (DNA-directed RNA polymerase II subunit), a gene found altered in about 6% of meningiomas [42]. From another perspective, inactivating somatic and germline mutations or gene deletions in the BAP1 tumor suppressor gene are explicitly found within high-grade rhabdoid meningioma [45]. Also, the loss of BAP1 is correlated with tumor aggressiveness and decreased time to progression. Alterations in the SWI/SNF pathway, specifically mutations in ARID1A, were recently found in 12% of high-grade meningiomas. Other components of this canonical pathway, including SMARCB1, SMARCA4, and PBRM1, are altered in up to 15% of patients with non-NF2-dependent meningiomas [46].

3. Epigenetics

Through whole-genome analysis, global DNA methylation profiling has demonstrated that higher methylation levels are associated with increased tumor aggressiveness and risk of recurrence. DNA methylation is an epigenetic change hypothesized to contribute to genomic instability by silencing genes involved with DNA repair and control of cell cycling. Evidence suggests that methylation status may predict tumor behavior more accurately than the current WHO classification, thus, DNA methylation status has been proposed as an alternative classification system for MNs [47]. The most important genes involved in the DNA methylation of MNs are tissue inhibitors of metalloproteinase 3 (TIMP3), cyclin-dependent kinase inhibitor 2A (CDKN2A), and tumor protein 73 (TP73), which are hypermethylated in at least 10% of cases [48]. TIMP3 hypermethylation results in transcriptional downregulation and inhibits its tumor suppressor properties [49]. In addition, TIMP3 is frequently hypermethylated in higher-grade MNs (40–60%) and is related to a decrease in relapse-free time and increased biological aggressiveness [50]. Notably, TIMP3 is found on chromosome 22q12, and almost all cases with gene hypermethylation had a concurrent allelic loss of 22q. About 60–80% of high-grade meningiomas carry TP73 promoter methylation, a queue event not common in grade I tumors, suggesting its potential use as a marker for high-grade lesions [51].

Recently, several studies highlighted the importance of global methylation profiles in the molecular subclassification of meningiomas [52], Olar et al. demonstrated that unsupervised clustering of DNA methylation data classified meningiomas into two distinct subgroups associated with recurrence-free survival. A statistically significant association between DNA methylation subclasses and tumor recurrence was maintained after adjusting for clinical factors, such as WHO grade and Simpson grade [41]. Similarly, Sahm et al. identified two major groups and six subgroups of meningiomas based on unsupervised clustering of DNA methylation data, with significantly different genomic makeup and clinical behaviors. Interestingly, most non-NF2 meningiomas clustered together into a single benign subgroup [53]. These initial efforts suggest that epigenetic signatures may have solid clinical associations with tumor recurrence, to a more significant extent than can be correlated with mutational genetic analysis and could be used clinically to stratify patients. An additional manifestation of the importance of epigenetic changes in meningioma clinical behavior was recently shown, describing an increased risk of recurrence in tumors that show a loss of histone H3K27 trimethylation [54].

3.1 Protein expression

Classically, the identification of meningiomas using immunohistochemistry has been done using the expression of the progesterone receptor (PR) and the epithelial membrane antigen (EMA). However, over the last few years, it has been found that the specificity of RP for the diagnosis of high-grade meningiomas is low, especially when trying to differentiate between clear cell, fibrous, and microcystic subtypes. Likewise, EMA expression correctly identifies ~90% of grade I meningiomas, but only 75% of grade III, with even lower specificity rates for secretory and microcystic subtypes [55]. Due to these markers' poor performance, the expression of somatostatin receptor 2A (SSTR2A) in combination with EMA was included, a profile that provides a sensitivity of 100% and specificity of 95%, regardless of tumor grade. Likewise, recent work suggests that the absence of Sox10 and STAT6 [56, 57] are superior approaches to distinguishing meningioma from schwannoma, solitary fibrous tumor, and synovial sarcoma.

In addition, marking for lymphocyte infiltration can contribute to the grading of meningiomas and the prediction of response to some interventions. Most low-grade meningiomas possess a high percentage of CD-3+ T-lymphocytes but relatively few CD20+ B cells; however, across tumor grades, these populations are greatly enriched compared to those seen in peripheral blood mononuclear cells (PBMC) [58]. Flow cytometry analysis reveals evidence of class switching in B cells, an increased percentage of CD8+ cells compared to CD4+ T cells, and a prevalence of CD45RO+/CD45RA− effector cells compared to naive T cells [59]. This information allows predicting that tumor-infiltrating immune cells have had exposure to various tumor antigens despite low BMR. Among high-grade meningiomas and particularly anaplastic tumors, there is a reduction in the count of CD4+, CD8+, and PD-1+ T cells, and an increase in the number of FoxP3+ T-regulatory cells (Tregs) [60]. This immune cell phenotype, also observed in other tumor types, is associated with tumor-mediated evasion of the immune system.

Du et al. report high levels of PD-L1 mRNA, which correlated to protein expression levels, in ~40% of grade I, 60% of grade II, and 77–88% of grade III meningiomas [59]. Nevertheless, Everson et al. only identified PD-L1 expression in 25% of grade III cases, with no expression detected in grade I or II cases [25]. The controversy has been amplified since PD-L1 does not predict outcomes. However, in the future, the expression of TIM-3 and LAG-3 could be helpful to consider the use of agonist monoclonal antibodies [58]. Another potential biomarkers that could

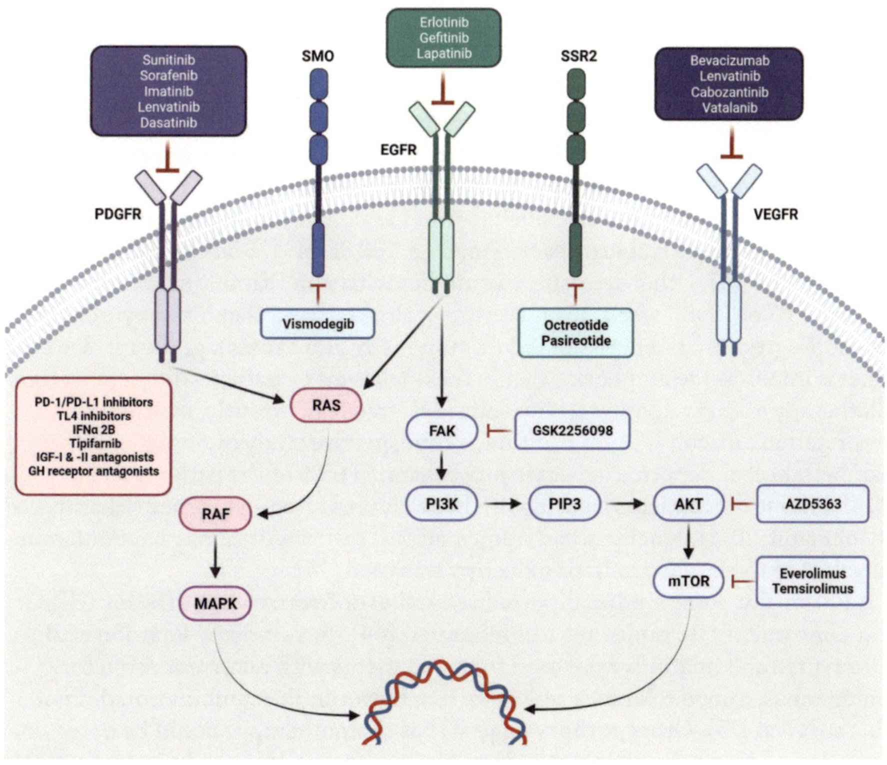

Figure 2.
Signaling pathways and potential targets implicated in high-grade meningiomas.

predict the response to targeted therapies are EGFR expression, which is present in up to 90% of meningiomas [25]. Furthermore, the expression of TOP2A (35% of the samples) is associated with a higher tumor grade and could be useful to assess the usefulness of anthracyclines or trabectedin. Likewise, TOP1 over-expression is observed in 29% of meningiomas and correlates with sensitivity to irinotecan and topotecan, while elevated levels of PDGFR and c-MET are observed in more than 20% of cases [25] (**Figure 2**).

4. Medical treatment for meningioma

The classical first-line treatment for all MNs is surgery. However, high grade meningiomas have a high recurrence rate; up to 60% of tumors may recur after 15 years of complete resection [12, 61]. Unfortunately, at the moment there are no standard effective treatments determined because of lack of existent evidence [12]. The use of systemic treatments as standard care remains experimental and is reserved for cases of recurrent/progressive disease not suitable for surgery or radiotherapy [62]. Hereafter we are going to present some of the systemic strategies currently in used and under study. A summary of the main therapies that have shown some benefit in MN treatment can be seen in **Table 1**, and a summary of current active clinical trials is shown in **Table 2.**

4.1 Chemotherapy

It is known that chemotherapy is poorly effective as adjuvant treatment after surgery and radiotherapy. Some clinical trials and case series have shown a minimal or no impact in patients' outcomes. However, some agents are being tested in several clinical trials [63].

Hydroxyurea is a ribonucleotide reductase inhibitor that was initially developed to treat myeloproliferative disorders and chronic myelogenous leukemia [64]. It induces apoptosis in meningioma cells, arresting meningioma cells in the S-phase of the cell cycle [63]. In pre-clinical trials from Schrell et al., they demonstrated that hydroxyurea prevent recurrence for 24 months in patients who had complete resection [65, 66]. However, clinical trials, failed to provide similar results showing that 50% of the patients achieve stable disease, a median PFS of 44–176 weeks and acceptable toxicity [63, 65–71]. Other retrospective studies with small sample sizes, have shown a median PFS of 10–80 weeks [64]. Weston et al. also found that hydroxyurea may prevent progression, but does not reduce tumor size and causes significant side effects [72]. It is important to emphasize that in these trials many patients did not received radiotherapy or that radiotherapy was administered concurrently, making data interpretation difficult [73]. In addition, a retrospective study of 60 patients from Chamberlain et al. reported a disease progression in 65% of the patients and a median PFS of 4 months in patients treated with hydroxyurea after recurrence (Chamberlain and Johnston, 2011). Finally, some studies suggest hydroxyurea may have outcomes equivalent to those when radiation therapy was used [74].

Additionally, some studies reported reduction of hydroxyurea efficacy when other concomitant therapies are administrated [64]. In a study by Reardon et al., hydroxyurea and imatinib were used to treat patients with recurrent refractory meningiomas, a good tolerance was reported; however, the combination did not affect survival [75]. Other authors suggest that chemotherapy should be based on expression of drug resistance genes, in patients whose mRNA analysis predicted sensitivity to chemotherapy. In these cases, a concomitant treatment with mitoxantrone and hydroxyurea reported long-term efficacy [61]. Currently, some investigators are

Type of agent	Medication	Mechanism of action
Chemotherapy	Temozolomide	Alkylating agent
	Irinotecan	Topoisomerase 1 inhibitor
	Hydroxyurea	Ribonucleotide reductase inhibitor
	Trabectedin	Mechanism unclear
Plant-derived agents	AKBA	Induction of apoptosis and antiinflammatory
	Curcumin	Interaction with multiple cell signaling proteins
EGFR antagonists	Gefitinib	EGFR antagonist
	Erlotinib	EGFR antagonist
	Monoclonal antibodies	Humanized antibodies to EGFR
PDGFR antagonists	Imatinib	PDGFR antagonist
	Satinib	PDGFR inhibitors
	Nilotinib	PDGFR inhibitors
mTOR inhibitors	Temsirolimus	mTOR inhibitor
	Vistusertib	mTOR inhibitor
	Everolimus	mTOR inhibitor
VEGFR antagonists	Bevacizumab	Humanized monoclonal antibody to VEGFR
	Cediranib	VEGFR antagonist
Combination antagonists	Sorafenib	VEGFR and PDGFR antagonist
	Sunitinib	VEGFR and PDGFR antagonist
	Vatalanib	VEGFR and PDGFR antagonist
Hormonal agents	Megestrol Mifepristone	Progesterone receptor partial agonist Progesterone receptor competitive antagonist
	Tamoxifen	Estrogen receptor antagonist
	Octreotide Pasireotide	Somatostatin mimetic Somatostatin mimetic
	Pegvisomant	Growth hormone receptor antagonist
	Lutathera	Somatostatin receptor afinity and radiation β- emission
	Fenretinide	Synthetic retinoid induces apoptosis
Immunomodulators	IFNα 2B	Antiproliferative and antiangiogenic
	Nivolumab Pembrolizumab Aveoumab Sintilimab	PD-1 receptor and ligand inhibitors
	Trametinib	Inhibits MEK1 and MEK2
	Alpelisib	PI3K inhibitor
	Ipililumab	CTLA-4 blockade
Oncolytic virus	Adenovirus	Antineoplastic effect against the malignant meningioma and significant tumor regression
	Herpes virus	Replication of adenovirus and oncolysis at high dose and at a lower dose meningioma cells killing
Farnesyl transferase inhibitors	Tipifarnib	Farnesyl transferase inhibitor

Type of agent	Medication	Mechanism of action
Possible adjunctive agents	Calcium channel blockers	Reduction of intracellular calcium concentrations
	Statins	MAPK pathway inhibition
	Antiretrovirals	Protein downregulation
RNAi		Antisense abrogation of mRNA strands

Table 1.
A summary of different agents with promising evidence in the treatment of high-grade meningioma.

ClinicalTrials.gov Identifier	Status	Intervention	Arms	Outcomes
NCT03071874	Active, not recruiting	AZD2014 a dual mTORC1/mTORC2 inhibitor	Experimental: AZD2014	PFS OS Radiographic response rate Duration of radiographic response Frequency of adverse events
NCT02648997	Recruiting	Nivolumab 240 mg every 2 weeks Nivolumab 480 mg once every 4 weeks	Experimental: Cohort 1 (original cohort): Nivolumab Monotherapy	PFS Median PFS Median OS Objective radiologic response rate Adverse events
		Ipilimumab 1 mg/kg every 3 weeks Nivolumab 480 mg once every 4 weeks Nivolumab 3 mg/kg every 3 weeks External Beam RT	Experimental: Cohort 2: Nivolumab in Combination with Ipilimumab	PFS Median PFS Median OS Objective radiologic response rate Adverse events
NCT03279692	Active, not recruiting	Pembrolizumab	Experimental: Pembrolizumab	PFS OS Toxicity Intracraneal response
NCT04997317	Recruiting	177Lu-DOTA-JR11 (Phase 0); Cycle 1 and Cycle 2 (cross-over) 177Lu-DOTATOC (Phase 0); Cycle 1 and Cycle 2 (cross-over), Cycle 3 and 4	Active Comparator: Phase 0: Group A	Change in Tumor-to-dose limiting organ dose ratio T-to-bone marrow Change in Tumor-to-dose limiting organ dose ratio T-to-kidney Assessment of treatment safety (phase I/II) by number of AEs graded according to CTCAE v5.0
		177Lu-DOTA-JR11 (Phase 0); Cycle 1 and Cycle 2 (cross-over) 177Lu-DOTATOC (Phase 0); Cycle 1 and Cycle 2 (cross-over), Cycle 3 and 4	Active Comparator: Phase 0: Group B	
		177Lu-DOTA-JR11 (Phase I/II)	Active Comparator: Phase I/II	
NCT03971461	Recruiting	Lutathera	Experimental: Lutathera	PFS at 6 months Objective response rate OS at 12 months PFS OS

ClinicalTrials.gov Identifier	Status	Intervention	Arms	Outcomes
NCT04082520	Recruiting	Gallium Ga 68-DOTATATE Lutetium Lu 177 Dotatate Magnetic Resonance Imaging Positron Emission Tomography Quality-of-Life Assessment Questionnaire Administration	Treatment (gallium Ga 68-DOTATATE PET/MRI, Lutathera)	PFS at 6 months OS PFS Adverse events incidence Change in quality of life Local control Duration of local control Objective response to treatment Response rate by volumetric analysis
NCT03016091	Recruiting	Pembrolizumab	Experimental: Arm 1 IV Pembrolizumab	PFS at 6 months PFS at 12 months OS
NCT03604978	Recruiting	Ipilimumab Nivolumab Stereotactic Radiosurgery	Patients receive nivolumab	Maximum tolerated combination of radiosurgery and nivolumab plus or minus ipilimumab Incidence of adverse event profile Objective response rate Objective radiological response PFS OS Changes of peripheral T-cells
NCT02333565	Unknown	Everolimus Octreotide	Experimental: Combinaison everolimus and octreotide	PFS rate
NCT04501705	Recruiting	Apatinib mesylate	Experimental: test group	PFS-6% ORR OS
NCT03267836	Recruiting	Avelumab Proton surgery	Experimental: Avelumab + proton therapy	Immunogenicity Safety of therapy Pathologic response PFS OS
NCT04728568	Recruiting	Sintilimab	Experimental: Sintilimab	PFS at 6 months OS
NCT03631953	Recruiting	Trametinib Alpelisib	Experimental: Alpelisib in combination with Trametinib administered	Dose Limiting Toxicity (DLT) rate of combination Alpelisib and Trametinib
NCT00904735	Unknown	Hydroxyurea Imatinib mesylate	Experimental: Arm I Patients receive hydroxyurea and imatinib	PFS Survival Response rate according to MacDonald criteria Toxicity as assessed by NCI CTCAE v. 3.0
		Hydroxyurea	Experimental: Arm II Patients receive hydroxyurea	

Table 2.
A summary of currently ongoing clinical trials that assess the effectiveness and safety of different systemic therapies in high-grade meningiomas.

looking for the role of hydroxyurea as an adjunct to other therapies, such as calcium channel blockers, as calcium channel antagonists have an inhibitory effect on meningioma growth in culture [76]. For this matter, Ragel et al. reported that calcium channel antagonists can block stimulatory effects of growth factors on meningioma cell cultures and increase hydroxyurea effectiveness [77]. Evidence of hydroxyurea treatment in patients with high grade meningioma varies widely across patients. Demonstrating that this treatment is generally well-tolerated but evidence in tumor control is not conclusive to establish a standard treatment in high-grade MNs.

Trabectedin it is an alkylating agent used in soft tissue sarcomas. It inhibits transcription, its mechanism is not completely understood but some studies reported decreased cell proliferation, induction of apoptosis and inhibition of transcription factor binding by binding to the minor groove of the DNA helix [78]. In the randomized phase II clinical trial NCT02234050 by EORTC Brain Tumor Group (EORTC-1320-BTG), treatment with trabectidin in grade II/III meningiomas did not improve PFS or OS and it was associated with significantly higher toxicity as compared to local standard care. A median PFS of 4.17 months was reported in the local standard care arm and of 2.43 months in the trabectedin arm (hazard ratio [HR] for progression, 1.42; 80% CI, 1.00–2.03; $p = 0.204$). Also, the median OS was 10.61 months in the local standard care arm and was 11.37 months in the trabectedin arm (HR for death, 0.98; 95% CI, 0.54–1.76; $p = 0.94$). In 44.4% of the local standard care arm patients occurred adverse events (4 serious adverse events, 0 lethal events) and 59% of the trabectidin arm presented adverse events (57 serious adverse events and 2 toxic deaths) [79]. Trabectedin did not improve PFS and OS and was associated with significantly higher toxicity. Evidence is not conclusive to establish a standard treatment in high grade meningiomas. However, the data future clinical trials are needed.

Temozolomide another alkylating agent, used as standard care in management of glioma. It does not prolong PFS in clinical trials of recurrent meningioma [80]. It is believed that the no effect on meningioma could be due to intact activity of the DNA repair enzyme O6-methylguanine DNA methyltransferase (MGMT) [63, 81, 82].

Chamberlain et al. reported a median time tumor progression of 4.6 years and median OS of 5.3 years in patients treated with cyclophosphamide, doxorubicin, and vincristine. They also reported high toxicity and very low response. However, without a control group the results are difficult to interpret [83]. Some small case series also reported results by administrating cyclophosphamide, adriamycin, vincristine, isofosfamide/mesna or adriamycin/dacarbazine, but the evidence is limited [84]. In some in vitro an in vivo animal studies, was reported that irinotecan has an anti-meningioma effect. However, it did not show benefits in phase II clinical trials [81, 82, 85].

Finally, some preclinical studies evaluated the response of Plant-Derived Chemotherapeutic Agents. Curic et al. described an antitumorigenic properties from curcumin (from the spice plant *Curcuma longa*) [86]. Additionally, Park et al. reported a cytotoxic effect of acetyl-11-keto-beta-boswellic acid (substance isolated from the *Boswellia serrata*), by inhibition of microsomal prostaglandin E synthase–1 and the serine protease cathepsin G [87]. Overall, traditional chemotherapy has demonstrated limited clinical efficacy in treating meningiomas. Additionally, it may lead to complications as immunosuppression, myelosuppression, gastrointestinal distress, organ damage, and fatigue [88].

5. Targeted therapy

Unlike other solid tumors, MN presents with a low mutation rate of approximately 3.5 mutations per megabase [25]. However, the case of high-grade MNs has been evaluated recently. Bi et al. analyzed 39 samples of high-grade MN and found an average of 23 (range 1–223) nonsynonymous coding alterations. This number of alterations is similar to that of craniopharyngioma and thyroid cancer, but considerably lower than other aggressive tumors like head and neck carcinoma, colorectal carcinoma and melanoma [34]. Because of its relatively low mutational burden, very few potential molecular targets have been identified. Interestingly, Bi et al. found that non-NF2 driver mutations in high-grade MN was considerably lower than in low grade MN, which reduces the number of possible targets than can be addressed. In the other hand, NF2 is usually altered in high-grade MN (80% of cases) more frequently than in low grade MN (40%). Most of genetic and regulatory alterations that have been described in high grade MN occur downstream to a disrupted NF2 protein. Some of the pathways altered might involve Rac1/Cdc42, Ras/JNK and the master regulator AP-1 [89]. Furthermore, one of the main pathways associated with NF2 is the mTOR signaling cascade. NF2 naturally acts as a repressor of the mTORC1 and mTORC2, and when it is mutated, unregulated activation of this pathway occurs. Based on this, mTOR and some of its upstream/downstream effectors (Akt/PI3K) have been identified as potential targets. Other pathways regulated by receptor tyrosine kinases (RTKs) like EGFR, PDGFR and VEGFR (angiogenesis) are also being studied.

6. Epidermal Growth Factor Receptor (EGFR) inhibitors

The EGFR pathway has been demonstrated to play a role in the tumorigenesis of a great proportion of meningioma cases. Torp et al. demonstrated that EGFR expression is not detectable in healthy and injured adult human meninges, but is expressed in cases of meningioma [90]. Arnli et al. also showed that EGFR was absent in healthy meninges but present in MN [91]. Narla et al. analyzed 79 samples of MN using immunohistochemistry, to detect EGFR expression. They found that EGFR was expressed in all different grades of MN, but its expression was considerably higher in grade I MN (82.93%), than grade II MN (35.71%) and grade III MN (20%) ($p < 0.0001$) [92]. When analyzed as a general population, the expression of EGFR in MN ranges between 50% and 89% [93]. Even though EGFR is a potentially targetable molecule, its significance in meningioma might not be prognostic [94]. Caltabiano et al. analyzed MN samples using immunohistochemistry and FISH. They found that the expression of EGFR was not associated with outcomes like OS and PFS. Interestingly, they also found that progression from low grade MN to higher grades was associated with an increase in the level of EGFR expression (not the proportion of expression) [95].

Similar results were published by Wernicke et al. who found in a cohort of 89 MN samples that EGFR expression was more common in grade I MN than in other grades. They also showed that the staining percentage (SP) of immunoreactive cells was associated with histopathologic subtypes ($p = 0.029$), with anaplastic MN having the highest average SP [96]. EGFR expression in MN is also accompanied by a demonstrated receptor activation [93]. In the cell line IOMM-Lee, EGFR was found to play a role in radiation-induced progression of MN. Furthermore, EGFR is involved in the regulation of certain intracellular pathways including the MAPK, the PI3K/Akt and phospholipase C pathways, which have been seen to be activated in meningioma [37, 97].

In 2010, results from a phase II trial of erlotinib and gefitinib for the treatment of MN were published. Erlotinib is an orally available, reversible TKI directed against EGFR. Its use has been approved in different neoplastic disorders including non-small cell lung cancer (NSCLC) and pancreatic cancer [98]. Gefitinib is a first-generation

EGFR-TKI also approved for the treatment of locally advanced and advanced NSCLC [99]. In 2010, a clinical trial enrolled patients with recurrent histologically confirmed MN that were treated with no more than 2 chemotherapy regimens.

The study evaluated 25 patients with a median age of 57 years. From this cohort, 16 patients received gefitinib and 9 received erlotinib. Nine patients had atypical MN and 8 had anaplastic MN. PFS and OS were assessed at 6 and 12 months. For patients with low-grade histology, PFS-6 was 25%, PFS12 was 13%, OS-6 was 63% and OS12 50%. In the other hand, high-grade meningiomas seemed to respond a little better with a PFS6 of 29%, PFS-12 18%, OS6 71% and OS-12 65%. When statistical analysis was done no significant difference between low-grade and high-grade MN was seen [100]. Survival outcomes were not significantly better than that of standard treatment.

In 2020 Ferluga et al. found that STAT1 is overexpressed and present a constitutive phosphorylation in MN. They also found that this overactivation was not associated with the JAK-STAT pathway but instead it was induced by the constitutive phosphorylation of EGFR. They even demonstrated that STAT1 knockdown models presented a significant reduction of cellular proliferation as well as a deactivation of AKT and ERK1/2. The most interesting finding of this study was that the researchers used BM-1 cells and exposed them to three different EGFR inhibitors, two from second generation (canertinib and afatinib) and one first generation (erlotinib). After exposure to canertinib and afatinib, a decrease in about 60% of STAT1 expression was seen as well as an almost complete elimination of phosphorylated forms of STAT1, this effect was not seen after exposure to erlotinib.

Lapatinib is a dual EGFR/ErbB2 inhibitor currently approved for the treatment of advanced breast cancer with ErbB2 (HER2) expression [101]. There is preclinical evidence of lapatinib efficacy in decreasing tumoral growth in NF2-related Schwannomas. Ammoun et al. demonstrated that when NF2 is mutated or lost, there is an upregulation of different RTKs in Schwannoma, with EGFR and HER2 being two of the highest expressed [102]. Similar results have been seen in NF2-related MN. When the researchers added lapatinib at 5 and 10 μM concentrations to cultures of Schwannoma cells derived from patients' samples, they found that lapatinib successfully induced inhibition of the intracellular pathways downstream HER2, including ERK 1/2 and Akt. They also showed that after 24 h of exposure to lapatinib, cell viability decreased in a dose-dependent manner, with statistically significant differences between both concentrations of lapatinib to baseline, and from lapatinib 5 μM to lapatinib 10 μM [102].

The same group of researchers also tested lapatinib during a phase II clinical trial, with good results in terms of volumetric response, progression-free survival and safety profile [103]. Six years after this trial, the authors did a retrospective analysis of patients presenting with NF2-related meningiomas from the same cohort of patients with Schwannoma. Eight patients fulfilled criteria for analysis. After two months under treatment with lapatinib, the best volumetric response achieved was 26.1%. It is important to mention that in the group that was receiving lapatinib, two tumors increased in volume by more than 20%. Results from this analysis were confusing, with no clear benefit of lapatinib, however, the sample was extremely small, and the analysis was retrospective. This study might influence the development of future, prospective, larger clinical trials specifically for patients with MN [104].

In 2001, Crombet et al. published their results on the efficacy of a mouse anti-human neutralizing monoclonal antibody against EGFR (ior egf/r3). They performed a phase I clinical trial using this antibody in 9 patients with high-grade brain tumors that persisted or relapsed after surgery. Only one of the patients had MN (hemangiopericytic). The patient had 48 years old and a Karnofsky Performance

Score of 90. She received four doses of 160 mg of antibody. At the end of the study, no objective response was seen in any of the patients, however the remained with stable disease until 6 months after the last antibody dose [105]. Even though EGFR inhibition has revolutionized cancer care in neoplasms with high incidence like NSCLC and colorectal cancer, these effects have not been seen in brain tumors, even when EGFR upregulation has been proved. Further studies must be performed with newer and more effective EGFR inhibitors, including monoclonal antibodies.

7. Platelet-Derived Growth Factor Receptor (PDGFR) inhibitors

PDGFR is another RTK whose expression is critical during development, as well as in the growth and differentiation of certain cell lineages. Its role in multiple chronic diseases have been studied, and it is considered a possible target in conditions like cancer, fibrosis, neurological disorders and atherosclerosis. The PDGF/PDGFR axis promotes cell proliferation, survival and migration primarily in cells of mesenchymal origin [106]. The ligands for PDGFR are four different polypeptide chains (PDGF-A, PDGF-B, PDGF-C and PDGF-D) which can be organized in an array of dimers that behave as functional growth factors (PDGF-AA, PDGF-BB, PDGF-AB, PDGF-CC and PDGF-DD [107]. These ligands have two different receptors, PDGFRα and PDGFRβ. The different ligands bind to the receptors with a differential specificity. PDGF-A, -B and -C will bind strongly to PDGFRα while the others will bind to PDGFRβ [106].

It has been demonstrated that MN expresses different forms of PDGF ligands, namely PDGF-AA and PDGF-BB, and expresses considerable levels of PDGFRβ. It has been shown that the PDGF/PDGFR axis might play a key role in the tumorigenesis of MN. Black et al. proved that PDGFRβ in MN cells derived from patients are susceptible to the stimulation with PDGF-BB ligands, with a shown increased in the activation of MAPK [21] and c-fos, a critical part of the master regulator AP-1, and a recognized proto-oncogene [108, 109]. Unlike EGFR expression, PDGFR levels appear to be higher in atypical and anaplastic MN than in grade I MN. In those MN that express PDGFR and the aforementioned PDGF ligands, there is an autocrine loop that supports maintenance and cell growth [109]. Todo et al. demonstrated that there is a considerable decrease in meningioma cells proliferation when these cells are given a neutralizing antibody against PDGF-BB. They saw a similar but less potent behavior when an anti-PDGF-AA antibody, also suggesting that the PDGF-BB pathway is the most important for meningioma maintenance [110].

Imatinib, a potent PDGF inhibitor currently used in different conditions (mainly chronic myeloid leukemia), has also been proven in MN patients. Imatinib possess a very low IC50 of 0.1 μM, this is especially important in MN as the blood-brain-barrier might decrease the flux of imatinib and other drug particles into the brain. In the NABTC 01–08 study, 23 patients with MN were enrolled, with 13 patients bearing low grade tumors, five with atypical MN and five with anaplastic MN. Response was only evaluated in 19 patients from whom 10 patients experienced disease progression. The rest of the patients remained disease stable. Median PFS was only 2 months, with a PFS6 of 29.4%. When analyzed separately, PFS for grade I MN was 3 months and PFS6 was as high as 45%. In the case of high-grade MN, PFS was 2 months but PFS6 was 0%.

The current landscape of PDGF inhibition is somewhat promising. Other agents like sunitnib, MLN518, dasatinib, AMN 107, pazopanib, sorafenib, CP673451 and CHIR 265 have been studied [111]. Furthermore, combination therapies using imatinib and other different agents like hydroxyurea [112], which has showed some benefit in the treatment of glioblastoma in a Phase I/II trial [113].

8. mTOR inhibitors

The mTORC1 (mammalian target of rapamycin complex 1) pathway has been reported to interact with merlin as a negative regulator of cell growth control [114]. mTOR is a serine/threonine kinase involved in cell signaling controlling transcription, actin cytoskeleton organization, translational activation, and metabolism in response to environmental cues [9]. The protein exists in two distinct multiprotein complexes. The rapamycin-sensitive complex mTORC1 regulates cell growth and proliferation in response to growth factors and metabolic conditions, whereas the rapamycin-insensitive mTORC2 regulates locally restricted growth processes within a cell and is involved in cell migration. Merlin was shown to enhance the kinase activity of mTORC2 [115].

Previously, Pachou et al. [116] found that mTORC1 is activated in the majority of MNs (7–10%) and that systemic mTORC1 inhibition can impair meningioma tumor formation in vivo. In addition, Akt is well known to be an upstream element of mTORC1 and to be activated in meningioma cells by platelet-derived growth factor [117]. PDGF also induces phosphorylation of p70S6K, the expression of which was reported to be increased in malignant MNs [118].

Several groups analyzed the biological effects of everolimus and temsirolimus on meningioma cell viability. They could clearly show that both inhibitors were effective in reducing meningioma cell viability and proliferation [114]. Moreover, evidence was found that the NF2 gene status may affect the response to both inhibitors but differentially activated mTOR pathways could not explain this result in isogenic meningioma cell lines with and without merlin expression [119]. Further, octreotide was shown to augment the inhibitory effect on the mTOR pathway in meningioma cell lines because mTOR inhibition increases the hyperphosphorylation of AKT which thereby increases cell proliferation [120].

In 2020, Graillon et al. reported the results of the CEVOREM trial, a phase II open label study that evaluated the combination of everolimus and octreotide in 20 high-grade MNs patients. Furthermore, four patients harbored NF2 germline mutation [121]. The overall PFS6 was 55% (95% CI 31.3–73.5%), and 6- and 12-month OS rates were 90% (95% CI 65.6–97.4%) and 75% (95% CI 50.0–88.7%), respectively. A decrease >50% was observed in the growth rate at 3 months in 78% of tumors. In addition, the median tumor growth rate decreased from 16.6%/3 months before inclusion to 0.02%/3 months at 3 months ($p < 0.0002$) and 0.48%/3 months at 6 months after treatment ($p < 0.0003$) [120].

In a small trial, everolimus has also been studied in conjunction with bevacizumab without finding any objective tumor response but showing a slight increase in PFS for those with high-grade MNs (NCT00972335) [122]. In this study, 88% of the 18 patients showed SD for a median duration of 10 months (2–29 months). Nevertheless, overall median PFS was 22 months (95% CI 4.5–26.8), higher for patients with WHO grade II and III than grade I tumors (22.0 months vs. 17.5 months). Four patients discontinued treatment due to toxicity (proteinuria, 2; colitis, 1, thrombocytopenia, 1), but another grade 3 toxicity was uncommon, and no patient had grade 4 toxicity. The interesting improvement in higher histological grade MNs could be due to their increased vasculature and the increased dependence on the mTOR pathway of these lesions [122].

There is currently a phase 0, single group assignment, trial for everolimus in NF2 mutant MNs and vestibular schwannomas (NCT01880749). There are two single group assignment phase II trials of another mTOR inhibitor, AZD2014; NCT03071874 for recurrent grade II/III MNs and NCT02831257 for NF2 patients with MNs. These trials will help determine the efficacy of mTOR inhibition in patients with these challenging lesions. Besides, a case report of a female patient with metastatic meningotheliomatous meningioma involving the brain and the lung was treated with the pan-AKT inhibitor, AZD5363 for AKT1E17K mutation, showed a favorable and durable response [123]. Ex vivo cultured meningioma cells revealed sensitivity to the drug as shown by pan-AKT accumulation on immunoblots. The patient has been treated for more than a year with a response which warrants further research [123].

9. Anti-angiogenesis

Angiogenesis depends on the balance between angiogenic and anti-angiogenic regulators [124]. Among the former, VEGF has been demonstrated to play an essential role in stimulating angiogenesis by promoting the migration, proliferation, and tube formation of endothelial cells. VEGF upregulation has been shown in MNs, suggesting its role as a pro-angiogenic factor responsible for edema formation in these tumors [125–127].

Neoangiogenesis in MNs is regulated by the balance between concentrations of both VEGF and semaphorin 3A (SEMA3A) in the tumor's microenvironment rather than by VEGF alone [125]. Accordingly, neo-angiogenesis would be blocked or stimulated depending on the prevalence of VEGF or SEMA3A with a high ratio between VEGF and SEMA3A as a negative predictor of recurrences [125]. Additionally, VEGF expression in MNs seems to be enhanced by hypoxia-inducible factor 1-alpha [128] and EGF [129], and reduced by dexamethasone.

Caveolin-1 (cav-1), which is a 20-KDa protein mainly expressed by fibroblasts, endothelial cells, myocytes, and adipocytes, seems to be involved in the oncogenesis and progression of several neoplasms, including MNs [130]. Similar to what has been reported in several solid tumors, a significant correlation has been shown between tumor-cell-derived cav-1 and microvascular density (MVD) in MNs [131], suggesting that this protein behaves as a pro-angiogenic factor. Consistent with this hypothesis, cav-1 has been shown to regulate endothelial cell growth and differentiation and to stimulate capillary tubule formation in vitro [132]. Moreover, VEGF-mediated pathological angiogenesis is strikingly reduced in cav-1 knock-out mice [133]. On the other hand, the association between cav-1 expression and MVD may also be related to factors regulating both the MNs neo-angiogenesis and cav-1 expression. Indeed, cav-1 may function as a pro-tumorigenic factor that can stimulate cell proliferation, following its tyrosine-14 phosphorylation by Src kinase [134].

Endothelin-1 (ET-1) has been demonstrated to play a role in the mechanism of meningioma tumorigenesis via the ETA receptor [135]. ET-1 expression/upregulation may contribute to meningioma growth by inducing the formation of new blood vessels. Indeed, a significant correlation has been shown between the expression of ET-1 and that of VEGF or MVD in MNs, in agreement with its proangiogenic action in these tumors.

Following these biological considerations, several angiogenesis inhibitors, such as bevacizumab, sunitinib, and vatalanib, have been evaluated in phase II trials with promising results [136]. The efficacy and safety of bevacizumab were evaluated in grades II and III MNs, finding a PFS6 of 43.8%. In addition, a review of 22 additional case reports for a total of 92 patients revealed a PFS of 16.8 months with 6 months PFS of 73% in those exposed to bevacizumab [137]. A phase II trial designed for all grades recurrent MNs that included 15 patients (15, 22, and 13 grade I, II, and III, respectively) showed stability of the disease in 100% of benign tumors and 82–85% among those with high-grade injuries. In addition, the PFS6, the median PFS, and OS, were 87%, 22.5 months, and 35.6 months for patients with grade I tumors, while this distribution was 77%, 15.3 months, and not reached for grade II, and 46%, 3.7 months, and 12.4 months for grade III, respectively [138]. There is an ongoing phase II trial evaluating bevacizumab in recurrent and progressive MNs (NCT01125046).

Kaley et al. reported a prospective, multicenter single-arm phase 2 trial that investigated the efficacy of sunitinib, a tyrosine kinase inhibitor that inhibits VEGF and PDGF receptors, which are over-expressed in MNs [139]. Thirty-six patients with grade II and III recurrent or progressive MNs were enrolled. They were heavily pre-treated (median five recurrences) and received sunitinib at 50 mg per day for days 1–28 of a 42-day cycle. The PFS6 was 42%, the median PFS was 5.2 months (95% CI 2.8–8.3), and the median overall survival was 24.6 months (16.5–38.4). Adverse events included four (8%) intratumoral hemorrhages, of which one was fatal, one (2%) grade 4 thrombotic microangiopathy, and one (2%) grade 3 gastrointestinal perforation. MRI perfusion in the exploratory group indicated that sunitinib is an active agent, and expression of VEGFR2 predicted PFS with a median of 1.4 months in VEGFR2-negative patients versus 6.4 months in VEGFR2- positive patients ($p = 0.005$) [139]. More recently, Cardona et al. reported a PFS of 9.1 months (95% CI 6.8–16.8) in a cohort of patients with high-grade MNs treated with sunitinib [140].

10. Hormonal therapy

Evidence suggests that meningioma growth could be hormone dependent because of the female predominance specially after puberty and reproductive years. Additionally, that 30% of the meningiomas are estrogen receptor positive and 70% are progesterone receptor positive [76]. It is also known, that high grade meningiomas express more estrogen receptors whereas benign meningiomas express more progesterone receptors [141]. It is also important to add, that approximately 90% of meningiomas express somatostatin receptors [142]. Therefore, hormonal therapies have been utilized in high grade meningioma treatment.

Due to estrogen receptors low expression, treatment with tamoxifen (estrogen receptor antagonist) has not shown effective results. Additionally, there is not any reports of androgen receptor antagonists in meningiomas [143]. In 1993 Goodwin et al. in a retrospective case series of 21 patients with meningioma treated with tamoxifen, they reported response in only 1 patient and disease progression in 10 patients [144]. Additionally, in a case study from Markwalder et al. a small group of patients with inoperable meningiomas that received tamoxifen were studied and only two patients show radiographical partial response [145].

Currently, due to the lack of evidence of anti-estrogenic agents' effect on meningioma no recommendation is available. Mifepristone is a progesterone receptor inhibitor. In a study published in 1991 by Wolfsberger et al., they used mifepristone as treatment of unresectable meningioma patients, they reported that five patients showed reduction of tumor size on neuroimaging and visual field improvement; in addition, three patients experienced headache relief and improvement in extraocular muscle function. No toxicities were reported [141]. Other study by Lamberts et al. reported stable disease in three patients, tumor size reduction in other three patients and no toxicities were reported [146]. These studies were limited because of the small sample size and tumor stage wasn't described in any of them. Therefore, more studies are needed to conclude the effect of mifeprisotne in high grade meningiomas. Other trial by Ji et al. reported a median PFS of 10 months and a median OS of 31 months in the mifepristone arm of patients with recurrent meningioma [147]. Additionally, in 2006 Grunberg et al. reported a reduction of less than 10% of the tumor area without clinical improvement in eight patients with unresectable meningioma who received mifepristone [148].

Megestrol acetate is an oral progesterone agonist that was used in a small trial. However no response was observed in high grade meningiomas [76]. So far there is no evidence that supports the use of progesterone receptor inhibitors in high grade meningiomas.

Somatostatin is important in regulation and proliferation of normal cells and tumor cells. It is known that meningiomas report the highest frequency of somatostatin receptor expression in brain tumors, especially the sst2A subtype. It is also reported that somatostatin inhibits meningioma growth in vitro in most studies, but increases meningioma proliferation in some [76].

Chamberlan et al. reported that 31% of patients demonstrated a partial radiographic response and 44% achieved PFS at 6 months with minimal toxicity in patients treated with octreotide (a somatostatin agonist). Furthermore, one-third of patients showed stable disease after treatment [149]. Therefore, somatostatin analogs are recommended for systemic treatment of unresectable or radiorefractory relapsed meningiomas [150]. The phase II CEVOREM trial explored the efficacy of the combination of everolimus (an mTOR inhibitor) and octreotide in high grade meningiomas treatment. The trial reported that the 6-month progression-free survival rate was 55% and the 6-month overall survival was 90% and 12-month survival rate was 90%. Additionally, a decrease of more than 50% was observed in the growth rate at 3 months in 78% of the tumors. That happens because, octreotide suppressed AKT activation during everolimus treatment and synergistically reduced expression of downstream proteins [121]. The previous results suggest that the combination of everolimus and octreotide could be a very good option to treat high grade meningiomas, however more studies are needed. In other phase II trial by Johnson et al. only 2 of 12 high grade cases experience long progression-free intervals, but at the end all patients experienced disease progression with median time of 17 weeks; a median survival 2.7 years was reported and octreotide was well-tolerated [151]. Additionally, an in- vitro study by Graillon et al. reported a significant anti-proliferative effects octreotide, but no apoptotic response [152].

Parasoreotide (SOM230C) is an intramuscularly long-acting somatostatin analogue. In the phase II trial by Norden et al., they reported that pasireotide has limited activity in recurrent meningiomas, a PFS-6 of 17% and median PFS of 15 weeks were reported. Furthermore, expression of somatostatin receptor was predictive of favorable response. However the findings in this trial require further investigation [153]. These findings are promising, nevertheless, larger randomized studies should be conducted to make a solid conclusion.

Growth hormone is secreted by the pituitary gland, and it induces production of insulin-like growth factor-I (IGF-I-), these hormones influence normal growth and metabolism [73]. There is existent evidence that reports abuntant growth hormone receptors expression in meningioma cells. There is also reported that inhibition of these receptors represents a decreased meningioma cell proliferation [154]. McCutcheon et al. reported that administration of pegvisomant reduces meningioma growth and in some cases causes tumor regression. Pegvisomant blocks growth hormone receptors and induces downregulation of the GH/IGF-I axis [155]. In other study, Puduvalli et al. reported that fenretinide, a synthetic retinoid, induced apoptosis in meningioma primary cells tested, it also increases levels of the death receptor DR5 and causes mitochondrial membrane depolarization. They also reported eradication of IGF-I proliferation in the meningioma cells [156].

Finally, insulin-like growth factor-II acts like IGF-I. In multiple studies have reported that the invasiveness of meningiomas is correlated to levels of IGF-II expression [157]. However, several studies are needed to establish IGF-II blockade could be an option to treat patients with meningiomas. These results provide preliminary evidence, but further studies are needed to explore these options as treatment against meningioma.

11. Interferons

Existent evidence, shows that recombinant interferon-α (INF-α) is a biologic agent able to inhibit DNA synthesis, it binds to the interferon-a/b receptor and is involved in cell resistance to viral infection [64]. In 1991 in vitro studies also reported that interferon-alpha inhibits tumor cells growth [158].

In 1997 Kaba et al., reported a minor reduction of tumor size in one patient and a stable disease that lasted up to 14 months in four of six patients with recurrent unresectable meningioma who received INF-α 2b [159]. Other study in 2001, reported a stable disease that lasted up to eight years in nine of twelve patients treated with INF-α [160]. In 2008 Chamberlain and Glantz, reported in a phase II study that 26 of 35 patients that received treatment with INF-α demonstrated stable disease after the first 3 cycles and that 9 patients developed progressive disease. Additionally, a PFS rate was 54% at 6 months and 31% at 12 months were reported, median time to tumor progression was 7 months and median survival was 8 months. Furthermore, no patient demonstrated neuroradiographic complete or partial response, fatigue, anemia and leukopenia were the most common toxicities but overall, the drug was safe. A limitation form this study is that it was conducted only in patients with refractory grade I meningiomas [161]. Currently, these options are used as therapy for recurrent meningiomas or progression following surgery and radiation. It is also used for meningiomas that no respond to standard treatment options. Nevertheless, evidence that supports the use of interferons for meningiomas is poor.

12. Oncolytic virus

Oncolytic viruses are biologic anti-tumor agents that selectively kill tumor cells leaving non tumoral cells intact [63]. A lot of oncolytic viruses have been investigated in different clinical trials, however no clinical trials have been conducted in meningiomas [162].

There are a few preclinical trials conducted in meningioma models. In 2005 Grill et al. evaluated the efficacy of conditionally replicating adenovirus (Ad) for oncolysis of meningiomas of 12 patients. Four different Ads were constructed and tested on meningioma cells and spheroids: Ad with an E1ACR2 deletion (Ad.d24), Ad with complete E1 region (Ad.E1+), Ad encoding the luciferase marker gene (Ad.Luc) and Ad encoding the luciferase gene in the E3 region (Ad.E1Luc). They demonstrated replication of adenovirus and oncolysis in primary cell cultures of meningioma cells at high dose (greater than 50 plaque-forming units per cell). Additionally, they also reported that at a lower dose (5 plaque-forming units per cell), Ad.d24 kills meningioma cells more efficiently than Ad.E1+ in benign, atypical, and malignant meningiomas [163].

Herpes virus it has a large dsDNA with more than 30 kb making the virus encoding for nonessential genes, this feature allows for genetic manipulation. Additionally, herpesviruses have a good safety profile, because they replicate in the nucleus without causing insertional mutagenesis [164].

In 1992, Market et al. added thymidine kinase-negative herpes simplex-I mutant virus, d/sptk, to meningioma cell cultures. They reported an antineoplastic effect against the malignant meningioma and significant tumor regressions [165]. In the study from Yazaki et al., reported that mutant herpes simplex virus (termed G207) can replicate and kill cells from human malignant meningiomas in cell culture. They also reported tumor growth reduction in nude mice harboring human malignant meningioma [166]. Additionally, it is reported that efficacy of oncolytic herpes simplex viruses (HSV) as single agent is unsatisfactory; so in 2006 Liu et al. demonstrated that oncolytic HSV encoding dnFGFR enhances antitumor efficacy [167]. In 2016 Nigim et al., reported that G47Δ, an oncolytic HSV derived from G207, was able to replicate and kill several human primary meningioma cultures in vitro. They also reported that this treatment prolonged survival, with 20% of mice surviving more than160 days. Furthermore, a lack of signs of encephalitic associated with G47Δ treatment was reported [168]. In 2018, they also reported that the mechanism of action of oHSV enables killing NF2 intact and mutant meningiomas and meningiomas that harbor other mutations [63].

Several studies have demonstrated the ability of oncolytic viruses to recruit T cells and induce immune responses against virus and tumor. Furthermore, some studies have demonstrated that oncolytic viruses combined with other cancer therapies, create synergistic effects in brain cancer treatment. Although many questions remain to be answered to fully exploit the therapeutic potential of oncolytic viruses against meningiomas [169].

13. Immune checkpoint inhibitors

Several studies have aimed to characterize the interactions between MNs and the immune system. Specifically, studies of the immune microenvironment in MNs have revealed that NY-ESO-1, PD-L1, PD-L2, B7-H3, and CTLA-4 are expressed in MNs and may be at least partly responsible for the suppression of the anti-tumor immune response [170, 171]. PD-L1 is expressed in MNs, and expression levels are higher for higher-grade tumors [172]. The expression of these proteins has been associated with tumor progression, recurrence, and poor survival outcomes. Fang et al. extensively characterized the immune infiltrate in MNs and found that the immune cells infiltrating MNs are mainly antigen-experienced T cells and B cells [58]. In their study, B cells were activated and underwent immunoglobulin class switching, somatic hypermutation, and clonal expansion. T-cells demonstrated evidence of antigen exposure and increased expression of PD-1 and TIM-3, which can be a sign of an exhausted phenotype. Tumor-infiltrating lymphocytes in MNs are mainly T-cells. Interestingly in anaplastic MNs, the number of CD4 and CD8 T-cells is low. At the same time, the proportion of Tregs is increased [59]. These data support the notion that an immunosuppressive microenvironment in MNs may contribute to tumor progression.

In a mouse model of meningioma, infusion of anti-PD1 antibody avelumab plus highly-active NK cells (HaNK) led to increased survival, showing the importance of innate NK cell activity [173]. Currently there are two case reports on PD-L1 checkpoint inhibition for recurrent MNs [174, 175]. The cases report disease-free recurrence for >2 years in one patient and > 6 months in another patient, with both having reductions in tumor volume, cerebral edema, and patient-reported symptoms following nivolumab treatment. Based on the existing evidence on PD-L1 expression in recurrent MNs, five clinical trials are enrolling patients with to receive anti-PD1 antibodies nivolumab, avelumab, or pembrolizumab. An ongoing phase II trial is designed to compare nivolumab alone to combination therapy with the anti-CTLA-4 antibody ipilimumab (NCT02648997). A phase Ib trial will investigate the preoperative use of avelumab in combination with hypo-fractionated proton radiotherapy for 3 months to evaluate its effect on the size of unresected MNs (NCT03267836). The other trials are recruiting patients with recurrent MNs to receive adjuvant immunotherapy as PD1 blockade.

14. CAR-T cell therapy

Chimeric Antigen Receptor (CAR) T cell therapies are a novel therapeutic approach to cancer. The standard treatment consists in the leukapheresis of autologous peripheral blood mononuclear cells from the patient bearing the tumor. After successful leukapheresis, T cell isolation is performed. T cells are then grown in culture and are further transduced with a lentiviral vector carrying an integrative plasmid that encodes the CAR, which is essentially a fusion protein containing a single-chain variable fragment derived from a full antibody, plus a transmembrane domain and different array of intracellular co-receptor and co-stimulatory domains that will trigger the intracellular signaling necessary for T cell activation [176].

CAR-T cell therapies were initially approved in 2017 (axi-cel and tisa-cel) for the treatment of relapsed/refractory diffuse large B cell lymphoma and relapsed/refractory B-cell acute lymphoblastic leukemia [177]. Unfortunately, the landscape of CAR-T cell therapies in solid tumors has not been promising, mainly due to different resistance from typical features of the tumor microenvironment like high acidity, immune effector exhaustion induction and the extracellular matrix. Different workaround strategies have been explored to address these problems and currently, highly engineered cells and very complex therapies (CAR-Ts in combination with checkpoint inhibition, or small molecules, or chemotherapy, or immunomodulators) are under study in different clinical trials [178].

Brain tumors have not been an exception in CAR-T development, with glioblastoma being the most attacked condition. Tang et al. reported a case of a patient with an anaplastic MN that underwent three surgical resections and had an Ommaya device implanted. IHC from her tumor sample showed a high expression of B7-H3, also known as CD276 ([179], p. 3). The researchers prepared CAR-Ts from autologous PBMCs, and during CAR-T development patient recur and CAR-Ts were administered in three doses via the Ommaya device. A fourth surgical treatment was performed as patient was progressing quickly, and unfortunately the patient died one day after surgery. Post-mortem analysis of the tumor sample showed that CAR-T indeed penetrated the tumor and successfully targeted some cells expressing B7-H3, however, as not all the tumor was expressing this molecule, antigen loss and selection of other cells with a different transcriptome occurred [180]. Even though results were not as expected, this case marks an important step toward the development of cell therapies of different natures, to treat brain tumors, especially those of high recurrency and aggressiveness.

15. Conclusions

Treatment in MN has remained similar since some decades ago. Major improvements in survival are achieved mainly by surgery and radiation therapy. Most cases of MN will respond to these conventional therapies, however, transformation of low-grade MN to high-grade MN, or de novo high-grade MN are highly recurrent and impose a very low survivability. For these tumors, surgery and radiation therapy are less than enough. With the era of genomic analysis and a better understanding of the genetic basis of cancer, different molecular targets and new therapeutic approaches have been studied for high-grade MN treatment. In this review we went through the main critical advancements in evidence that suggests that molecular targeting might be the future of high-grade MN treatment. To the date, all these molecular approaches are still under study, a conventional management is still the mainstay, but we hope in the following years, new evidence of the clinical relevance of these therapies is available and introduction of them into the therapeutic arsenal could be a true.

Author details

Juan Esteban Garcia-Robledo[1], Camila Ordóñez-Reyes[2,3], Alejandro Ruiz-Patiño[2,3], Álvaro Muñoz[4], Oscar Arrieta[5], Enrique Jiménez[7], Fernando Hakim[7], Diego Gómez[7], Juan Fernando Ramón[7] and Andrés F. Cardona[2,3,6]*

1 Division of Hematology/Oncology, Mayo Clinic, Phoenix, AZ, United States

2 Foundation for Clinical and Applied Cancer Research—FICMAC, Bogotá, Colombia

3 Molecular Oncology and Biology Systems Research Group (Fox-G), Universidad El Bosque, Bogotá, Colombia

4 Radiation Oncology Department, Carlos Ardila Lülle Cancer Institute—ICCAL, Fundación Santa Fe de Bogotá, Bogotá, Colombia

5 Thoracic Oncology Unit and Personalized Oncology Laboratory, National Cancer Institute (INCan), México City, Mexico

6 Direction of Research and Education, Luis Carlos Sarmiento Angulo Cancer Treatment and Research Center (CTIC), Bogotá, Colombia

7 Neurosurgery Department, Fundación Santa Fe de Bogotá, Bogotá, Colombia

*Address all correspondence to: andres.cardona@clinicadelcountry.com; a_cardonaz@yahoo.com

References

[1] Kalamarides M, Stemmer-Rachamimov AO, Niwa-Kawakita M, Chareyre F, Taranchon E, Han ZY, et al. Identification of a progenitor cell of origin capable of generating diverse meningioma histological subtypes. Oncogene. 2011;**30**:2333-2344. DOI: 10.1038/onc.2010.609

[2] Huntoon K, Toland AMS, Dahiya S. Meningioma: A review of clinicopathological and molecular aspects. Frontiers in Oncology. 2020;**10**:1-14. DOI: 10.3389/fonc.2020.579599

[3] Ostrom QT, Cioffi G, Gittleman H, Patil N, Waite K, Kruchko C, et al. CBTRUS statistical report: Primary brain and other central nervous system tumors diagnosed in the United States in 2012-2016. Neuro-Oncology. 2019;**21**: V1-V100. DOI: 10.1093/neuonc/noz150

[4] Holleczek B, Zampella D, Urbschat S, Sahm F, von Deimling A, Oertel J, et al. Incidence, mortality and outcome of meningiomas: A population-based study from Germany. Cancer Epidemiology. 2019;**62**:101562. DOI: 10.1016/j.canep.2019.07.001

[5] Wen PY, Huse JT. 2016 World Health Organization Classification of central nervous system tumors. Continuum: Lifelong Learning in Neurology. 2017;**23**:1531-1547. DOI: 10.1212/CON.0000000000000536

[6] Magill ST, Young JS, Chae R, Aghi MK, Theodosopoulos PV, McDermott MW. Relationship between tumor location, size, and WHO grade in meningioma. Neurosurgical Focus. 2018;**44**:E4. DOI: 10.3171/2018.1.FOCUS17752

[7] Moliterno J, Cope WP, Vartanian ED, Reiner AS, Kellen R, Ogilvie SQ, et al. Survival in patients treated for anaplastic meningioma. Journal of Neurosurgery. 2015;**123**:23-30. DOI: 10.3171/2014.10.JNS14502

[8] Wang YC, Chuang CC, Wei KC, Chang CN, Lee ST, Wu CT, et al. Long term surgical outcome and prognostic factors of atypical and malignant meningiomas. Scientific Reports. 2016;**6**:35743. DOI: 10.1038/srep35743

[9] Perry A, Scheithauer BW, Stafford SL, Lohse CM, Wollan PC. "Malignancy" in meningiomas: A clinicopathologic study of 116 patients, with grading implications. Cancer. 1999;**85**:2046-2056. DOI: 10.1002/(SICI)1097-0142(19990501)85:9<2046::AID-CNCR23>3.0.CO;2-M

[10] Brodbelt AR, Barclay ME, Greenberg D, Williams M, Jenkinson MD, Karabatsou K. The outcome of patients with surgically treated meningioma in England: 1999-2013. A cancer registry data analysis. British Journal of Neurosurgery. 2019;**33**:641-647. DOI: 10.1080/02688697.2019.1661965

[11] Negroni C, Hilton DA, Ercolano E, Adams CL, Kurian KM, Baiz D, et al. GATA-4, a potential novel therapeutic target for high-grade meningioma, regulates miR-497, a potential novel circulating biomarker for high-grade meningioma. eBioMedicine. 2020;**59**:102941. DOI: 10.1016/j.ebiom.2020.102941

[12] Al-Rashed M, Foshay K, Abedalthagafi M. Recent advances in meningioma immunogenetics. Frontiers in Oncology. 2020;**9**:1472. DOI: 10.3389/fonc.2019.01472

[13] Louis DN, Perry A, Reifenberger G, von Deimling A, Figarella-Branger D, Cavenee WK, et al. The 2016 World Health Organization classification of tumors of the central nervous system:

A summary. Acta Neuropathologica. 2016;**131**:803-820. DOI: 10.1007/s00401-016-1545-1

[14] Pham MH, Zada G, Mosich GM, Chen TC, Giannotta SL, Wang K, et al. Molecular genetics of meningiomas: A systematic review of the current literature and potential basis for future treatment paradigms. Neurosurgical Focus. 2011;**30**:E7. DOI: 10.3171/2011.2.FOCUS1117

[15] Preusser M, Brastianos PK, Mawrin C. Advances in meningioma genetics: Novel therapeutic opportunities. Nature Reviews. Neurology. 2018;**14**:106-115. DOI: 10.1038/nrneurol.2017.168

[16] Ragel BT, Jensen RL. Aberrant signaling pathways in meningiomas. Journal of Neuro-Oncology. 2010;**99**:315-324. DOI: 10.1007/s11060-010-0381-8

[17] Bi WL, Greenwald NF, Abedalthagafi M, Wala J, Gibson WJ, Agarwalla PK, et al. Genomic landscape of high-grade meningiomas. NPJ Genomic Medicine. 2017;**2**:15. DOI: 10.1038/s41525-017-0014-7

[18] Lerner C, Ketter R, Linsler S, Henn W, Oertel J, Urbschat S. Establishment of a molecular cytogenetic analysis for native tumor tissue of meningiomas-suitable for clinical application. Molecular Cytogenetics. 2014;**7**:12. DOI: 10.1186/1755-8166-7-12

[19] Williams EA, Santagata S, Wakimoto H, Shankar GM, Barker FG, Sharaf R, et al. Distinct genomic subclasses of high-grade/progressive meningiomas: NF2-associated, NF2-exclusive, and NF2-agnostic. Acta Neuropathologica Communications. 2020;**8**:171. DOI: 10.1186/s40478-020-01040-2

[20] Barbera S, Miguel TS, Gil-Benso R, Muñoz-Hidalgo L, Roldan P, Gonzalez-Darder J, et al. Genetic changes with prognostic value in histologically benign meningiomas. Clinical Neuropathology. 2013;**32**:311-317. DOI: 10.5414/NP300580

[21] Ruttledge MH, Sarrazin J, Rangaratnam S, Phelan CM, Twist E, Merel P, et al. Evidence for the complete inactivation of the NF2 gene in the majority of sporadic meningiomas. Nature Genetics. 1994;**6**:180-184. DOI: 10.1038/ng0294-180

[22] Sulman EP, White PS, Brodeur GM. Genomic annotation of the meningioma tumor suppressor locus on chromosome 1p34. Oncogene. 2004;**23**:1014-1020. DOI: 10.1038/sj.onc.1206623

[23] Liu ZY, Wang JY, Liu HH, Ma XM, Wang CL, Zhang XP, et al. Retinoblastoma protein-interacting zinc-finger gene 1 (RIZ1) dysregulation in human malignant meningiomas. Oncogene. 2013;**32**:1216-1222. DOI: 10.1038/onc.2012.155

[24] Goutagny S, Yang HW, Zucman-Rossi J, Chan J, Dreyfuss JM, Park PJ, et al. Genomic profiling reveals alternative genetic pathways of meningioma malignant progression dependent on the underlying *NF2* status. Clinical Cancer Research. 2010;**16**:4155-4164. DOI: 10.1158/1078-0432.CCR-10-0891

[25] Everson RG, Hashimoto Y, Freeman JL, Hodges TR, Huse J, Zhou S, et al. Multiplatform profiling of meningioma provides molecular insight and prioritization of drug targets for rational clinical trial design. Journal of Neuro-Oncology. 2018;**139**:469-478. DOI: 10.1007/s11060-018-2891-8

[26] Nassiri F, Liu J, Patil V, Mamatjan Y, Wang JZ, Hugh-White R, et al. A clinically applicable integrative molecular classification of meningiomas. Nature. 2021;**597**:119-125. DOI: 10.1038/s41586-021-03850-3

[27] Clark VE, Erson-Omay EZ, Serin A, Yin J, Cotney J, Ozduman K, et al.

Genomic analysis of non-NF2 meningiomas reveals mutations in TRAF7, KLF4, AKT1, and SMO. Science. 2013;**339**:1077-1080. DOI: 10.1126/science.1233009

[28] Sahm F, Schrimpf D, Olar A, Koelsche C, Reuss D, Bissel J, et al. TERT promoter mutations and risk of recurrence in meningioma. Journal of the National Cancer Institute. 2016;**108**: djv377. DOI: 10.1093/jnci/djv377

[29] Spiegl-Kreinecker S, Lötsch D, Neumayer K, Kastler L, Gojo J, Pirker C, et al. *TERT* promoter mutations are associated with poor prognosis and cell immortalization in meningioma. Neuro-Oncology. 2018;**20**:1584-1593. DOI: 10.1093/neuonc/noy104

[30] Biczok A, Kraus T, Suchorska B, Terpolilli NA, Thorsteinsdottir J, Giese A, et al. TERT promoter mutation is associated with worse prognosis in WHO grade II and III meningiomas. Journal of Neuro-Oncology. 2018;**139**: 671-678. DOI: 10.1007/s11060-018-2912-7

[31] AlSahlawi A, Aljelaify R, Magrashi A, AlSaeed M, Almutairi A, Alqubaishi F, et al. New insights into the genomic landscape of meningiomas identified FGFR3 in a subset of patients with favorable prognoses. Oncotarget. 2019;**10**:5549-5559. DOI: 10.18632/oncotarget.27178

[32] Yuzawa S, Nishihara H, Tanaka S. Genetic landscape of meningioma. Brain Tumor Pathology. 2016;**33**:237-247. DOI: 10.1007/s10014-016-0271-7

[33] Zotti T, Scudiero I, Vito P, Stilo R. The emerging role of TRAF7 in tumor development: TRAF7 in tumor development. Journal of Cellular Physiology. 2017;**232**:1233-1238. DOI: 10.1002/jcp.25676

[34] Brastianos PK, Horowitz PM, Santagata S, Jones RT, McKenna A, Getz G, et al. Genomic sequencing of meningiomas identifies oncogenic SMO and AKT1 mutations. Nature Genetics. 2013;**45**:285-289. DOI: 10.1038/ng.2526

[35] Boetto J, Bielle F, Sanson M, Peyre M, Kalamarides M. SMO mutation status defines a distinct and frequent molecular subgroup in olfactory groove meningiomas. Neuro-Oncology. 2017;**14**:now276. DOI: 10.1093/neuonc/now276

[36] Abedalthagafi M, Bi WL, Aizer AA, Merrill PH, Brewster R, Agarwalla PK, et al. Oncogenic PI3K mutations are as common as *AKT1* and *SMO* mutations in meningioma. Neuro-Oncology. 2016;**18**:649-655. DOI: 10.1093/neuonc/nov316

[37] Mawrin C, Sasse T, Kirches E, Kropf S, Schneider T, Grimm C, et al. Different activation of mitogen-activated protein kinase and Akt signaling is associated with aggressive phenotype of human meningiomas. Clinical Cancer Research. 2005;**11**:4074-4082. DOI: 10.1158/1078-0432.CCR-04-2550

[38] Tang H, Zhu H, Wang X, Hua L, Li J, Xie Q, et al. KLF4 is a tumor suppressor in anaplastic meningioma stem-like cells and human meningiomas. Journal of Molecular Cell Biology. 2017;**9**:315-324. DOI: 10.1093/jmcb/mjx023

[39] Reuss DE, Piro RM, Jones DTW, Simon M, Ketter R, Kool M, et al. Secretory meningiomas are defined by combined KLF4 K409Q and TRAF7 mutations. Acta Neuropathologica. 2013;**125**:351-358. DOI: 10.1007/s00401-013-1093-x

[40] Schuetz A, Nana D, Rose C, Zocher G, Milanovic M, Koenigsmann J, et al. The structure of the Klf4 DNA-binding domain links to self-renewal and macrophage differentiation. Cellular and Molecular Life Sciences.

2011;**68**:3121-3131. DOI: 10.1007/s00018-010-0618-x

[41] Proctor DT, Ramachandran S, Lama S, Sutherland GR. Towards molecular classification of meningioma: Evolving treatment and diagnostic paradigms. World Neurosurgery. 2018;**119**:366-373. DOI: 10.1016/j.wneu.2018.08.019

[42] Clark VE, Harmancı AS, Bai H, Youngblood MW, Lee TI, Baranoski JF, et al. Recurrent somatic mutations in POLR2A define a distinct subset of meningiomas. Nature Genetics. 2016;**48**:1253-1259. DOI: 10.1038/ng.3651

[43] Gerkes EH, Fock JM, den Dunnen WFA, van Belzen MJ, van der Lans CA, Hoving EW, et al. A heritable form of SMARCE1-related meningiomas with important implications for follow-up and family screening. Neurogenetics. 2016;**17**:83-89. DOI: 10.1007/s10048-015-0472-y

[44] Smith MJ, Wallace AJ, Bennett C, Hasselblatt M, Elert-Dobkowska E, Evans LT, et al. Germline SMARCE1 mutations predispose to both spinal and cranial clear cell meningiomas. The Journal of Pathology. 2014;**234**:436-440. DOI: 10.1002/path.4427

[45] Shankar GM, Abedalthagafi M, Vaubel RA, Merrill PH, Nayyar N, Gill CM, et al. Germline and somatic BAP1 mutations in high-grade rhabdoid meningiomas. Neuro-Oncology. 2016;**19**(4):535-545. DOI: 10.1093/neuonc/now235

[46] Collord G, Tarpey P, Kurbatova N, Martincorena I, Moran S, Castro M, et al. An integrated genomic analysis of anaplastic meningioma identifies prognostic molecular signatures. Scientific Reports. 2018;**8**:13537. DOI: 10.1038/s41598-018-31659-0

[47] Gao F, Shi L, Russin J, Zeng L, Chang X, He S, et al. DNA methylation in the malignant transformation of meningiomas. PLoS One. 2013;**8**:e54114. DOI: 10.1371/journal.pone.0054114

[48] Bello MJ, Amiñoso C, Lopez-Marin I, Arjona D, Gonzalez-Gomez P, Alonso ME, et al. DNA methylation of multiple promoter-associated CpG islands in meningiomas: Relationship with the allelic status at 1p and 22q. Acta Neuropathologica. 2004;**108**:413-421. DOI: 10.1007/s00401-004-0911-6

[49] He S, Pham MH, Pease M, Zada G, Giannotta SL, Wang K, et al. A review of epigenetic and gene expression alterations associated with intracranial meningiomas. Neurosurgical Focus. 2013;**35**:E5. DOI: 10.3171/2013.10.FOCUS13360

[50] Barski D, Wolter M, Reifenberger G, Riemenschneider MJ. Hypermethylation and transcriptional downregulation of the TIMP3 gene is associated with allelic loss on 22q12.3 and malignancy in meningiomas. Brain Pathology. 2010;**20**:623-631. DOI: 10.1111/j.1750-3639.2009.00340.x

[51] Nakane Y, Natsume A, Wakabayashi T, Oi S, Ito M, Inao S, et al. Malignant transformation-related genes in meningiomas: Allelic loss on 1p36 and methylation status of p73 and RASSF1A. Journal of Neurosurgery. 2007;**107**:398-404. DOI: 10.3171/JNS-07/08/0398

[52] Olar A, Wani KM, Wilson CD, Zadeh G, DeMonte F, Jones DTW, et al. Global epigenetic profiling identifies methylation subgroups associated with recurrence-free survival in meningioma. Acta Neuropathologica. 2017;**133**:431-444. DOI: 10.1007/s00401-017-1678-x

[53] Sahm F, Schrimpf D, Stichel D, Jones DTW, Hielscher T, Schefzyk S, et al. DNA methylation-based classification and grading system for meningioma: A multicentre, retrospective analysis. The Lancet Oncology. 2017;**18**:682-694. DOI: 10.1016/S1470-2045(17)30155-9

[54] Katz LM, Hielscher T, Liechty B, Silverman J, Zagzag D, Sen R, et al. Loss of histone H3K27me3 identifies a subset of meningiomas with increased risk of recurrence. Acta Neuropathologica. 2018;**135**:955-963. DOI: 10.1007/s00401-018-1844-9

[55] Boulagnon-Rombi C, Fleury C, Fichel C, Lefour S, Marchal Bressenot A, Gauchotte G. Immunohistochemical approach to the differential diagnosis of meningiomas and their mimics. Journal of Neuropathology and Experimental Neurology. 2017;**76**:289-298. DOI: 10.1093/jnen/nlx008

[56] Berghoff AS, Kresl P, Bienkowski M, Koelsche C, Rajky U, Hainfellner JA, et al. Validation of nuclear STAT6 immunostaining as a diagnostic marker of meningeal solitary fibrous tumor (SFT)/hemangiopericytoma. Clinical Neuropathology. 2017;**36**:56-59. DOI: 10.5414/NP300993

[57] Ng J, Celebre A, Munoz DG, Keith JL, Karamchandani JR. Sox10 is superior to S100 in the diagnosis of meningioma. Applied Immunohistochemistry & Molecular Morphology. 2015;**23**:215-219. DOI: 10.1097/PAI.0000000000000072

[58] Fang L, Lowther DE, Meizlish ML, Anderson RCE, Bruce JN, Devine L, et al. The immune cell infiltrate populating meningiomas is composed of mature, antigen-experienced T and B cells. Neuro-Oncology. 2013;**15**:1479-1490. DOI: 10.1093/neuonc/not110

[59] Du Z, Abedalthagafi M, Aizer AA, McHenry AR, Sun HH, Bray M-A, et al. Increased expression of the immune modulatory molecule PD-L1 (CD274) in anaplastic meningioma. Oncotarget. 2015;**6**:4704-4716. DOI: 10.18632/oncotarget.3082

[60] Zou W. Regulatory T cells, tumour immunity and immunotherapy. Nature Reviews. Immunology. 2006;**6**:295-307. DOI: 10.1038/nri1806

[61] Apra C, Peyre M, Kalamarides M. Current treatment options for meningioma. Expert Review of Neurotherapeutics. 2018;**18**:241-249. DOI: 10.1080/14737175.2018.1429920

[62] Maggio I, Franceschi E, Tosoni A, Nunno VD, Gatto L, Lodi R, et al. Meningioma: Not always a benign tumor. A review of advances in the treatment of meningiomas. CNS Oncology. 2021;**10**:CNS72. DOI: 10.2217/cns-2021-0003

[63] Nigim F, Wakimoto H, Kasper E, Ackermans L, Temel Y. Emerging medical treatments for meningioma in the molecular era. Biomedicine. 2018;**6**:86. DOI: 10.3390/biomedicines6030086

[64] Karsy M, Guan J, Cohen A, Colman H, Jensen RL. Medical management of meningiomas. Neurosurgery Clinics of North America. 2016;**27**:249-260. DOI: 10.1016/j.nec.2015.11.002

[65] Schrell UMH, Rittig MG, Anders M, Kiesewetter F, Marschalek R, Koch UH, et al. Hydroxyurea for treatment of unresectable and recurrent meningiomas. I. Inhibition of primary human meningioma cells in culture and in meningioma transplants by induction of the apoptotic pathway. Journal of Neurosurgery. 1997;**86**:845-852. DOI: 10.3171/jns.1997.86.5.0845

[66] Schrell UMH, Rittig MG, Anders M, Koch UH, Marschalek R, Kiesewetter F, et al. Hydroxyurea for treatment of unresectable and recurrent meningiomas. II. Decrease in the size of meningiomas in patients treated with hydroxyurea. Journal of Neurosurgery. 1997;**86**:840-844. DOI: 10.3171/jns.1997.86.5.0840

[67] Hahn BM, Schrell UMH, Sauer R, Fahlbusch R, Ganslandt O, Grabenbauer GG. Prolonged oral hydroxyurea and concurrent 3d-conformal radiation in patients with

progressive or recurrent meningioma: Results of a pilot study. Journal of Neuro-Oncology. 2005;**74**:157-165. DOI: 10.1007/s11060-004-2337-3

[68] Loven D, Hardoff R, Bar Sever Z, Steinmetz AP, Gornish M, Rappaport ZH, et al. Non-resectable slow-growing meningiomas treated by hydroxyurea. Journal of Neuro-Oncology. 2004;**67**:221-226. DOI: 10.1023/B:NEON.0000021827.85754.8e

[69] Mason WP, Gentili F, Macdonald DR, Hariharan S, Cruz CR, Abrey LE. Stabilization of disease progression by hydroxyurea in patients with recurrent or unresectable meningiomas. Journal of Neurosurgery. 2002;**97**:341-346. DOI: 10.3171/jns.2002.97.2.0341

[70] Newton H, Scott S, Volpi C. Hydroxyurea chemotherapy for meningiomas: Enlarged cohort with extended follow-up. British Journal of Neurosurgery. 2004;**18**:495-499. DOI: 10.1080/02688690400012392

[71] Rosenthal MA, Ashley DL, Cher L. Treatment of high risk or recurrent meningiomas with hydroxyurea. Journal of Clinical Neuroscience. 2002;**9**:156-158. DOI: 10.1054/jocn.2001.1019

[72] Weston G, Martin A, Mufti G, Strong A, Gleeson M. Hydroxyurea treatment of meningiomas: A pilot study. Skull Base. 2006;**16**:157-160. DOI: 10.1055/s-2006-949518

[73] Moazzam AA, Wagle N, Zada G. Recent developments in chemotherapy for meningiomas: A review. Neurosurgical Focus. 2013;**35**:E18. DOI: 10.3171/2013.10.FOCUS13341

[74] Kim J, Kim KH, Kim YZ. The clinical outcome of hydroxyurea chemotherapy after incomplete resection of atypical meningiomas. Brain Tumor Research and Treatment. 2017;**5**:77. DOI: 10.14791/btrt.2017.5.2.77

[75] Reardon DA, Norden AD, Desjardins A, Vredenburgh JJ, Herndon JE, Coan A, et al. Phase II study of Gleevec® plus hydroxyurea (HU) in adults with progressive or recurrent meningioma. Journal of Neuro-Oncology. 2012;**106**:409-415. DOI: 10.1007/s11060-011-0687-1

[76] Chamberlain MC. The role of chemotherapy and targeted therapy in the treatment of intracranial meningioma. Current Opinion in Oncology. 2012;**24**:666-671. DOI: 10.1097/CCO.0b013e328356364d

[77] Ragel BT, Couldwell WT, Wurster RD, Jensen RL. Chronic suppressive therapy with calcium channel antagonists for refractory meningiomas. Neurosurgical Focus. 2007;**23**:E10. DOI: 10.3171/FOC-07/10/E10

[78] Preusser M, Spiegl-Kreinecker S, Lötsch D, Wöhrer A, Schmook M, Dieckmann K, et al. Trabectedin has promising antineoplastic activity in high-grade meningioma: Trabectedin in meningioma. Cancer. 2012;**118**:5038-5049. DOI: 10.1002/cncr.27460

[79] Preusser M, Silvani A, Le Rhun E, Soffietti R, Lombardi G, Sepulveda J, et al. PL3.2 Trabectedin for recurrent WHO grade II or III meningioma: A randomized phase II study of the EORTC Brain Tumor Group (EORTC-1320-BTG). Neuro-Oncology. 2019;**21**:iii2-iii3. DOI: 10.1093/neuonc/noz126.005

[80] Gupta S, Bi WL, Dunn IF. Medical management of meningioma in the era of precision medicine. Neurosurgical Focus. 2018;**44**:E3. DOI: 10.3171/2018.1.FOCUS17754

[81] Shao Z, Liu L, Zheng Y, Tu S, Pan Y, Yan S, et al. Molecular mechanism and approach in progression of meningioma. Frontiers in Oncology. 2020;**10**:538845. DOI: 10.3389/fonc.2020.538845

[82] Wilson TA, Huang L, Ramanathan D, Lopez-Gonzalez M, Pillai P, De Los Reyes K, et al. Review of atypical and anaplastic meningiomas: Classification, molecular biology, and management. Frontiers in Oncology. 2020;**10**:565582. DOI: 10.3389/fonc.2020.565582

[83] Chamberlain MC. Adjuvant combined modality therapy for malignant meningiomas. Journal of Neurosurgery. 1996;**84**:733-736. DOI: 10.3171/jns.1996.84.5.0733

[84] Chamberlain MC. Intracerebral meningiomas. Current Treatment Options in Neurology. 2004;**6**:297-305. DOI: 10.1007/s11940-004-0029-0

[85] Chamberlain MC, Tsao-Wei DD, Groshen S. Salvage chemotherapy With CPT-11 for recurrent meningioma. Journal of Neuro-Oncology. 2006;**78**:271-276. DOI: 10.1007/s11060-005-9093-x

[86] Curic S, Wu Y, Shan B, Schaaf C, Utpadel D, Lange M, et al. Curcumin acts anti-proliferative and pro-apoptotic in human meningiomas. Journal of Neuro-Oncology. 2013;**113**:385-396. DOI: 10.1007/s11060-013-1148-9

[87] Park YS, Lee JH, Bondar J, Harwalkar JA, Safayhi H, Golubic M. Cytotoxic action of acetyl-11-keto-β-boswellic acid (AKBA) on meningioma cells. Planta Medica. 2002;**68**:397-401. DOI: 10.1055/s-2002-32090

[88] König M, Osnes T, Bruland Ø, Sundby Hall K, Bratland Å, Meling TR. The role of adjuvant treatment in craniofacial malignancy: A critical review. Frontiers in Oncology. 2020;**10**:1402. DOI: 10.3389/fonc.2020.01402

[89] Dai J, Ma Y, Chu S, Le N, Cao J, Wang Y. Identification of key genes and pathways in meningioma by bioinformatics analysis. Oncology Letters. 2018;**15**:8245-8252. DOI: 10.3892/ol.2018.8376

[90] Torp SH, Helseth E, Dalen A, Unsgaard G. Expression of epidermal growth factor receptor in human meningiomas and meningeal tissue. APMIS. 1992;**100**:797-802. DOI: 10.1111/j.1699-0463.1992.tb04002.x

[91] Arnli MB, Backer-Grøndahl T, Ytterhus B, Granli US, Lydersen S, Gulati S, et al. Expression and clinical value of EGFR in human meningiomas. PeerJ. 2017;**2017**:215-222. DOI: 10.7717/peerj.3140

[92] Narla S, Uppin MS, Saradhi MV, Sahu BP, Purohit AK, Sundaram C. Assessment of expression of epidermal growth factor receptor and p53 in meningiomas. Neurology India. 2014;**62**:37-41. DOI: 10.4103/0028-3886.128276

[93] Bujko M, Kober P, Tysarowski A, Matyja E, Mandat T, Bonicki W, et al. EGFR, PIK3CA, KRAS and BRAF mutations in meningiomas. Oncology Letters. 2014;**7**:2019-2022. DOI: 10.3892/ol.2014.2042

[94] Burnett BA, Womeldorff MR, Jensen R. Meningioma: Signaling pathways and tumor growth. In: Handbook of Clinical Neurology. Amsterdam: Elsevier; 2020. pp. 137-150. DOI: 10.1016/B978-0-12-804280-9.00009-3

[95] Caltabiano R, Barbagallo GMV, Castaing M, Cassenti A, Senetta R, Cassoni P, et al. Prognostic value of EGFR expression in de novo and progressed atypical and anaplastic meningiomas: An immunohistochemical and fluorescence in situ hybridization pilot study. Journal of Neurosurgical Sciences. 2013;**57**:139-151

[96] Wernicke AG, Dicker AP, Whiton M, Ivanidze J, Hyslop T,

Hammond EH, et al. Assessment of Epidermal Growth Factor Receptor (EGFR) expression in human meningioma. Radiation Oncology. 2010;**5**:46. DOI: 10.1186/1748-717X-5-46

[97] Johnson M, Toms S. Mitogenic signal transduction pathways in meningiomas: Novel targets for meningioma chemotherapy? Journal of Neuropathology and Experimental Neurology. 2005;**64**:1029-1036. DOI: 10.1097/01.jnen.0000189834.63951.81

[98] Tang PA, Tsao MS, Moore MJ. A review of erlotinib and its clinical use. Expert Opinion on Pharmacotherapy. 2006;**7**:177-193. DOI: 10.1517/14656566.7.2.177

[99] Dhillon S. Gefitinib: A review of its use in adults with advanced non-small cell lung cancer. Targeted Oncology. 2015;**10**:153-170. DOI: 10.1007/s11523-015-0358-9

[100] Norden AD, Raizer JJ, Abrey LE, Lamborn KR, Lassman AB, Chang SM, et al. Phase II trials of erlotinib or gefitinib in patients with recurrent meningioma. Journal of Neuro-Oncology. 2010;**96**:211-217. DOI: 10.1007/s11060-009-9948-7

[101] Opdam FL, Guchelaar H-J, Beijnen JH, Schellens JHM. Lapatinib for advanced or metastatic breast cancer. The Oncologist. 2012;**17**:536-542. DOI: 10.1634/theoncologist.2011-0461

[102] Ammoun S, Cunliffe CH, Allen JC, Chiriboga L, Giancotti FG, Zagzag D, et al. ErbB/HER receptor activation and preclinical efficacy of lapatinib in vestibular schwannoma. Neuro-Oncology. 2010;**12**:834-843. DOI: 10.1093/neuonc/noq012

[103] Karajannis MA, Legault G, Hagiwara M, Ballas MS, Brown K, Nusbaum AO, et al. Phase II trial of lapatinib in adult and pediatric patients with neurofibromatosis type 2 and progressive vestibular schwannomas. Neuro-Oncology. 2012;**14**:1163-1170. DOI: 10.1093/neuonc/nos146

[104] Osorio DS, Hu J, Mitchell C, Allen JC, Stanek J, Hagiwara M, et al. Effect of lapatinib on meningioma growth in adults with neurofibromatosis type 2. Journal of Neuro-Oncology. 2018;**139**:749-755. DOI: 10.1007/s11060-018-2922-5

[105] Crombet T, Torres O, Rodríguez V, Menéndez A, Stevenson A, Ramos M, et al. Phase I clinical evaluation of a neutralizing monoclonal antibody against epidermal growth factor receptor in advanced brain tumor patients: Preliminary study. Hybridoma. 2001;**20**:131-136. DOI: 10.1089/02724570152057634

[106] Papadopoulos N, Lennartsson J. The PDGF/PDGFR pathway as a drug target. Molecular Aspects of Medicine. 2018;**62**:75-88. DOI: 10.1016/j.mam.2017.11.007

[107] Fredriksson L, Li H, Eriksson U. The PDGF family: Four gene products form five dimeric isoforms. Cytokine & Growth Factor Reviews. 2004;**15**:197-204. DOI: 10.1016/j.cytogfr.2004.03.007

[108] Black PM, Carroll R, Glowacka D, Riley K, Dashner K. Platelet-derived growth factor expression and stimulation in human meningiomas. Journal of Neurosurgery. 1994;**81**:388-393. DOI: 10.3171/jns.1994.81.3.0388

[109] Candeliere GA, Glorieux FH, Prud'homme J, St-Arnaud R. Increased expression of the c-fos proto-oncogene in bone from patients with fibrous dysplasia. The New England Journal of Medicine. 1995;**332**:1546-1551. DOI: 10.1056/NEJM199506083322304

[110] Todo T, Adams EF, Fahlbusch R, Dingermann T, Werner H. Autocrine growth stimulation of human

meningioma cells by platelet-derived growth factor. Journal of Neurosurgery. 1996;**84**:852-858; discussion 858-859. DOI: 10.3171/jns.1996.84.5.0852

[111] Norden AD, Drappatz J, Wen PY. Targeted drug therapy for meningiomas. Neurosurgical Focus. 2007;**23**:E12. DOI: 10.3171/FOC-07/10/E12

[112] Reardon DA, Egorin MJ, Quinn JA, Rich JN, Gururangan I, Vredenburgh JJ, et al. Phase II study of imatinib mesylate plus hydroxyurea in adults with recurrent glioblastoma multiforme. Journal of Clinical Oncology. 2005;**23**: 9359-9368. DOI: 10.1200/JCO.2005. 03.2185

[113] Wen PY, Yung WKA, Lamborn KR, Dahia PL, Wang Y, Peng B, et al. Phase I/II study of imatinib mesylate for recurrent malignant gliomas: North American brain tumor consortium study 99-08. Clinical Cancer Research. 2006;**12**:4899-4907. DOI: 10.1158/1078-0432.CCR-06-0773

[114] James MF, Han S, Polizzano C, Plotkin SR, Manning BD, Stemmer-Rachamimov AO, et al. NF2/merlin is a novel negative regulator of mTOR complex 1, and activation of mTORC1 is associated with meningioma and schwannoma growth. Molecular and Cellular Biology. 2009;**29**:4250-4261. DOI: 10.1128/MCB.01581-08

[115] Ryskalin L, Lazzeri G, Flaibani M, Biagioni F, Gambardella S, Frati A, et al. mTOR-dependent cell proliferation in the brain. BioMed Research International. 2017;**2017**:7082696. DOI: 10.1155/2017/ 7082696

[116] Pachow D, Andrae N, Kliese N, Angenstein F, Stork O, Wilisch-Neumann A, et al. mTORC1 inhibitors suppress meningioma growth in mouse models. Clinical Cancer Research. 2013;**19**:1180. DOI: 10.1158/ 1078-0432.CCR-12-1904

[117] Johnson MD, Okedli E, Woodard A, Toms SA, Allen GS. Evidence for phosphatidylinositol 3-kinase-Akt-p7S6K pathway activation and transduction of mitogenic signals by platelet-derived growth factor in meningioma cells. Journal of Neurosurgery. 2002;**97**:668-675. DOI: 10.3171/jns.2002.97.3.0668

[118] Cai DX, James CD, Scheithauer BW, Couch FJ, Perry A. PS6K amplification characterizes a small subset of anaplastic meningiomas. American Journal of Clinical Pathology. 2001;**115**:213-218. DOI: 10.1309/ FVNU-7UBY-DXE3-77MT

[119] Corona AM, Di L, Shah AH, Crespo R, Eichberg DG, Lu VM, et al. Current experimental therapies for atypical and malignant meningiomas. Journal of Neuro-Oncology. 2021;**153**:203-210. DOI: 10.1007/s11060-021-03759-x

[120] Graillon T, Defilles C, Mohamed A, Lisbonis C, Germanetti A-L, Chinot O, et al. Combined treatment by octreotide and everolimus: Octreotide enhances inhibitory effect of everolimus in aggressive meningiomas. Journal of Neuro-Oncology. 2015;**124**:33-43. DOI: 10.1007/s11060-015-1812-3

[121] Graillon T, Sanson M, Campello C, Idbaih A, Peyre M, Peyrière H, et al. Everolimus and octreotide for patients with recurrent meningioma: Results from the Phase II CEVOREM Trial. Clinical Cancer Research. 2020;**26**: 552-557. DOI: 10.1158/1078-0432. CCR-19-2109

[122] Shih KC, Chowdhary S, Rosenblatt P, Weir AB, Shepard GC, Williams JT, et al. A phase II trial of bevacizumab and everolimus as treatment for patients with refractory, progressive intracranial meningioma. Journal of Neuro-Oncology. 2016;**129**: 281-288. DOI: 10.1007/s11060-016-2172-3

[123] Weller M, Roth P, Sahm F, Burghardt I, Schuknecht B, Rushing EJ, et al. Durable control of metastatic AKT1-mutant WHO Grade 1 meningothelial meningioma by the AKT inhibitor, AZD5363. Journal of the National Cancer Institute. 2017;**109**. DOI: 10.1093/jnci/djw320

[124] Pistolesi S, Boldrini L, Gisfredi S, De Ieso K, Camacci T, Caniglia M, et al. Angiogenesis in intracranial meningiomas: Immunohistochemical and molecular study. Neuropathology and Applied Neurobiology. 2004;**30**: 118-125. DOI: 10.1046/j.0305-1846. 2003.00516.x

[125] Barresi V, Tuccari G. Increased ratio of vascular endothelial growth factor to semaphorin3A is a negative prognostic factor in human meningiomas. Neuropathology: Official Journal of the Japanese Society of Neuropathology. 2010;**30**:537-546. DOI: 10.1111/j.1440-1789.2010.01105.x

[126] Barresi V, Tuccari G. Evaluation of neo-angiogenesis in a case of chordoid meningioma. Journal of Neuro-Oncology. 2009;**95**:445-447. DOI: 10.1007/s11060-009-9942-0

[127] Guevara P, Escobar-Arriaga E, Saavedra-Perez D, Martinez-Rumayor A, Flores-Estrada D, Rembao D, et al. Angiogenesis and expression of estrogen and progesterone receptors as predictive factors for recurrence of meningioma. Journal of Neuro-Oncology. 2010;**98**:379-384. DOI: 10.1007/s11060-009-0086-z

[128] Jensen RL, Soleau S, Bhayani MK, Christiansen D. Expression of hypoxia inducible factor-1 alpha and correlation with preoperative embolization of meningiomas. Journal of Neurosurgery. 2002;**97**:658-667. DOI: 10.3171/jns.2002. 97.3.0658

[129] Tsai JC, Hsiao YY, Teng LJ, Shun CT, Chen CT, Goldman CK, et al. Regulation of vascular endothelial growth factor secretion in human meningioma cells. Journal of the Formosan Medical Association = Taiwan yi zhi. 1999;**98**:111-117

[130] Barresi V, Cerasoli S, Paioli G, Vitarelli E, Giuffrè G, Guiducci G, et al. Caveolin-1 in meningiomas: Expression and clinico-pathological correlations. Acta Neuropathologica. 2006;**112**:617-626. DOI: 10.1007/ s00401-006-0097-1

[131] Barresi V, Cerasoli S, Tuccari G. Correlative evidence that tumor cell-derived caveolin-1 mediates angiogenesis in meningiomas. Neuropathology: Official Journal of the Japanese Society of Neuropathology. 2008;**28**:472-478. DOI: 10.1111/ j.1440-1789.2008.00902.x

[132] Massimino ML, Griffoni C, Spisni E, Toni M, Tomasi V. Involvement of caveolae and caveolae-like domains in signalling, cell survival and angiogenesis. Cellular Signalling. 2002;**14**:93-98. DOI: 10.1016/ s0898-6568(01)00232-7

[133] Chang S-H, Feng D, Nagy JA, Sciuto TE, Dvorak AM, Dvorak HF. Vascular permeability and pathological angiogenesis in caveolin-1-null mice. The American Journal of Pathology. 2009;**175**:1768-1776. DOI: 10.2353/ ajpath.2009.090171

[134] Li S, Seitz R, Lisanti MP. Phosphorylation of caveolin by src tyrosine kinases. The alpha-isoform of caveolin is selectively phosphorylated by v-Src in vivo. The Journal of Biological Chemistry. 1996;**271**:3863-3868

[135] Knowles J, Loizidou M, Taylor I. Endothelin-1 and angiogenesis in cancer. Current Vascular Pharmacology. 2005;**3**:309-314. DOI: 10.2174/ 1570161054329462

[136] Kim L. A narrative review of targeted therapies in meningioma. Chinese Clinical Oncology. 2020;**9**: 76-76. DOI: 10.21037/cco-2020-mbt-01

[137] Lou E, Sumrall AL, Turner S, Peters KB, Desjardins A, Vredenburgh JJ, et al. Bevacizumab therapy for adults with recurrent/ progressive meningioma: A retrospective series. Journal of Neuro-Oncology. 2012;**109**:63-70. DOI: 10.1007/s11060-012-0861-0

[138] Grimm SA, Kumthekar P, Chamberlain MC, Schiff D, Wen PY, Iwamoto FM, et al. Phase II trial of bevacizumab in patients with surgery and radiation refractory progressive meningioma. Journal of Clinical Oncology. 2015;**33**:2055-2055. DOI: 10.1200/jco.2015.33.15_ suppl.2055

[139] Kaley TJ, Wen P, Schiff D, Ligon K, Haidar S, Karimi S, et al. Phase II trial of sunitinib for recurrent and progressive atypical and anaplastic meningioma. Neuro-Oncology. 2015;**17**:116-121. DOI: 10.1093/neuonc/nou148

[140] Cardona AF, Ruiz-Patiño A, Zatarain-Barrón ZL, Hakim F, Jiménez E, Mejía JA, et al. Systemic management of malignant meningiomas: A comparative survival and molecular marker analysis between Octreotide in combination with Everolimus and Sunitinib. PLoS One. 2019;**14**:e0217340. DOI: 10.1371/journal. pone.0217340

[141] Wolfsberger S, Doostkam S, Boecher-Schwarz H-G, Roessler K, van Trotsenburg M, Hainfellner JA, et al. Progesterone-receptor index in meningiomas: Correlation with clinico-pathological parameters and review of the literature. Neurosurgical Review. 2004;**27**:238-245. DOI: 10.1007/ s10143-004-0340-y

[142] Arena S, Barbieri F, Thellung S, Pirani P, Corsaro A, Villa V, et al. Expression of somatostatin receptor mRNA in human meningiomas and their implication in in vitro antiproliferative activity. Journal of Neuro-Oncology. 2004;**66**:155-166. DOI: 10.1023/B:N EON.0000013498.19981.55

[143] Zhao L, Zhao W, Hou Y, Wen C, Wang J, Wu P, et al. An overview of managements in meningiomas. Frontiers in Oncology. 2020;**10**:1523. DOI: 10.3389/fonc.2020.01523

[144] Goodwin JW, Crowley J, Eyre HJ, Stafford B, Jaeckle KA, Townsend JJ. A phase II evaluation of tamoxifen in unresectable or refractory meningiomas: A southwest oncology group study. Journal of Neuro-Oncology. 1993;**15**:75-77. DOI: 10.1007/ BF01050266

[145] Markwalder T-M, Seiler RW, Zava DT. Antiestrogenic therapy of meningiomas—A pilot study. Surgical Neurology. 1985;**24**:245-249. DOI: 10.1016/0090-3019(85)90030-8

[146] Lamberts SW, Tanghe HL, Avezaat CJ, Braakman R, Wijngaarde R, Koper JW, et al. Mifepristone (RU 486) treatment of meningiomas. Journal of Neurology, Neurosurgery, and Psychiatry. 1992;**55**:486-490. DOI: 10.1136/jnnp.55.6.486

[147] Ji Y, Rankin C, Grunberg S, Sherrod AE, Ahmadi J, Townsend JJ, et al. Double-blind phase III randomized trial of the antiprogestin agent mifepristone in the treatment of unresectable meningioma: SWOG S9005. Journal of Clinical Oncology. 2015;**33**:4093-4098. DOI: 10.1200/ JCO.2015.61.6490

[148] Grunberg SM, Weiss MH, Russell CA, Spitz IM, Ahmadi J, Sadun A, et al. Long-term administration of mifepristone (RU486): Clinical tolerance during extended treatment of meningioma.

Cancer Investigation. 2006;**24**:727-733. DOI: 10.1080/07357900601062339

[149] Chamberlain MC, Glantz MJ, Fadul CE. Recurrent meningioma: Salvage therapy with long-acting somatostatin analogue. Neurology. 2007;**69**:969-973. DOI: 10.1212/01.wnl.0000271382.62776.b7

[150] Foiani G, Guelfi G, Chiaradia E, Mancini F, Trivelli C, Vitellozzi G, et al. Somatostatin receptor 2 expression in canine meningioma. Journal of Comparative Pathology. 2019;**166**:59-68. DOI: 10.1016/j.jcpa.2018.11.002

[151] Johnson DR, Kimmel DW, Burch PA, Cascino TL, Giannini C, Wu W, et al. Phase II study of subcutaneous octreotide in adults with recurrent or progressive meningioma and meningeal hemangiopericytoma. Neuro-Oncology. 2011;**13**:530-535. DOI: 10.1093/neuonc/nor044

[152] Graillon T, Romano D, Defilles C, Saveanu A, Mohamed A, Figarella-Branger D, et al. Octreotide therapy in meningiomas: In vitro study, clinical correlation, and literature review. Journal of Neurosurgery. 2017;**127**:660-669. DOI: 10.3171/2016.8.JNS16995

[153] Norden AD, Ligon KL, Hammond SN, Muzikansky A, Reardon DA, Kaley TJ, et al. Phase II study of monthly pasireotide LAR (SOM230C) for recurrent or progressive meningioma. Neurology. 2015;**84**:280-286. DOI: 10.1212/WNL.0000000000001153

[154] Friend KE, Radinsky R, McCutcheon IE. Growth hormone receptor expression and function in meningiomas: Effect of a specific receptor antagonist. Journal of Neurosurgery. 1999;**91**:93-99. DOI: 10.3171/jns.1999.91.1.0093

[155] McCutcheon IE, Flyvbjerg A, Hill H, Li J, Bennett WF, Scarlett JA, et al. Antitumor activity of the growth hormone receptor antagonist pegvisomant against human meningiomas in nude mice. Journal of Neurosurgery. 2001;**94**:487-492. DOI: 10.3171/jns.2001.94.3.0487

[156] Puduvalli VK, Li JT, Chen L, McCutcheon IE. Induction of apoptosis in primary meningioma cultures by fenretinide. Cancer Research. 2005;**65**:1547-1553. DOI: 10.1158/0008-5472.CAN-04-0786

[157] Nordqvist AC, Peyrard M, Pettersson H, Mathiesen T, Collins VP, Dumanski JP, et al. A high ratio of insulin-like growth factor II/insulin-like growth factor binding protein 2 messenger RNA as a marker for anaplasia in meningiomas. Cancer Research. 1997;**57**:2611-2614

[158] Koper JW, Zwarthoff EC, Hagemeijer A, Braakman R, Avezaat CJJ, Bergström M, et al. Inhibition of the growth of cultured human meningioma cells by recombinant interferon-α. European Journal of Cancer & Clinical Oncology. 1991;**27**:416-419. DOI: 10.1016/0277-5379(91)90375-N

[159] Kaba SE, DeMonte F, Bruner JM, Kyritsis AP, Jaeckle KA, Levin V, et al. The treatment of recurrent unresectable and malignant meningiomas with interferon alpha-2B. Neurosurgery. 1997;**40**:271-275.DOI:10.1097/00006123-199702000-00007

[160] Muhr C, Gudjonsson O, Lilja A, Hartman M, Zhang ZJ, Långström B. Meningioma treated with interferon-alpha, evaluated with [(11)C]-L-methionine positron emission tomography. Clinical Cancer Research: An Official Journal of the American Association for Cancer Research. 2001;**7**:2269-2276

[161] Chamberlain MC, Glantz MJ. Interferon-α for recurrent World Health Organization grade 1 intracranial

meningiomas. Cancer. 2008;**113**: 2146-2151. DOI: 10.1002/cncr.23803

[162] Ning J, Wakimoto H. Oncolytic herpes simplex virus-based strategies: Toward a breakthrough in glioblastoma therapy. Frontiers in Microbiology. 2014;**5**. DOI: 10.3389/fmicb. 2014.00303

[163] Grill J, Lamfers MLM, van Beusechem VW, van der Valk P, Huisman A, Sminia P, et al. Oncolytic virotherapy of meningiomas in vitro with replication-competent adenovirus. Neurosurgery. 2005;**56**:146-154. DOI: 10.1227/01.NEU.0000146207.55774.69

[164] Aldrak N, Alsaab S, Algethami A, Bhere D, Wakimoto H, Shah K, et al. Oncolytic Herpes simplex virus-based therapies for cancer. Cell. 2021;**10**: 1541. DOI: 10.3390/cells10061541

[165] Markert JM, Coen DM, Malick A, Mineta T, Martuza RL. Expanded spectrum of viral therapy in the treatment of nervous system tumors. Journal of Neurosurgery. 1992;77:590-594. DOI: 10.3171/jns.1992.77.4.0590

[166] Yazaki T, Manz HJ, Rabkin SD, Martuza RL. Treatment of human malignant meningiomas by G207, a replication-competent multimutated herpes simplex virus 1. Cancer Research. 1995;**55**:4752-4756

[167] Liu T-C, Zhang T, Fukuhara H, Kuroda T, Todo T, Canron X, et al. Dominant-negative fibroblast growth factor receptor expression enhances antitumoral potency of oncolytic Herpes simplex virus in neural tumors. Clinical Cancer Research. 2006;**12**: 6791-6799. DOI: 10.1158/1078-0432. CCR-06-0263

[168] Nigim F, Esaki S, Hood M, Lelic N, James MF, Ramesh V, et al. A new patient-derived orthotopic malignant meningioma model treated with oncolytic herpes simplex virus. Neuro-Oncology. 2016;**18**:1278-1287. DOI: 10.1093/neuonc/now031

[169] de Sostoa J, Dutoit V, Migliorini D. Oncolytic viruses as a platform for the treatment of malignant brain tumors. International Journal of Molecular Sciences. 2020;**21**:7449. DOI: 10.3390/ ijms21207449

[170] Deng J, Ma M, Wang D, Zhu H, Hua L, Sun S, et al. Expression and clinical significance of immune checkpoint regulator B7-H3 (CD276) in human meningioma. World Neurosurgery. 2020;**135**:e12-e18. DOI: 10.1016/j.wneu.2019.10.044

[171] Proctor DT, Patel Z, Lama S, Resch L, van Marle G, Sutherland GR. Identification of PD-L2, B7-H3 and CTLA-4 immune checkpoint proteins in genetic subtypes of meningioma. OncoImmunology. 2019;**8**:e1512943. DOI: 10.1080/2162402X.2018.1512943

[172] Han SJ, Reis G, Kohanbash G, Shrivastav S, Magill ST, Molinaro AM, et al. Expression and prognostic impact of immune modulatory molecule PD-L1 in meningioma. Journal of Neuro-Oncology. 2016;**130**:543-552. DOI: 10.1007/s11060-016-2256-0

[173] Giles AJ, Hao S, Padget M, Song H, Zhang W, Lynes J, et al. Efficient ADCC killing of meningioma by avelumab and a high-affinity natural killer cell line, haNK. JCI Insight. 2019;**4**:e130688. DOI: 10.1172/jci.insight.130688

[174] Dunn IF, Du Z, Touat M, Sisti MB, Wen PY, Umeton R, et al. Mismatch repair deficiency in high-grade meningioma: A rare but recurrent event associated with dramatic immune activation and clinical response to PD-1 blockade. JCO Precision Oncology. 2018:1-12. DOI: 10.1200/PO.18.00190

[175] Gelerstein E, Berger A, Jonas-Kimchi T, Strauss I, Kanner AA, Blumenthal DT, et al. Regression of

intracranial meningioma following treatment with nivolumab: Case report and review of the literature. Journal of Clinical Neuroscience. 2017;**37**:51-53. DOI: 10.1016/j.jocn.2016.11.011

[176] June CH, Sadelain M. Chimeric antigen receptor therapy. The New England Journal of Medicine. 2018;**379**:64-73. DOI: 10.1056/NEJMra1706169

[177] Zheng P-P, Kros JM, Li J. Approved CAR T cell therapies: Ice bucket challenges on glaring safety risks and long-term impacts. Drug Discovery Today. 2018;**23**:1175-1182. DOI: 10.1016/j.drudis.2018.02.012

[178] Marofi F, Motavalli R, Safonov VA, Thangavelu L, Yumashev AV, Alexander M, et al. CAR T cells in solid tumors: Challenges and opportunities. Stem Cell Research & Therapy. 2021;**12**:81. DOI: 10.1186/s13287-020-02128-1

[179] Yang S, Wei W, Zhao Q. B7-H3, a checkpoint molecule, as a target for cancer immunotherapy. International Journal of Biological Sciences. 2020;**16**:1767-1773. DOI: 10.7150/ijbs.41105

[180] Tang X, Liu F, Liu Z, Cao Y, Zhang Z, Wang Y, et al. Bioactivity and safety of B7-H3-targeted chimeric antigen receptor T cells against anaplastic meningioma. Clinical & Translational Immunology. 2020;**9**:e1137-e1137. DOI: 10.1002/cti2.1137

Chapter 3

Meninges Outside the Meninges: Ectopic Meningiomas and Meningothlelial Proliferations

John A. Ozolek

Abstract

Extracranial meningiomas have been reported for decades now and have been described in the head and neck; calvarial, nasal cavity, paranasal sinuses, nasopharynx, parotid gland and in various remote anatomical locations systemically. The presence of microanatomical structures for all intents and purposes resembling and having the histopathological characteristics of meninges outside of the central nervous system meninges is uncommon but well-documented. Typically, these lesions are found in the lung or part of hamartomatous/choristomatous lesions and frequently occur in the head and neck anatomical region. The lesion first described by Suster and Rosai termed "hamartoma of the scalp with ectopic meningothelial elements" is the prototypical example of lesions with meningothelial elements. We have described recently a similar hamartomatous lesion with meningothelial elements occurring in the tongue. In this chapter, we will review the clinicopathological features of ectopic meningiomas and lesions that contain meningothelial elements and their possible pathogenesis.

Keywords: ectopic, meningioma, meningothelial, hamartoma, choristoma, pathology

1. Introduction

This chapter will cover, in brief, clinical and pathological characteristics of what are known as primary ectopic meningiomas (PEM) and the presence of tissue histomorphologically and immunophenotypically consistent with meningeal tissue (meningothelial) occurring in other organs or as part of teratomas or hamartomas/choristomas. PEMs, that is, those that occur outside of the central nervous system (CNS) can occur as a result of direct extension of a primary CNS meningioma (through calvarial bone into adjacent soft tissue), as a metastatic lesion, or as a primary ectopic meningioma [1]. Cutaneous meningiomas or primary cutaneous meningiomas describe a subset of PEMs mostly found in the scalp and have a classification system delineated by whether lesions are congenital or acquired and whether they have connection to a primary intracranial meningioma. Type I are congenital and may present as midline scalp cystic lesions (rudimentary meningoceles, acoelic meningeal hamartomas). Rarely sinus tracts have been found connecting these to the CNS. Type II are soft tissue meningiomas that have predilection for the nose, mouth, eyes, and ears and have no connection to an intracranial meningioma. Type III are soft tissue extensions of a primary intracranial meningioma [2]. Meningothelial tissue (not meningioma) can be seen most notably described in the lungs and rarely in hamartomas/choristomas (lesions composed of tissue types arranged haphazardly but indigenous to the location; hamartoma or not indigenous to location; choristoma) particularly in the head and neck location. PEM have been described in teratomas and meningothelial tissue is not an infrequent component of mature neuroglial tissues in teratomas (tumors composed of tissues derived from all three primordial germ layers). This review will focus on those some aspects of meningiomas that occur outside the CNS; the primary ectopic meningiomas and lesions where meningothelial tissue has been found with particular focus on pulmonary and gonadal (in the context of gonadal mature teratomas) meningiomas and meningothelial proliferations and separately hamartomas/choristomas particularly of the head and neck. It is these latter lesions that the author has the most familiarity from practicing in the discipline of pediatric pathology.

2. Developmental aspects of meninges pertinent to primary ectopic meningiomas and ectopic meningothelial tissue

This will be a brief section and by no means an exhaustive treatment of the embryological, morphological and molecular genetics aspects of meninges development. For a more thorough review of meninges development, the reader is directed to the excellent reviews by Dasgupta and Jeong [3] and Lopes [4]. However, here, we will attempt to highlight elements of what is known about the embryological and particularly molecular pathways involved in meninges development as it may relate to the development of meningiomas and the presence of meningothelial tissues in other anatomical locations outside of the central nervous system (CNS) proper.

In contrast to other areas of CNS development, relatively little is known about the molecular characteristics of meninges development. In a broad sense, however, the meninges increasingly are being shown to be critical to proper calvarial and underlying brain development. It is noted that the cranial meninges are derived from two cellular pools; the neural crest (ectoderm) and mesoderm. Neural crest derived cells can be found in the three layers of meninges covering the forebrain cerebral hemispheres but not in the meninges covering midbrain or hindbrain. Calvarial development closely parallels meninges development in that the frontal bones are primarily neural crest derived while the parietal bones are of mesodermal origin. Foxc1 is a key and ubiquitously expressed transcription factor in meninges development with noted early upregulation in the primary meninx. Its prominent role is demonstrated by lack of apical arachnoid and dura mater formation as well as lack of apical calvarial development in Foxc1 mutant mice. Parietal bone development appears to depend on the underlying meninges (derived from neural crest) expressing transforming growth factor beta 2 receptor (Tgfbr2) as Tgfbr2 mutant mice show severe defects in both parietal bone and underlying meninges development. The dura or outer dense layer of the meninges becomes closely apposed to the underside of the bony calvarium and is the de facto periosteal layer. The mesenchyme around the developing brain is divided into layers that include a dermal layer (dermis of scalp), skeletogenic layer (skull), and then the meningeal primordium. By extension, it can be plausible that ectopic meningiomas can arise (and indeed do) in the bones of the calvarium and scalp. It has been proposed that arachnoid cells or precursors can migrate with cranial nerves as they exit their foramina during development and be the forerunners of primary ectopic meningiomas in anatomic regions such as the orbit, ear, and neck [1]. Meninges appear to play crucial roles in brain development including providing trophic factors for neuronal survival, migration/positioning of neurons, neuronal generation from neuronal progenitors, blood vessel development, corpus callosum development, and may provide a niche for neural stem cells [5].

Again, by extension, it is not implausible to think that since much of the structures comprising the head and neck are derived from neural crest (and mesenchymal) cells, cells with multipotent capabilities, that some of these cells could be dormant and later directed down a path of meningeal differentiation in aberrant locations.

3. Primary ectopic (extracranial) meningiomas

To begin this section with an aside, the designation of ectopic meningiomas as "primary" necessarily implies that there may be other categories of meningiomas as "secondary", "tertiary" and so on. The terminology "primary ectopic meningioma" (PEM for brevity sake) then designates those meningiomas that are outside of the CNS that develop presumably from separate meningeal precursor cells; either ectopic arachnoid cells or perhaps cells that are multipotent (e.g. neural crest) as we have briefly noted. In some sense, this terminology is redundant since if the meningioma (or any lesion) is designated as "ectopic" that lesion is not indigenous to its normal anatomic location and would therefore be "primary". So called "secondary extracranial meningiomas" are defined as those lesions that are an extension of an intracranial meningioma. The author has not seen further designations of meningiomas beyond secondary and it is difficult to conjure a scenario where the designation of "tertiary extracranial meningioma" would be applicable. In addition, in perusing this literature, the terminology is a bit confusing because different names have been applied descriptively to lesions that probably ultimately fall under an umbrella category (see above description of Type I cutaneous meningioma). Some have described extracranial meningothelial proliferations in four categories: 1) extracranial extension of intracranial meningioma, 2) extracranial meningioma, 3) the aforementioned primary cutaneous meningioma, and 4) metastatic meningioma [6]. We already see that category 1 is what has been referenced as a Type III cutaneous meningioma and 3 presumably encompasses the spectrum of cutaneous meningiomas that include Type III. In this author's simplistic way of thinking and since this is a review, primary ectopic meningioma is not an unreasonable designation because the terms denote a meningioma that is outside the CNS as a "stand alone" or primary tumor in that location. If the designation were only "ectopic meningioma" then extracranial extensions of intracranial meningiomas could technically be under that rubric. Additionally, and similarly, the term "meningothelial" seems to imply tissue that is by all standards meningeal but not a tumor (more later). Meningothelial tissue or proliferations would seem by definition to be primary and ectopic since intracranial meningothelial proliferations are really not a diagnostic category of CNS lesions except for the possibility of meningeal tissue as part of another tumor.

That aside, it is interesting when trying to quell cases of PEM from the searchable medical literature, the variety of names given to these lesions as hinted at, and the ensuing difficulty that arises in attempting to exactly define the numbers and types of PEM reported. As Gibson and Prayson aptly alert the reader in their excellent chapter on this subject [7], a variety of designations have been used when reporting these lesions including ectopic, extracranial, extraneuraxial, extradural, cutaneous, intraosseous, calvarial etc. In addition, case reports may designate one of these categories to describe the lesion, but indeed the lesion may actually represent a secondary extracranial meningioma, or the patient may have had a previous remote intracranial meningioma.

Combined with a previous review of 178 reported cases from the English language medical literature by Lang et al. [8], Gibson cited an additional 100 cases of PEM at the time of publication of their chapter (2009). In this author's brief survey of the entire medical literature not restricted to the English language from 1/1/2008 to the present, approximately 184 cases of PEM are noted after using search terms that Gibson identified as descriptors for PEMs such as "ectopic", "extracranial", "extraneuraxial", "extradural", "cutaneous", "calvarial", "intraosseous" and "meningioma". By far, the most cases are reported from the head/neck anatomic location with intraosseous PEM by far exceeding any other location in the head and neck or elsewhere outside of the head and neck (**Table 1**). The most common site/location for PEM outside the head and neck was interestingly pulmonary followed by spinal/mediastinal/thoracic (**Table 2**).

It should not be terribly surprising that from a teleological perspective and given the developmental biology of meninges that the most commonly cited location of PEM is in the head and neck location and more specifically in the calvarial/skull bones. The intimate association of mesenchymal and/or neural crest cells in the development of the calvarial bones and meninges, particularly the dura which is directly apposed to the bone, makes this causative possibility very plausible. Likewise could be said for the greater number of cases of PEM found in the spinal/mediastinal/thoracic location. In children, certain tumors particularly neuroblastoma and its variants, can be found in this paraxial location along the sympathetic chain where neuroblasts are migrating during development.

PEM are quite uncommon as might be expected and the multiple reviews all cite basically the same incidence of approximately 1–2% of all meningiomas. Several

Site	N
Intraosseous (skull)	62
Intraosseous (mandible)	5
Intraosseous (maxilla)	1
Scalp	13
Lacrimal/orbital	11
Sinonasal	10
Parapharyngeal/neck	9
Middle ear	2
Soft tissue	2
Cheek	1
	N = 117

Table 1.
Approximate location and number of primary ectopic meningiomas in the head and neck from 2008 to present.

Site	N
Pulmonary	34
Spinal/mediastinal/thoracic	21
Cutaneous	5
Intraosseous (hip/pelvis)	3
Adrenal gland	1
Brachial plexus	1
Kidney (hilum)	1
Soft tissue (thigh)	1
	N = 67

Table 2.
Approximate location and number of primary ectopic meningiomas outside the head and neck from 2008 to present.

excellent reviews have been published identifying the clinical and pathological characteristics of PEM in general and in specific locations including intraosseous (calvarial) [9], ear and temporal bone [10], sinonasal tract [11], and pulmonary [12–15]. In addition, PEMs have been reported in skin, kidney, retroperitoneum, mediastinum, extremities, adrenal gland, ovary (mature cystic teratoma) [7], In general, for PEM, in contrast to CNS meningiomas, there is only a slight female predominance in incidence with the exception of perhaps those presenting in the ear and temporal bone where at least in the series by Rushing et al., the M:F ratio (1,2) more closely approximated the M:F ratio for CNS meningiomas in adults [16]. PEM arising in the ear and temporal bone are particularly troublesome for the pathologist as they can have a broad differential diagnosis in a location that is not the genesis of a comparatively large number of specimens that might traverse a general pathologist's microscope. This differential diagnosis includes entities such as paraganglioma, schwannoma, melanoma, middle ear adenoma or carcinoid, and carcinoma. The middle ear was the most common location for these PEMs with a relatively high association with cholesteatoma (9/36 cases). A smattering of histological subtypes were identified in these PEM and this is the case for PEM in general. The most common histological subtype identified by far is meningothelial (range 47% to over 90% depending on site) followed at a significant distance by atypical or psammomatous [16]. As an aside, in searching our pathology archives for cases of meningioma, we found approximately 730 cases of meningioma over 20 years, with less than 5 PEMs found that were either intraosseous (calvarial) or middle ear (mastoid) (**Figure 1**) and no cases of extracranial soft tissue, visceral, or pulmonary PEMs.

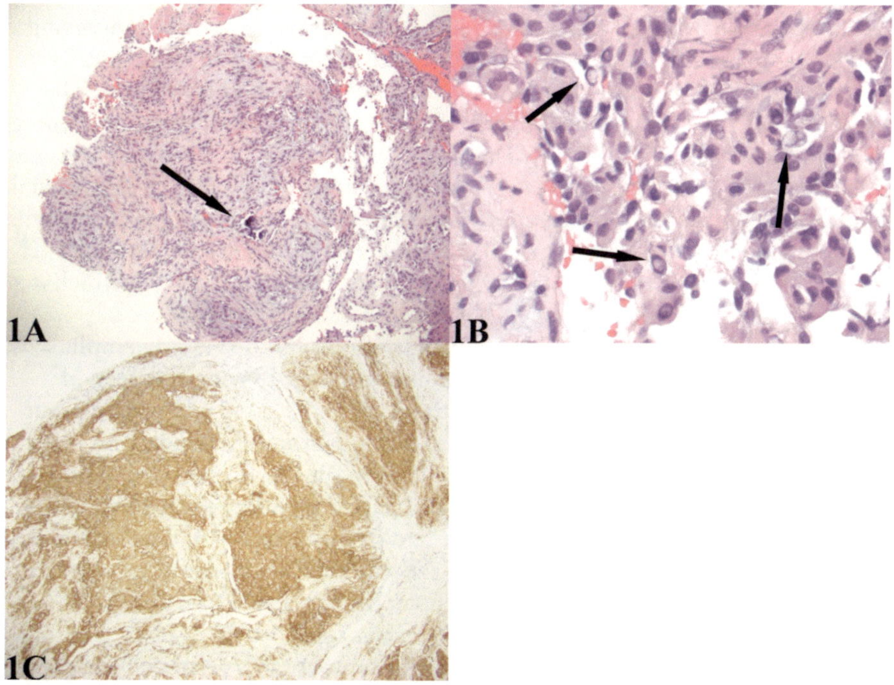

Figure 1.
Meningothelial meningioma of the mastoid presenting with tinnitus in a 46-year-old woman. No connection to the CNS was seen by imaging or intraoperatively. A: Low magnification view of meningioma composed of spindled and epitheliod cells in a whirling pattern with areas of more concentrated fibrous tissue. Scattered psammoma bodies were seen throughout the biopsy pieces (arrow, HE 40X). B: High magnification view of the relatively bland appearing nuclei with numerous pseudoinclusions, a hallmark nuclear feature of meningiomas (arrow, HE 600X). C: Diffuse staining of the meningeal lesional cells with epithelial membrane antigen (EMA 100X).

A few reviews have been published specifically addressing primary pulmonary meningiomas (PPM), that is, meningiomas that occur in the lung parenchyma as cited. Three of the four reviews included part of the time span included in the review here [12, 14, 15]. Our review provides perhaps more emphasis on the pathological phenotypes and concurrence with other tumors than other reviews.

PPMs are interesting entities for several reasons. One, their pathogenesis might not be as teleologically obvious compared to PEMs that occur say in the head and neck. Two, pulmonary meningothelial proliferations/nodules are not a terribly uncommon finding incidentally in lung resections and will be the subject of the latter part of this review as part of the spectrum of extracranial/extraneuraxial lesions of meningothelial lineage. Three, there are multiple case reports of concurrent CNS and pulmonary meningiomas [17] as well as reports of concurrent PEMs in lung and bone [18], metastases from CNS meningiomas to the lung [19] in particular, and metastases from other tumors into CNS meningiomas [20] and even metastases from PEMs to the lung [21]. Four, PPM can be mimickers of a primary lung cancer, now the second most common cancer in both men and women in the United States and therefore should be considered (albeit somewhat down the differential diagnostic list) by every pathologist who looks at lung biopsies and resections [22]. Five, pulmonary meningothelial proliferations, either sporadic or diffuse, may even be more troublesome for the pathologist. These interesting categories in the spectrum of meningiomas cannot, unfortunately, be further elucidated in this brief review.

Table 3 represents a review of the medical literature (English and non-English) searched in PubMed using the search terms "pulmonary" or "lung" and "meningioma" contained in the title/abstract from January 1, 2008 to August 16, 2021 (roughly corresponding to the last cases of PEM reported by Gibson et al. as noted). This search yielded 407 results of which 34 case reports were included reporting PPM [12–15, 18, 22–50]. One patient had two case reports approximately 10 years apart and one article published in a Spanish journal could not be obtained. The clinical characteristics (age, gender, location, size, recurrence rate) are in keeping with other reviews of PPM [12–15]. The immunohistochemical profiles were also in line with other reviews with most PPMs demonstrating staining with epithelial membrane antigen (EMA), progesterone receptor (PR), and vimentin. This review demonstrated perhaps higher numbers of both WHO grades II and III tumors (if presuming the remainder of the undesignated cases were WHO grade I which is a reasonably safe assumption).

An interesting aspect in the review of these cases and not overly emphasized in other reviews is the seemingly high number of patients with a history of other malignancies; almost one-third of the patients (10/34) with one patient having multiple (3) other tumors (osteosarcoma, fibrous dysplasia, and giant cell tumor of bone). This patient had a somatic mutation in the giant cell tumor of H3.3A and a germline mutation of BRCA2. Of course, one must be careful in drawing conclusions from a small dataset and in this case the patients with other malignancies were all in the age range where other malignancies are not uncommon (mean age 65 years, range 52–80). The malignancies in this group included buccal (1) (presumably squamous cell carcinoma), breast (2), gastric adenocarcinoma (1), papillary thyroid carcinoma (1), thymoma (1)/renal cell carcinoma (1)(same patient), rectal adenocarcinoma (1), concurrent lung adenocarcinoma (1) and teratoma (1) (immature and mature teratoma of the ovary and retroperitoneum, respectively). With the exception of the teratomas and thymoma, the other tumors are not uncommonly seen in this age group. As an aside, the PPM in the patient with teratomas does raise the remote possibility of a meningothelial/meningioma metastases from one of the teratomas particularly since one teratoma was designated as immature.

Characteristic	**N = 34 cases**
Age at presentation (years) (n = 34)	
Mean (SD)	57.1 (17.8)
Range	18–108
Median	60
Gender (M:F)	9:25 (1:2.8)
Symptoms at presentation	11 (23- no designation)
Follow-up (n = 17)	
Disease free/no recurrence	17
Mean (years) (SD)	3.2 (4.5)
Range	0.17–20
Patients with history of other malignancies	10/34
Multiple PPM	3/34
Site (R/L)	19:15
Size (cm) (n = 31)	
Mean (SD)	2.4 (2.6)
Range	0.45–15
Histological type (n = 29)	
Malignant	3
Atypical	1
WHO I	2
Transitional	5
Chordoid	2
Fibrous	1
Meningothelial	1
Psammomatous	1
Rhabdoid	1
Intrapulmonary metastases	1
No designation	17
WHO grade (I, II, III)	28/3/4*
Psammoma bodies	11/15
No designation	20
Epithelial membrane antigen/EMA +	30/30 (5-no designation)
Progesterone receptor (PR) +	17/18 (17-no designation)
Vimentin +	20/20 (15-no designation)
S100 +	6/14 (21-no designation)
Cytokeratins +	0/16 (19-no designation)
Ki-67 (≥ 10%)	3/14 (15-no designation)
≥ 10%	3
< 10%	13
No designation	19

*- *One patient had two asynchronous tumors.*

Table 3.
Review of clinical and pathological characteristics of primary pulmonary meningioma 2008–2021.

A 21-year-old female with Diamond-Blackfan anemia was included in this cohort who presented with a chordoid histology PPM [39]. Diamond-Blackfan anemia (DBA) is an inherited bone marrow failure syndrome that has approximately 20 known genetic aberrations in genes encoding small/large subunit associated ribosomal proteins (RPS and RPL genes) [51]. A cursory review shows no definitive RPS or RPL genes to be associated with any of the non-neurofibromatosis, type 2 (NF2) associated genes known to be mutated in meningiomas [52–54]. While DBA is associated with higher rates of other cancers including osteosarcoma, vaginal squamous cell carcinomas, esophageal cancer, colon adenocarcinoma, and myeloid leukemias, increased risk for meningiomas have not been seen in patients with DBA to date [51]. However, subsequent to the publication of this young patient with DBA and chordoid meningioma, she was found to have a mutation of the RSP19 gene [51].

As noted, one patient in this cohort had papillary thyroid carcinoma (PTC). An interesting epidemiological study by Sughrue et al. [55] showed that compared to the expected prevalence for a similar population, patients with meningioma had a statistically higher incidence of papillary thyroid cancer and acute leukemia. From a pathology perspective, it is also interesting that both tumors share at least one characteristic histopathological feature; psammoma bodies. Psammoma bodies can be seen characteristically in several tumors including PTC, meningiomas, serous cystadenocarcinoma of the ovary, and melanotic schwannoma (one of the tumors with high prevalence in Carney syndrome). The pathogenesis of psammoma bodies is still controversial with theories involving vascular thrombosis of papillae, followed by calcification and endothelial necrosis. More recently, osteopontin (OPN), a calcium-binding glycophosphotein has been implicated in the formation of psammoma bodies being expressed in CD68 positive macrophages along with other factors that include alkaline phosphatase, osteocalcin, metalloproteinases, bone sialoprotein, and others [56]. OPN expression has been shown to be increased in meningiomas compared to normal meninges, correlates with histological grade, and is a predictor of recurrence in WHO grade I tumors [57, 58].

The pathogenesis of PPM and PEM particularly those outside of the head and neck, of course, remains speculative as do many aspects of normal meninges development as noted earlier. Hypotheses regarding the origin of PEMs have included ectopic arachnoid cells that are present in cranial and peripheral nerve sheaths and in cranial sutures, misplacement of arachnoid cells during development, pluripotent mesenchymal cells, perineurial cells of peripheral nerves, and entrapped meninges at sites of trauma [7, 16]. Meningiomas, arachnoid cap cells (cells making up the outer layer of the arachnoid mater and villi), and spindle cells within perineurium express EMA that is detected immunohistochemically. While nearly all meningiomas and perineuriomas express EMA, only about one-third of meningiomas express glucose transporter-1 (GLUT-1) while most perineuriomas express GLUT-1. Similarly, SSTR2 and PR are expressed in a high percentage of meningiomas compared to perineuriomas while the reverse is true for claudin-1 [59]. Indirect support for pluripotent mesenchymal cells as the cell of origin for PEMs derives from the fact that meningiomas can exhibit histologically other tissue types including bone, cartilage, muscle, vascular, and other tissues. With regards to PPM specifically, two theories have arisen regarding their pathogenesis. The first is similar to what has been proposed for PEMs elsewhere; pluripotent mesenchymal cells that reside in the subpleural region or from "precursor" lesions known as minute pulmonary meningothelial nodules (MPMN, more on these later) [12]. Both PPM and MPMN share some similar phenotypes particularly the expression of similar immunohistochemical markers (EMA, PR, vimentin) but it is certainly unclear if MPMNs are truly precursors of PPM. Indeed, there seems to be some discrepancy in incidence of MPMN and meningiomas in autopsy series leading some to conclude that MPMN cannot be a precursor lesion [12]. Some have argued that MPMN are not precursor lesions based on genotyping studies demonstrating higher frequencies of loss of heterozygosity (LOH) and LOH affecting different loci in meningiomas compared to MPMN [60]. It is interesting that a progression of increasing frequency of LOH was noted from solitary MPMN to meningotheliomatosis to meningioma. Weissferdt et al. demonstrated that MPMN do share some genotypic alterations with PPM and CNS meningioma particularly deletion of the NF2 gene and gains of chromosome 22q [61]. The distinction between the two has mostly been by somewhat arbitrary size criteria (≤ 3 mm for MPMN). PPMs also tend to form a "mass" displacing lung.

From the pathology perspective, PEMs present specific and diverse diagnostic challenges. This is largely due to the variable histomorphologies that have been described not only in CNS meningiomas but also in PEMs and the various locations that PEMs can occur which raise different differential diagnoses. The differential diagnoses for PEM in the middle ear and temporal bone has already been discussed. For all PEMs in the head and neck location, Rushing et al. found paraganglioma, schwannoma, and metastatic carcinomas to be the most frequent misdiagnoses for ear and temporal bone PEM; Carcinoma, melanoma, olfactory neuroblastoma, and aggressive psammomatoid ossifying fibroma for sinonasal tract PEM, and dermatofibroma, melanoma, fibrosarcoma, leimyosarcoma, and synovial sarcoma for soft tissue and skin PEM [16]. The differential diagnosis for PPMs brings a variety of entities that can occur in the lung and mediastinum. These include sarcomatoid mesothelioma, solitary fibrous tumor, spindle cell thymoma, spindle cell carcinomas, inflammatory myofibroblastic tumor, synovial sarcoma, epithelioid hemangioendothelioma, and of course metastases [12]. As noted, meningiomas can present with a wide range of histological features including meningothelial, fibrous, microcystic, transitional (spindle cell component) psammomatous, angiomatous, secretory, metaplastic (lipidized cells), lymphoplasmacytic rich (all WHO grade I), clear cell (mimicking clear cell renal cell carcinoma), chordoid, atypical (WHO grade II), and rhabdoid (cells with eccentric nuclei and abundant eosinophilic cytoplasm), papillary, and anaplastic (WHO grade III). There are several excellent reviews of the histopathology of meningiomas along with the criteria for atypical and anaplastic variants [52, 54, 62]. And as mentioned before, other tissue types can be seen occasionally within meningiomas (i.e. bone, cartilage/chondroid, muscle). The variety of tissue types and potential to produce other tissues speaks highly for a pluripotent cell of origin (neural crest, mesenchymal) and are reminiscent of some other tumors that have such potentially variable histological appearances (e.g. yolk sac/endodermal sinus tumor which is derived from a pluripotent cell). Suffice it to say that given these variations, the differential diagnoses become expanded and criteria for narrowing the diagnoses are critical. Most of the identified histological subtypes have been identified in PEMs. In the review by Rushing et al. of extracranial head and neck PEMs, meningothelial, psammomatous, clear cell, atypical, and anaplastic were noted [16]. In sinonasal tract meningiomas, meningothelial is the most common subtype and transitional, metaplastic, and psammomatous types have been identified [11]. In PPMs, as noted in this review and others, meningothelial, transitional, fibrous, chordoid, rhabdoid, psammomatous, atypical, and anaplastic have been reported. Transitional histology is reported as the most common histological subtype in PPMs [12]. As seen in our review and noted in many publications, the immunohistochemical trio of EMA, vimentin, and progesterone receptor is present in the majority of cases of meningioma including PPMs. A smattering of cases will show staining with CD34, S100, and CD68 but are almost always negative for cytokeratins. In cases where these stains and morphology still leave doubt, other markers should be included in the work-up panel. A cytokeratin stain (both high and low molecular weight or pankeratin) is very important in the exclusion of entities such as metastases from carcinoma, mesothelioma, and thymoma. Neural markers (chromogranin, synaptophysin) are usually negative in meningiomas and positive in paragangliomas for instance. CD56 has been shown to mark some meningiomas (4 positive cases in our series although most cases in the series did not perform or report this marker) but is also strongly positive in most paragangliomas. Since melanoma can be a great mimicker of many tumors, markers such as HMB-45, melan-A, MART1, and MITF are helpful in this distinction since these are almost always negative in meningiomas. S100 may be useful also in the distinction of melanocytic tumors and peripheral nerve sheath tumors (schwannoma) with usual strong diffuse staining of these entities. However, as seen, 6/14 cases that reported results of S100 staining in PPMs were positive in our series. While most did not report the extent or intensity of staining for S100, in general, it is probably not to the degree seen in melanocytic or peripheral nerve sheath tumors. Vascular markers, CD31 and CD34, can be helpful since most meningiomas are negative for these markers. These vascular markers should be positive in hemangioendothelioma. CD34 is usually positive in solitary fibrous tumor along with bcl-2 and is almost always negative for EMA. Bcl-2 is also useful for distinguishing synovial sarcoma. Muscle markers (smooth muscle actin, muscle specific actin, calponin and others) can helpful in the distinction of smooth muscle neoplasms and inflammatory myofibroblastic tumors along with ALK-1.

Another marker that demonstrates very high positive and negative predictive values for meningiomas is the monoclonal antibody to SSTR2a (somatostatin receptor 2a) [63]. This receptor is highly expressed in meningiomas as are other somatostatin receptors. Somatostatin ligand analogs such as DOTATOC and DOTATATE have been linked to ^{68}Ga and used in PET imaging of meningiomas with great success. ^{68}Ga-DOTATATE uptake correlates with SSTR2 expression and has high sensitivity for detecting active tumor in untreated and recurrent meningiomas [64]. In tissue specimens, the monoclonal antibody to SSTR2a has higher sensitivity than EMA or PR and did not stain with high intensity other lesions in the differential diagnoses including peripheral nerve sheath tumors (malignant and benign) and other carcinomas, mesenchymal tumors, or melanomas [63]. A high percentage of meningiomas also express p40 which is one isoform of p63 (p53 homolog gene) and the intensity of expression correlates with histological grade and recurrence [65].

All meningiomas are not sporadic. Multiple familial syndromes associated with specific genetic aberrations have increased risk for development of meningiomas. Neurofibromatosis 2 (NF2 gene, chromosome 22q12) has the highest lifetime risk for development of meningioma at 50%. Approximately 40% of sporadic meningiomas are driven by other genetic mutations other than NF2 [54]. **Table 4** highlights the known familial syndromes associated with varying degrees of increased risk of meningioma. As somewhat of an aside, patients with Werner syndrome (Progeria, premature aging syndrome) as noted have an increased risk of meningioma. In the excellent review by Lauper et al. [66], they noted 27 meningiomas in their cohort of 189 confirmed Werner syndrome patients. Eight of these tumors occurred in patients with multiple tumors and 5/9 patients with meningiomas also had thyroid neoplasia (1 PTC, 1 thyroid carcinoma NOS, 3 adenomas). Four of 5 patients had only meningioma and thyroid neoplasia as manifestation of their multiple tumors. Gardner/Turcot syndrome (APC-associated polyposis), PTEN hamartoma syndrome (Cowden, Bannayan-Riley-Ruvalcaba, Lhermitte-Duclos syndromes), MEN1 (Wermer syndrome), and Werner syndrome are familial inherited syndromes also highly associated with thyroid neoplasia [67]. Carney complex also has a high

Familial syndrome	Gene	Chromosome location	Risk %
Neurofibromatosis 2	NF2	22q12	>50
Multiple spinal meningiomas	SMARCE1	17q21.2	
BAP1 tumor predisposition	BAP1	3p21.1	2
Familial schwannomatosis	SMARCB1	22q11.23	
Gorlin syndrome	PTCH1	9q22.3	5
Cowden disease	PTEN	10q23.31	8
Familial multiple meningiomas	SUFU	10q24.32	
Li-Fraumeni	TP53/CHEK2	17p13.1/22q12.1	
Rubinstein-Taybi	CREBBP	16p13.3	
Gardner syndrome/Turcot syndrome	APC	5q21–22	
Multiple endocrine neoplasia I	MEN	11q13	
Werner syndrome	WRN (RECQL)	8p11.1–21.2	14
Von Hippel–Lindau	VHL	3p25.3	
Ataxia telangiectasia	ATM	11q22	

Table 4.
Familial syndromes associated with increased risk of meningioma.

association of thyroid neoplasia and has as a pathognomonic lesion the melanotic schwannoma, a tumor characterized by schwannian differentiation with the feature of psammoma bodies. Carney complex is known to result from mutations in PRKAR1A (chromosome 17q22–24) and CNC2 (2p16) while WHO grades II and III meningiomas have been shown to be associated with gains and amplification of 17q [53, 54, 67]. In addition, interestingly, Gardner/Turcot syndrome, Carney complex, and Werner syndrome all have various bone tumors as part of the manifestation/diagnostic criteria for their respective syndromes. In the review by Lauper et al. [66], 17/189 Werner syndrome patients had osteosarcoma with 7/19 osteosarcomas occurring in patients with multiple tumors and one of these patients had meningioma/thyroid adenoma/osteosarcoma as the manifestation of multiple neoplasia. Another association is the presence of neoplasia associated with derivatives of the neural crest (retinal epithelial hypertrophy, benign and malignant peripheral nerve sheath tumors, benign and malignant melanocytic lesions). Gardner/Turcot, Carney complex, PTEN hamartoma, Werner syndromes all have melanocytic lesions as part of their neoplasia spectrum.

These are very interesting associations and can and will lead us to further elucidation of unifying mechanisms of molecular and cellular origins of tumors and in this case meningiomas. It is worth noting here that there are very few reports of PEMs associated with a familial inherited syndrome. What was presented above was data for associations with primary CNS meningiomas. Very few reports of PEMs in patients with a familial syndrome can be found. One case report describes an ectopic meningioma of the right parapharyngeal space in a 14-year-old girl with NF2 [68]. A second report describes an intranodal meningothelial proliferation in a 55-year-old woman with confirmed Cowden syndrome [69]. There seems likely a true difference in familial genetic syndromes and association with PEMs since one would think that specific case reports would address this as part of the unique spectrum of individual presentations of PEM.

4. Meningothelial proliferations

I suppose a general definition of "meningothelial proliferation" would likely be in order. It was alluded to earlier in this review. I say "general" because as noted in the case of PPMs the distinction between what is a meningothelial nodule/proliferation and what is termed a meningioma may be a bit arbitrary and certainly subjective. In this review of PPM, for instance, 6/31 "meningiomas" were less than 1 cm in greatest dimension. In pathology, the distinction between what determines a proliferation and what determines a "tumor" is sometimes based on size with 1 cm being a threshold size for specific tumor designations. For instance, the distinction of papillary thyroid microcarcinoma and papillary thyroid carcinoma is based on the former being less than 1 cm in greatest dimension. In radiology, the standard threshold for detecting tumors has traditionally (although not as much now with improvements in imaging modalities) been less than or greater than 1 cm. In the practice of pathology, these distinctions are not always clear and other features in addition to size are considered in the diagnostic algorithm. An important feature is what the tumor is doing to the surrounding tissue. Is it "blending" in as in the cases, for example, of dominant hyperplastic nodules in the thyroid or nephroblastomatosis in the spectrum of Wilms tumor or it is replacing/pushing normal tissue.

With regards to meningothelial proliferations that occur outside the CNS, that is the presence of meningothelial or meningeal tissue that is not a tumor of meninges, these have been described in a few general settings (although not an exhaustive list) including heterotopic neuroglial proliferations, pulmonary meningothelial nodules (to include diffuse pulmonary meningotheliomatosis), teratomas, and rarely in choristomatous lesions particularly in the head and neck.

One of the reasons to include a review of PPM as cited above was that meningothelial proliferations are well-described in the lungs. In the older pathological literature, MPMNs were originally termed "minute pulmonary paragangliomas" or "chemodectomas" since their ontogeny was thought to be distal airway chemoreceptors [70]. However, subsequently, these have been shown not only morphologically but immunohistochemically and ultrastructurally to be meningothelial in origin. They present as a nested proliferation of spindled and epithelioid cells with bland nuclei around small veins in the lung and exhibit the characteristic EMA+, vimentin+, and PR+ immunophenotype. The incidence of MPMN is reported up to 5% in autopsy studies and in up to approximately 14% of surgical biopsy specimens and in nearly half of lobectomy specimens [70]. Interestingly, in the large series by Mukhopadhyay that included resections from patients in the pediatric age range and over 90 pediatric autopsies, no MPMN were seen in the pediatric population [71]. Radiographically, by CT, MPMN are round solid or partially solid nodules and can be multiple and have a "ground glass" appearance. They typically show low SUV (benign) values for FDG-avidity on ^{18}F-FDG PET-CT imaging [13]. Depending on the clinical scenarios (concurrent other lung lesions, history or concurrence of other tumors), metastases or synchronous tumors cannot be entirely excluded thus necessitating removal and pathological examination. Rarely, MPMN can occur in the setting of PPM; some of these cases being diagnosed as intrapulmonary metastases [14, 25].

Diffuse pulmonary meningotheliomatosis (DPM) is an interesting if not quite rare entity. These patients can present with symptoms of restrictive pulmonary disease with diffuse bilateral reticulonodular infiltrates that have the differential diagnoses including a variety of interstitial lung diseases, carcinomatosis, neuroendocrine tumorlets, metastatic meningioma, and pulmonary lymphangioleiomyomatosis (PLAM). The separation of these entities is relatively straightforward based on morphology and immunophenotyping. Metastatic meningiomas should be distinguished by clinical grounds (presence of a CNS tumor), involvement of the bronchovascular tree as opposed to DPM which is usually found centered around small veins, and more atypical appearance. Carcinomatosis, neuroendocrine tumorlets, and PLAM are distinguished by positivity for keratins, neuroendocrine markers (typically synaptophysin and chromogranin), and actins while similarly to MPMN and PPM, DPM lesions are EMA, vimentin, and PR positive [61, 71–73]. Primary pulmonary meningothelial lesions (MPMN, DPM, and PPM) are very interesting from developmental and genetic perspectives as lung meningothelial lesions seem to predominate the epidemiological landscape of meningothelial lesions outside of the CNS and head/neck and seem to have an extremely low prevalence in the pediatric population leading some to speculate that their origins may not be pluripotent mesenchymal cells but more related to environmental and age-related factors. Although, just because they are not found in the pediatric age group, should not totally discount that they arise from resting pluripotent stem cells or other dormant embryological remnants and their recrudescence as meningothelial lesions is stimulated by other factors. The lungs like other organs also have a "stem cell niche" that is triggered when there is bronchial epithelial injury for the purposes of regeneration/repair [74]. As we have also discussed there seems to be a spectrum of increasing mutations in MPMN and DPM raising the possibilities for a mutational spectrum or "hit" hypotheses in their pathogenesis.

Meningothelial tissue can occur as part of other pathological lesions. In this final section we will briefly touch on the presence of meningiomas and meningothelial tissue in teratomas and meningothelial elements as part of heterotopic/choristomatous/hamartomatous lesions. Somewhat surprisingly, very few cases of meningioma or meningothelial tissue in teratomas are described. A search of PubMed for "meningiomas" and "teratomas" yielded 8 results. One case was a posterior fossa tumor mimicking a meningioma and another case was teratoma and meningioma in the temporoparietal region. The remaining 6 cases were all gonadal teratomas with meningioma [75–82]. The clinical and pathological characteristics of these meningiomas is presented in **Table 5**. Two cases were in the pediatric age range (5-year-old male and 15-year-old female and all meningiomas were seen on gross examination to be whitish or brown firm nodular areas within the broader context of the mature

Characteristic	N = 6 cases
Teratoma type (T/O*)	
MCT** (T)	2
MCT (O)	4
Gender (M:F)	2:4
Age (years) (SD)	33.8 (20.7)
Range	5–60
Size (cm) (SD)	2.7 (1.2)
Psammoma bodies	5/6
Epithelial membrane antigen/EMA +	5 (1 with no designation)
Vimentin +	2 (4 with no designation)
Progesterone receptor (PR) +	2 (5 with no designation)

**T-testis, O-ovary.*
***MCT-mature cystic teratoma.*

Table 5.
Clinicopathological characteristics of meningiomas arising in gonadal teratomas.

cystic teratoma (MCT). Chen et al. searched for and characterized meningothelial proliferations in 25 consecutive ovarian MCT [83]. They found that 40% of their tumor had meningothelial proliferations that resembled what has been described in hamartoma of the scalp with ectopic meningothelial elements (more on this later). The meningeal nature of the tissue was confirmed morphologically and by EMA positivity. In all cases the meningothelial tissue was in close association with skin and mature glial tissue (ectodermally derived). Eight of 10 cases had pigmented cells and 3 had psammomatous calcifications. In the author's anecdotal experience, having microscopically examined numerous teratomas from children and adults and teratomas derived from the harvested embryonic stem cells from several species, the finding of meningeal tissue seems not that uncommon, although I have not encountered a meningioma tumor. A recent case of mine illustrates this from a 13-year-old girl with MCT. The meningeal tissue is intimately associated with mature neuroglial tissue and resembles arachnoid of the meninges (**Figure 2**).

Meningothelial tissue can be part of lesions described as heterotopias, particularly of the neuroglial flavor, hamartomas, and choristomas (tissues not indigenous to the anatomic location). In 2005, we reported a temporal glioneuronal heterotopia in a 19-month-old child without underlying connection to the CNS or calvarial defect. In our review of similar cases from the medical literature to that time, 11 infants were identified ranging in age from birth to 15-months. Six of 11 cases had no connection to the CNS (true heterotopias) and 2/6 had meningothelial elements as a component histologically [84]. In another review published at approximately

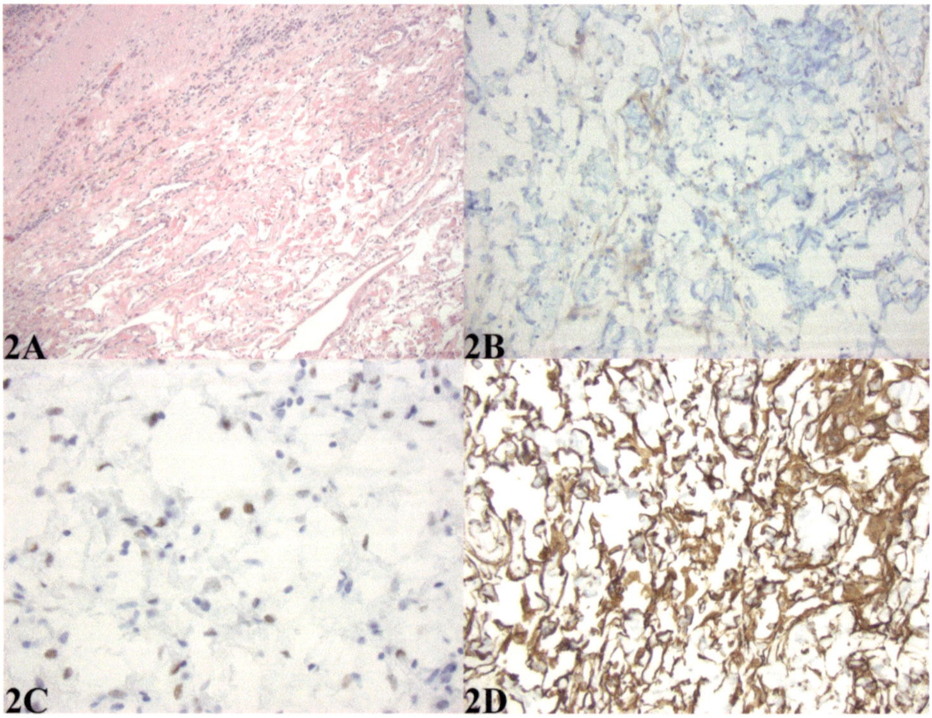

Figure 2.
Meningeal/meningothelial tissue within a mature cystic teratoma of the ovary in a 13-year-old girl. A: Low magnification view showing mature neuroglial tissue (upper left corner) adjacent to a proliferation of rarified, wispy anastomosing cords of fibrous tissue lined by bland small indistinct nuclei. In other areas of the teratoma, this pattern was also seen adjacent to skin and adnexal structures. This segregation of the meningothelial elements near skin and mature neuroglial is common. (HE, 40X). B: Weak by definite staining of the meningeal tissue with epithelial membrane antigen (EMA, 200X). C: Variably intense staining with progesterone receptor (PR, 400X). D: Diffuse strong intensity staining with vimentin (vimentin, 200X).

the same time by Rogers et al. from Boston Children's Hospital, they reported 11 patients with 12 tumors of the scalp ranging in age from 1-month to 20-months. Seven of the 12 tumors had no connection to the CNS and 5 of those 7 tumors had meningothelial tissue as a prominent component histologically [85].

Ectopic meningothelial tissues have been described that appear to arise entirely within the skin and often present in the neonate or infant (so called Type I cutaneous meningioma; defined in the beginning of this chapter). These have been previously termed "acoelic meningeal hamartoma" "cutaneous heterotopic meningeal nodules" and "rudimentary meningocele". In the series published in 1989 by Sibley and Cooper referenced earlier, they described 5 cases of what they termed "primary cutaneous meningioma". What they describe histologically is what is expected in meninges both morphologically and immunophenotypically including collagenous bodies and psammomatous calcifications. Some areas in the superficial dermis had a more rarified and lacy appearance with meningocytes wrapping around vessels and adnexa in intimate association similar to that described shortly thereafter by Suster and Rosai [86]. Their series described 5 patients who had pseudoinfiltrative lesions of the skin and subcutis by meningothelial elements that were in intimate association with the surrounding tissue elements (vessels, fat, connective tissue). In fact, they designated that the meningothelial elements were an interspersed component between a proliferation of connective tissue elements. Their designation for these lesions was "hamartoma of the scalp with ectopic meningothelial elements" and this has become the diagnostic term for such lesions. More recent reports in some cases have shortened the nomenclature to "meningothelial hamartoma". Suster and Rosai give the poignant perspective that the designation of these hamartomatous lesions with meningothelial elements are distinguished from primary cutaneous meningiomas by the association with other poorly arranged elements constituting a hamartoma. We have encountered similar tumors in the scalp (**Figure 3A** and **B**) and have published two cases in young children of tongue lesions with meningothelial elements (**Figure 3C** and **D**). Both tongue lesions were entirely composed of the typical anastomosing slit-like channels lined by bland flat-to-cuboidal cells expressing progesterone receptor and epithelial membrane antigen. Interestingly, but not surprisingly, meningothelial elements have been described occurring in the rare "teratoid" lesion of the palate known as hairy polyp [6]. These are pedunculated growths that can be composed of a variety of tissues derived predominantly from ectodermal and mesodermal (mesenchymal) germ layers. In the reported case, the presence of meningothelial tissue was confirmed by immunohistochemistry and ultrastructural examination demonstrating the characteristic interdigitating cytoplasmic processes connected by cell junctions, desmosomes, intermediate filaments (hence positive expression of vimentin).

In summary, CNS meningiomas are the most common primary CNS tumor and meningiomas and meningothelial tissue/proliferation occur in a multitude of extra-CNS sites and present in a diverse manner from isolated non-tumor proliferations to part of hamartomatous lesions to diffuse meningotheliomatosis to meningiomas tumors arising in multiple anatomic locations. Morphologically, immunophenotypically, ultrastructurally, and perhaps genetically, the meningeal tumors and proliferations outside the CNS are very similar to their CNS counterparts suggesting a common cellular origin. Because of the possibility of arising in diverse anatomic locations, they join a long list of differential diagnostic considerations for the practicing pathologist and should be entertained as possibilities particularly when the morphology could significantly overlap other tumors. In most cases, the immunohistochemical profile of EMA, vimentin, progesterone receptor, and SSTR2a (if available) is diagnostic in the proper morphological context. This panel should be included in diagnostically challenging cases.

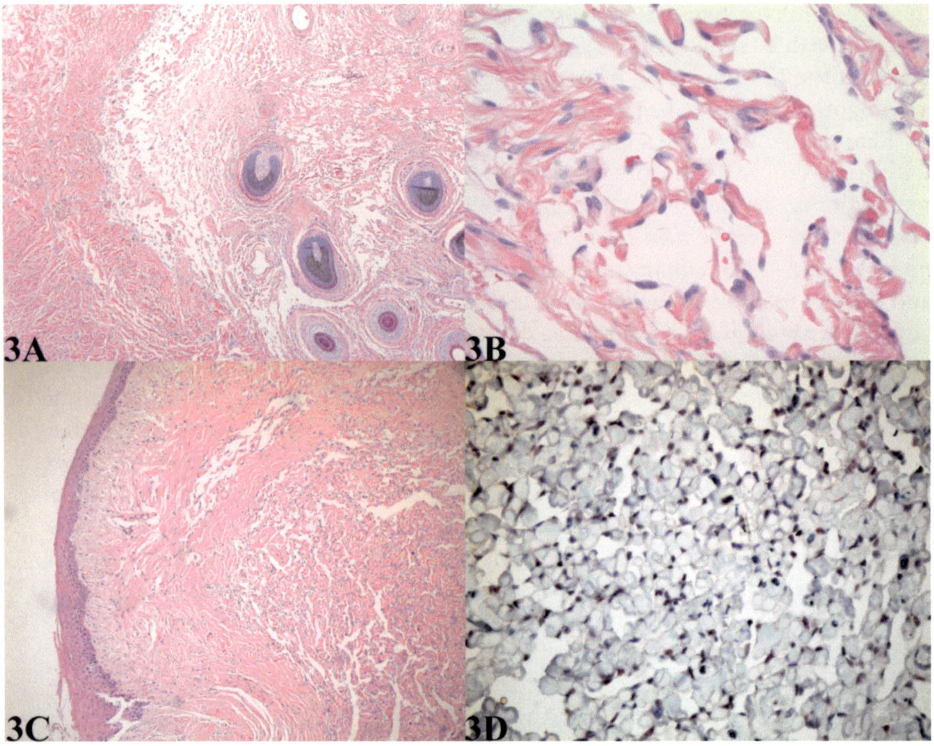

Figure 3.
Examples of ectopic meningothelial proliferations in the head and neck. A and B represent "hamartoma of the scalp with ectopic meningothelial elements" in a young child. 3A: Low magnification view of loose proliferation of anastomosing wispy fibrous cords lined by bland nuclei interdigitating around adnexal structures (HE, 40X). 3B: High magnification view of the microarchitecture of meningothelial proliferations. This pattern closely resembles vascular proliferations, particularly lymphatic malformations in children and must be excluded in the differential diagnosis (HE, 400X). C and D are from a nearly 2-year-old boy with a tongue mass. 3C: Less obvious than the previous case shown here yet the same microarchitectural pattern is appreciated below the surface epithelium of the tongue. This rarified pattern might be considered a "hemangiopericytomatous" pattern but in any case, is abnormal for the submucosa of the tongue (HE, 40X). 3D: This meningothelial proliferation show strong nuclear staining for progesterone receptor (PR, 400X).

Author details

John A. Ozolek
Department of Pathology, Anatomy, and Laboratory Medicine, West Virginia University, Morgantown, WV, USA

*Address all correspondence to: john.ozolek@hsc.wvu.edu; jclskpp@yahoo.com

References

[1] Sibley, D.A. and P.H. Cooper, *Rudimentary meningocele: a variant of "primary cutaneous meningioma".* J Cutan Pathol, 1989. **16**(2): p. 72-80.

[2] Miedema, J.R. and D. Zedek, *Cutaneous meningioma.* Arch Pathol Lab Med, 2012. **136**(2): p. 208-11.

[3] Dasgupta, K. and J. Jeong, *Developmental biology of the meninges.* Genesis, 2019. **57**(5): p. e23288.

[4] Lopes, M.B.S., *Meninges: Embryology*, in *Meningiomas*, J.H. Lee, Editor. 2009, Springer London: London. p. 25-29.

[5] Decimo, I., et al., *Meninges: from protective membrane to stem cell niche.* Am J Stem Cells, 2012. **1**(2): p. 92-105.

[6] Olivares-Pakzad, B.A., et al., *Oropharyngeal hairy polyp with meningothelial elements.* Oral Surg Oral Med Oral Pathol Oral Radiol Endod, 1995. **79**(4): p. 462-8.

[7] Gibson, S.E. and R.A. Prayson, *Primary Ectopic Meningiomas*, in *Meningiomas*, J.H. Lee, Editor. 2009, Springer London: London. p. 573-583.

[8] Lang, F.F., et al., *Primary extradural meningiomas: a report on nine cases and review of the literature from the era of computerized tomography scanning.* J Neurosurg, 2000. **93**(6): p. 940-50.

[9] Omofoye, O.A., et al., *Primary intraosseous meningioma of the calvarium: A systematic review.* Clin Neurol Neurosurg, 2020. **199**: p. 106283.

[10] Thompson, L.D., et al., *Primary ear and temporal bone meningiomas: a clinicopathologic study of 36 cases with a review of the literature.* Mod Pathol, 2003. **16**(3): p. 236-45.

[11] Thompson, L.D.R. and J.C. Fanburg-Smith, *Update on Select Benign Mesenchymal and Meningothelial Sinonasal Tract Lesions.* Head Neck Pathol, 2016. **10**(1): p. 95-108.

[12] Han, D., H. Deng, and Y. Liu, *Primary pulmonary meningiomas: report of two cases and review of the literature.* Pathol Res Pract, 2020. **216**(12): p. 153232.

[13] Incarbone, M., et al., *Primary pulmonary meningioma: report of a case and review of the literature.* Lung Cancer, 2008. **62**(3): p. 401-7.

[14] Masago, K., et al., *Is primary pulmonary meningioma a giant form of a meningothelial-like nodule? A case report and review of the literature.* Case Rep Oncol, 2012. **5**(2): p. 471-8.

[15] Ohashi-Nakatani, K., et al., *Primary pulmonary meningioma: A rare case report of aspiration cytological features and immunohistochemical assessment.* Diagn Cytopathol, 2019. **47**(4): p. 330-333.

[16] Rushing, E.J., et al., *Primary extracranial meningiomas: an analysis of 146 cases.* Head Neck Pathol, 2009. **3**(2): p. 116-30.

[17] Sathirareuangchai, S., et al., *Low grade intracranial meningioma presenting with pulmonary metastasis: Case report and literature review.* Pathol Res Pract, 2019. **215**(7): p. 152390.

[18] Tamura, H., et al., *Extracranial meningiomas concurrently found in the lung and vertebral bone: a case report.* J Med Case Rep, 2018. **12**(1): p. 279.

[19] Enomoto, T., et al., *WHO Grade I Meningioma Metastasis to the Lung 26 Years after Initial Surgery: A Case Report and Literature Review.* NMC Case Rep J, 2019. **6**(4): p. 125-129.

[20] Turner, N., A.H. Kaye, and I. Paldor, *Metastases to meningioma-review*

and meta-analysis. Acta Neurochir (Wien), 2021. **163**(3): p. 699-709.

[21] Murakami, K., et al., *A case report of resected ectopic malignant meningioma with lung metastasis.* Medicine (Baltimore), 2019. **98**(23): p. e15853.

[22] Fujikawa, R., et al., *A case of a primary pulmonary meningioma mimicking a metastasis from a papillary thyroid carcinoma due to a size reduction after radioactive iodine therapy.* Surg Case Rep, 2020. **6**(1): p. 57.

[23] Bae, S.Y., et al., *Primary Pulmonary Chordoid Meningioma.* Korean J Thorac Cardiovasc Surg, 2018. **51**(6): p. 410-414.

[24] Bercovici, D., et al., *[A rare pulmonary tumor].* Ann Pathol, 2017. **37**(5): p. 434-436.

[25] Chakrabarti, R. and D. Ghuman, *Diagnostic and Management Considerations in a Patient With Primary Pulmonary Meningioma With Associated Micro-Solid Nodules.* Cureus, 2021. **13**(6): p. e15700.

[26] Cimini, A., et al., *A Patient with a Benign and a Malignant Primary Pulmonary Meningioma: An Evaluation with 18F Fluorodeoxyglucose Positron Emission Tomography/Computed Tomography and Computed Tomography with Iodinated Contrast.* Indian J Nucl Med, 2019. **34**(1): p. 45-47.

[27] Fidan, A., et al., *Endobronchial primary pulmonary meningioma.* Saudi Med J, 2008. **29**(10): p. 1512-3.

[28] Gurcay, N., et al., *Primary pulmonary meningioma mimicking pulmonary metastasis: A rare case report.* Turk Gogus Kalp Damar Cerrahisi Derg, 2020. **28**(4): p. 699-701.

[29] Hong, S., et al., *Computed tomography findings of primary pulmonary meningioma: A case report.* Medicine (Baltimore), 2018. **97**(2): p. e9651.

[30] Huang, S., et al., *Primary pulmonary meningioma: A case report.* Medicine (Baltimore), 2017. **96**(19): p. e6474.

[31] Izumi, N., et al., *Primary pulmonary meningioma presenting with hemoptysis on exertion.* Ann Thorac Surg, 2009. **88**(2): p. 647-8.

[32] Jiang, M., et al., *A case report of primary pulmonary meningioma masquerading as lung metastasis in a patient with rectal carcinoma: role of (18) F-FDG PET/CT.* J Cardiothorac Surg, 2021. **16**(1): p. 153.

[33] Juan, C.M., et al., *Primary Pulmonary Meningioma Simulating a Pulmonary Metastasis.* Case Rep Pulmonol, 2016. **2016**: p. 8248749.

[34] Kim, Y.Y., et al., *Primary pulmonary meningioma: an unusual cause of a nodule with strong and homogeneous enhancement.* Clin Imaging, 2016. **40**(1): p. 170-3.

[35] Lepanto, D., et al., *Atypical primary pulmonary meningioma: a report of a case suspected of being a lung metastasis.* Ecancermedicalscience, 2014. **8**: p. 414.

[36] Luo, J.Z., et al., *Primary pulmonary meningioma mimicking lung metastatic tumor: a case report.* J Cardiothorac Surg, 2018. **13**(1): p. 99.

[37] Minami, Y., et al., *Malignant primary pulmonary meningioma with bone metastasis.* Oxf Med Case Reports, 2020. **2020**(2): p. omaa005.

[38] Oide, T., et al., *Primary Pulmonary Meningioma Presenting as a Coin Lesion.* Intern Med, 2017. **56**(15): p. 2073-2074.

[39] Petscavage, J.M., et al., *Primary chordoid meningioma of the lung.* J Thorac Imaging, 2011. **26**(1): p. W14-6.

[40] Sakai, K., et al., *[Multiple Primary Pulmonary Meningiomas]*. Kyobu Geka, 2019. **72**(9): p. 677-680.

[41] Satoh, Y. and Y. Ishikawa, *Multiple primary pulmonary meningiomas: 20-year follow-up findings for a first reported case confirming a benign biological nature.* Int J Surg Case Rep, 2017. **31**: p. 58-60.

[42] Tauziede-Espariat, A., et al., *[A pulmonary tumor that racks our brains!]*. Ann Pathol, 2021.

[43] Vaideeswar, P. and J. Chaudhari, *Primary pulmonary meningioma.* Indian J Pathol Microbiol, 2019. **62**(3): p. 486-487.

[44] Walter, J., et al., *Pulmonary meningioma and neurinoma associated with multiple CNS tumours in a patient with neurofibromatosis type 2.* Clin Neurol Neurosurg, 2009. **111**(5): p. 454-9.

[45] Wang, X., et al., *Intrapulmonary metastasis from primary pulmonary meningioma presenting as multiple cystic lesions: a case report.* BMC Pulm Med, 2019. **19**(1): p. 8.

[46] Weber, C., et al., *Primary pulmonary malignant meningioma with lymph node and liver metastasis in a centenary woman, an autopsy case.* Virchows Arch, 2013. **462**(4): p. 481-5.

[47] Xu, K.K., F. Tian, and Y. Cui, *Primary pulmonary meningioma presenting as a micro solid nodule: A rare case report.* Thorac Cancer, 2018. **9**(7): p. 874-876.

[48] Zhao, P., et al., *Rhabdoid Meningioma Arising Concurrent in Pulmonary and Intracranial with a Rare Malignant Clinical Progression: Case Report and Literature Review.* World Neurosurg, 2017. **107**: p. 1046 e17-1046 e22.

[49] Zhao, Z., et al., *Multiple primary tumors: a case report and review of the literature.* BMC Musculoskelet Disord, 2020. **21**(1): p. 394.

[50] Zulpaite, R., et al., *Primary Pulmonary Meningioma With Rhabdoid Features.* Int J Surg Pathol, 2019. **27**(4): p. 457-463.

[51] Vlachos, A., et al., *Increased risk of colon cancer and osteogenic sarcoma in Diamond-Blackfan anemia.* Blood, 2018. **132**(20): p. 2205-2208.

[52] Huntoon, K., A.M.S. Toland, and S. Dahiya, *Meningioma: A Review of Clinicopathological and Molecular Aspects.* Front Oncol, 2020. **10**: p. 579599.

[53] Lee, Y.S. and Y.S. Lee, *Molecular characteristics of meningiomas.* J Pathol Transl Med, 2020. **54**(1): p. 45-63.

[54] Ogasawara, C., B.D. Philbrick, and D.C. Adamson, *Meningioma: A Review of Epidemiology, Pathology, Diagnosis, Treatment, and Future Directions.* Biomedicines, 2021. **9**(3).

[55] Sughrue, M.E., et al., *Prevalence of previous extracranial malignancies in a series of 1228 patients presenting with meningioma.* J Neurosurg, 2010. **113**(5): p. 1115-21.

[56] Ferreira, L.B., et al., *Molecular Aspects of Thyroid Calcification.* Int J Mol Sci, 2020. **21**(20).

[57] Arikok, A.T., et al., *Osteopontin expressions correlate with WHO grades and predict recurrence in meningiomas.* Brain Tumor Pathol, 2014. **31**(2): p. 94-100.

[58] Li, H.Z., et al., *The role of osteopontin and its receptor in meningioma development and progression.* J Biol Regul Homeost Agents, 2018. **32**(1): p. 69-74.

[59] Agaimy, A., et al., *Comparative study of soft tissue perineurioma and*

meningioma using a five-marker immunohistochemical panel. Histopathology, 2014. **65**(1): p. 60-70.

[60] Ionescu, D.N., et al., *Pulmonary meningothelial-like nodules: a genotypic comparison with meningiomas.* Am J Surg Pathol, 2004. **28**(2): p. 207-14.

[61] Weissferdt, A., et al., *Pleuropulmonary Meningothelial Proliferations: Evidence for a Common Histogenesis.* Am J Surg Pathol, 2015. **39**(12): p. 1673-8.

[62] Backer-Grondahl, T., B.H. Moen, and S.H. Torp, *The histopathological spectrum of human meningiomas.* Int J Clin Exp Pathol, 2012. **5**(3): p. 231-42.

[63] Menke, J.R., et al., *Somatostatin receptor 2a is a more sensitive diagnostic marker of meningioma than epithelial membrane antigen.* Acta Neuropathol, 2015. **130**(3): p. 441-3.

[64] Rachinger, W., et al., *Increased 68Ga-DOTATATE uptake in PET imaging discriminates meningioma and tumor-free tissue.* J Nucl Med, 2015. **56**(3): p. 347-53.

[65] Guadagno, E., et al., *Expression of p40 (Np63) protein in meningiomas, an unexpected finding: immunohistochemical study and evaluation of its possible prognostic role.* J Neurooncol, 2016. **129**(3): p. 405-413.

[66] Lauper, J.M., et al., *Spectrum and risk of neoplasia in Werner syndrome: a systematic review.* PLoS One, 2013. **8**(4): p. e59709.

[67] Ozolek, J.A., *Selected Topics in the Pathology of the Thyroid and Parathyroid Glands in Children and Adolescents.* Head Neck Pathol, 2021. **15**(1): p. 85-106.

[68] Su, C.Q., et al., *Ectopic meningioma in a patient with neurofibromatosis Type 2: a case report and review of the literature.* BJR Case Rep, 2018. **4**(3): p. 20180007.

[69] Olofson, A., et al., *Intranodal meningothelial proliferation in a patient with Cowden syndrome: a case report.* Hum Pathol, 2017. **66**: p. 183-187.

[70] Morresi-Hauf, A.T., et al., *[Diffuse pulmonary meningotheliomatosis].* Pneumologie, 2015. **69**(9): p. 553-9.

[71] Mukhopadhyay, S., O.A. El-Zammar, and A.L. Katzenstein, *Pulmonary meningothelial-like nodules: new insights into a common but poorly understood entity.* Am J Surg Pathol, 2009. **33**(4): p. 487-95.

[72] Lin, D., et al., *Radiological manifestations, histological features and surgical outcomes of pulmonary meningothelial proliferation: a case series and rethinking.* Transl Lung Cancer Res, 2020. **9**(4): p. 1159-1168.

[73] Suster, S. and C.A. Moran, *Diffuse pulmonary meningotheliomatosis.* Am J Surg Pathol, 2007. **31**(4): p. 624-31.

[74] Wang, Y. and N. Tang, *The diversity of adult lung epithelial stem cells and their niche in homeostasis and regeneration.* Sci China Life Sci, 2021.

[75] Adams, H., et al., *[Meningothelial meningioma in a mature cystic teratoma of the ovary].* Pathologe, 2007. **28**(4): p. 278-80.

[76] Castro Pereira, F.M., et al., *A rare component of psammomatous meningioma in a testicular teratoma.* Case Rep Pathol, 2013. **2013**: p. 645415.

[77] Coulibaly, O., et al., *Mature posterior fossa teratoma mimicking infratentorial meningioma: a case report.* Neurochirurgie, 2012. **58**(1): p. 40-3.

[78] Lanuza, M., T.P. Poon, and A. Belmonte, *Mixed teratoma and meningioma in the temporoparietal region.* Surg Neurol, 1985. **23**(4): p. 399-402.

[79] Liu, Y.Y., et al., *Meningioma in mature cystic teratoma of the ovary: clinical and computed tomography findings.* Cancer Imaging, 2020. **20**(1): p. 15.

[80] Mandal, S., et al., *Rare growth of a psammomatous meningioma in a mature ovarian teratoma: a case report.* Pathol Res Pract, 2010. **206**(5): p. 322-4.

[81] Sinha, R., et al., *Meningothelial Meningioma Component in a Prepubertal Testicular Teratoma.* Case Rep Pathol, 2020. **2020**: p. 6495321.

[82] Takeshima, Y., et al., *Meningioma in mature cystic teratoma of the ovary.* Pathol Int, 2004. **54**(7): p. 543-8.

[83] Chen, E., C.D. Fletcher, and M.R. Nucci, *Meningothelial proliferations in mature cystic teratoma of the ovary: evidence for the common presence of cranially derived tissues paralleling anterior embryonic plate development. An analysis of 25 consecutive cases.* Am J Surg Pathol, 2010. **34**(7): p. 1014-8.

[84] Ozolek, J.A., et al., *Temporal soft tissue glioneuronal heterotopia in a child with a seizure disorder: case report and review of the literature.* Pediatr Dev Pathol, 2005. **8**(6): p. 673-9.

[85] Rogers, G.F., J.B. Mulliken, and H.P. Kozakewich, *Heterotopic neural nodules of the scalp.* Plast Reconstr Surg, 2005. **115**(2): p. 376-82.

[86] Suster, S. and J. Rosai, *Hamartoma of the scalp with ectopic meningothelial elements. A distinctive benign soft tissue lesion that may simulate angiosarcoma.* Am J Surg Pathol, 1990. **14**(1): p. 1-11.

Chapter 4

Overview of Radiosurgery for Intracranial Meningiomas

Tak Lap Poon and Ka Wing See

Abstract

Meningiomas are the second common Central Nervous System (CNS) neoplasm, and are the most common benign intracranial tumor. They approximately constitute up to 30% of all intracranial tumors. They arise from the arachnoidal coverings of brain. Presentation varies and depends on size, number and location of tumors. Symptoms include those related to increased in intracranial pressure, local irritative features including seizure and local pressure effect to eloquent areas, white matter tracts and cranial nerves. Management of meningiomsa is always challenging and multi-disciplinary approaches includes surgery, radiotherapy and possible chemotherapy and immunotherapy. Among radiation therapy treatment, stereotactic radiosurgery (SRS) or stereotactic radiosurgery (SRT) is getting the popularity compared to traditional conformal radiotherapy with comparable tumor control rate.

Keywords: intracranial meningioma, stereotactic radiosurgery, stereotactic radiotherapy, LINAC, Gamma Knife, CyberKnife

1. Introduction

Meningiomas are the second common Central Nervous System (CNS) neoplasm, and are the most common benign intracranial tumor. They approximately constitute up to 30% of all intracranial tumors. They arise from the arachnoidal coverings of brain. Presentation varies and depends on size, number and location of tumors. Symptoms include those related to increased in intracranial pressure, local irritative features including seizure and local pressure effect to eloquent areas, white matter tracts and cranial nerves. Management of meningiomsa is always challenging and multi-disciplinary approaches includes surgery, radiotherapy and possible chemotherapy and immunotherapy. Among radiation therapy treatment, stereotactic radiosurgery (SRS) or stereotactic radiosurgery (SRT) is getting the popularity compared to traditional conformal radiotherapy with comparable tumor control rate. This chapter is intended to discuss the overview of radiosurgery on management of intracranial meningiomas with more focus on the outcome related to location of tumors and different modalities of radiosurgery, and sharing of the local experience of our centre.

2. Epidemiology

The overall age-adjusted incidence is about 8.6 per 100,000 of all primary brain and spinal cord tumors. The incidence rates are correlated with ages, with a median age at diagnosis of 66 years. Tumors are reported to be 1.5 to 3 times more frequent in women. Under the World Health Organization (WHO) classification of brain tumors, majority of the tumors around 80–85% are grade I, around 15–20% are grade II, with 1–2% confirmed to be grade III malignant [1].

3. Classification

The WHO classification of brain tumors is the most popular classification system according to the histological molecular genetics. According to the 2016 WHO classification of tumors of CNS, there are totally 16 meningioma subtypes (**Table 1**) [2]. Meningiomas can also be classified according to their site of origin, and this classification method allows physician to predict the presenting signs and symptoms associated (**Table 2**).

Meningioma	**9530/0**
Meningothelial meningioma	9531/0
Fibrous meningioma	9532/0
Transitional meningioma	9537/0
Psammomatous meningioma	9533/0
Angiomatous meningioma	9534/0
Microcystic meningioma	9530/0
Secretory meningioma	9530/0
Lymphoplasmacyte-rich meningioma	9530/0
Metaplastic meningioma	9530/0
Chordoid meningioma	9538/1
Clear cell meningioma	9538/1
Atypical meningioma	9539/1
Papillary meningioma	9538/3
Rhabdoid meningioma	9538/3
Anaplastic (malignant) meningioma	9530/3

Table 1.
2016 World Health Organization (WHO) classification of meningiomas.

Location	**Typical symptoms**
Convexity – frontal	Affective disorders
Convexity – parietal	Seizures, motor or sensory disorder, hemiparesis
Convexity – temporal	Speech disorders, memory disturbance
Anterior cranial base	Loss of olfaction, affective disorders, loss of activity, visual field or acuity loss
Cavernous sinus meningioma	Diplopia, facial pain or numbness, ocular venous congestion
Orbital or optic nerve sheath	Exophthalmos, loss of vision
Sphenoid wing	Loss of vision, diplopia psychomotor seizures, schizoaffective
Ventricular	Isolated hydrocephalus
Tentorial	Hydrocephalus, seizures, visual field loss, ataxia
Posterior fossa	Ataxia, vertigo, hydrocephalus, symptoms related to brainstem compression, unilateral or bilateral cranial nerve palsies

Table 2.
Clinical presenting features according to location.

4. Treatment strategies

Treatment of intracranial meningiomas generally include observation, microsurgery, radiotherapy in terms of fractionated radiotherapy in terms of conventional radiotherapy, intensity-modulated radiotherapy (IMRT) or volumetric arch therapy (VMAT), proton therapy or stereotactic radiosurgery or radiotherapy (SRS/SRT) [3–5]. Chemotherapy is indicated in some selected refractory cases. Microsurgery remains the best option for symptomatic intracranial meningiomas if complete resection can be achieved with low morbidity. Based on the well-known Simpsons grading system, the extent of tumor resection correlates with the tumor recurrence rate (**Table 3**). Nevertheless, total excision together with dural origin is seldom possible, particularly in cases with involvement or encasement of important neurovascular structures around skull base.

Stereotactic radiosurgery or radiotherapy can be of curative intent when adopted as a primary treatment, in postoperative cases when there is residual disease or high risk of relapse especially in WHO grade II or III cases, or of palliative intent when the disease is beyond cure [6, 7]. European Association of Neuro-oncology (EANO) had published their suggested flowchart in treatment guidelines (**Figure 1**) [8]. There was a review of patients with meningioma between 2010 and 2012 under the National Cancer Database. A total of 802 patients were included, of which 173 patients received SRS/SRT (22%) and 629 patients (78%) received external beam

Grade	Definition	10-Year recurrence rate
I	Macroscopically complete removal with excision of dural attachment and abnormal bone	9%
II	Macroscopically complete removal with endothermy coagulation (Bovie or laser) of dural attachment	19%
III	Macroscopically complete removal without resection or coagulation of extradural extensions	29%
IV	Partial removal leaving intradural tumor in situ	40%
V	Simple decompression with or without biopsy	Not available

Table 3.
Simpson grading system on meningioma resection.

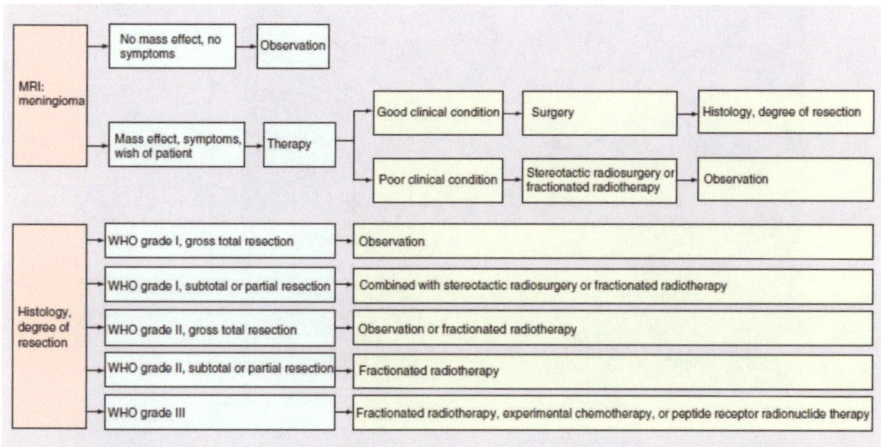

Figure 1.
The European Association of Neuro-oncology (EANO) treatment guideline flowchart for intracranial meningioma.

radiation therapy (EBRT). The 3-year overall survive rate of 2 treatments were similar (97.3% in SRS/SRT group and 93.4% in EBRT group) [9].

This chapter is intended to have an overview of radiosurgery as treatment of intracranial meningiomas.

5. Radiobiology of radiosurgery

Radiosurgery, invented by Prof. Lars Leksell, has been regarded as a significant treatment of choice in patients with intracranial neoplasm, since December 1967, when the first patient suffering from craniopharyngioma was treated with the prototype Gamma Knife at the Sophiahemmet Hospital in Stockholm, Sweden. Radiosurgery is the use of ionizing radiation to treat patients with neoplasm by delivering a precisely measured dose of irradiation to a defined tumor. The main aims include the followings:

1. to eradicate tumor

2. to arrest tumor progression

3. to relieve complaining symptom

4. to achieve better quality of life

5. to prolong survival

The difference between radiosurgery and radiotherapy generally is the size of the treatment volume, and the dose delivered during that single session. While volume is important, it is the radiosurgery team in achieving a precise and accurate radiation plan. Radiosurgery allow high dose per fraction which results in a higher biologically equivalent dose to the target without increasing the risk of complications in

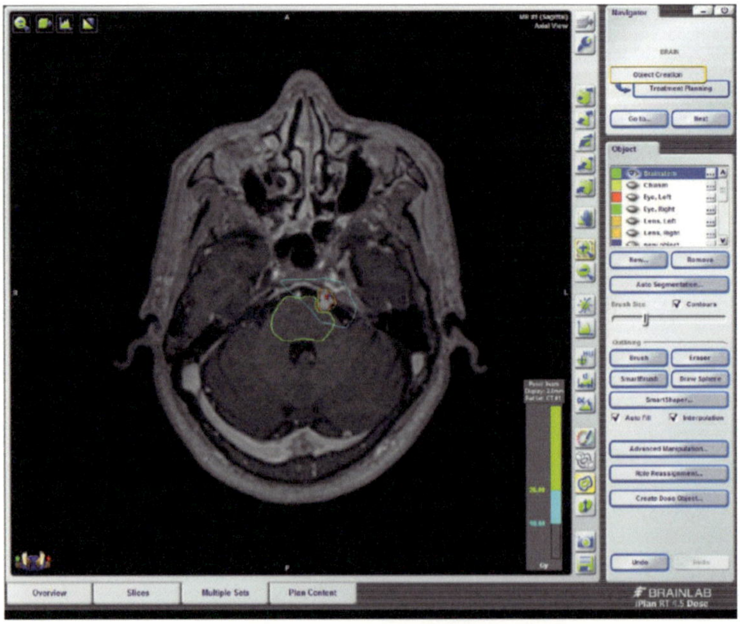

Figure 2.
LINAC stereotactic radiotherapy 25 Gy in 5 fractions for treatment of left petroclival meningioma in our centre.

Description	Constraint	1 fraction		3 fractions		5 fractions		8 fractions		Source	Did point (and magnitude of risk if previously quantified)
		Optimal (Gy)	Mandatory (Gy)	Optimal (Gy)	Mandatory (Gy)	Optimal (Gy)	Mandatory (Gy)	Optimal (Gy)	Mandatory (Gy)		
Optic pathway	DMax (0.1 cm^3)	—	<8	—	<15	—	<22.5	—	—	AAPM [13], Hiniker et al. [14]	AAPM: grade 3+ optic neuritis
											Hiniker et al.: 3 fraction: 0.8% and 5 fraction: 1.6% risk grade 4 radiation-induced optic neuropathy when limited to 0.05 cm^3
Cochlea	Mean	<4	<9	—	<17.1	—	<25	—	—	AAPM [13], Tamaru et al. [15]	AAPM: grade 3+ hearing loss
Brainstem (not medulla)	DMax (0.1 cm^3)	<10	<15	<18	<23.1	<23	<31	—	—	AAPM [13]	Grade 3+ cranial neuropathy
Spinal canal* (including medulla)	DMax (0.1 cm^3)	<10	<14	<18	<21.9	<23	<30	<25	<32	AAPM [13], Grimm et al. [16], UK SABR Consortium [17], LungTECH [18]	AAPM: grade 3+ myelitis

Description	Constraint	1 fraction		3 fractions		5 fractions		8 fractions		Source	Did point (and magnitude of risk if previously quantified)
		Optimal (Gy)	Mandatory (Gy)	Optimal (Gy)	Mandatory (Gy)	Optimal (Gy)	Mandatory (Gy)	Optimal (Gy)	Mandatory (Gy)		
											Grimm et al.: single and 3 fraction optimal doses to 0.1 cm^3 limit risk of grade 2–4 myelopathy to ≤0.4%
	D1 cm^3	<7	—	<12.3	—	<14.5	—	—	—		AAPM: grade 3+ myelitis
Cauda equina and sacral plexus	DMax (0.1 cm^3)	—	<16	—	<24	—	<32	—	—	AAPM [13]	Grade 3+ neuritis
	D5 cm^3	—	<14	—	<22	—	<30	—	—	AAPM [13]	Grade 3+ neuritis
Normal brain (whole brain – gross tumor volume)	D10 cm^3	<12	—	—	—	—	—	—	—	Group consensus	Radiation necrosis
	D50%	<5	—	—	—	—	—	—	—	Group consensus	Cognitive deterioration
Lens	DMax (0.1 cm^3)	<1.5	—	—	—	—	—	—	—	Group consensus	Cataract formation

Description	Constraint	1 fraction		3 fractions		5 fractions		8 fractions		Source	Did point (and magnitude of risk if previously quantified)
		Optimal (Gy)	Mandatory (Gy)	Optimal (Gy)	Mandatory (Gy)	Optimal (Gy)	Mandatory (Gy)	Optimal (Gy)	Mandatory (Gy)		
Orbit	DMax ($0.1\ cm^3$)	<8	—	—	—	—	—	—	—	Group consensus	Retinopathy

DMax is the near-point maximum dose, defined in this case as D0.1 cm^3, which is the minimum dose to the 0.1 cm^3 volume of the organ receiving the highest dose.
D1 cm^3, D5 cm^3 and D10 cm^3 are the minimum doses to the specified volume of the organ (1 cm^3, 5 cm^3, 10^3) that receive the highest doses.
*D50% is the median dose to the volume (equal to the minimum dose to the 50% of the volume receiving the highest doses).*For treatments of the spine itself, these constraints should be applied to the cord planning organ at risk volume (PRV).*

Table 4.
UK consensus on central nervous system dose constraints.

surrounding. Mechanism of radiation related tumoricidal activity include DNA injury together with induction of apoptosis and vascular endothelial damage [10]. The advantages compared to other radiotherapy modalities include maximal conformity, rapid dose fall-off at radiation beam edges and minimal spatial inaccuracies in patient set-up, with generally very low radiation related toxicity (**Figure 2**) [11].

In current radiosurgery principle, the generally applied prescription dose is 12–16 Gy to the tumor margin at 50% isodense line [12]. Treatment dose need to be balanced with the radiation tolerance thresholds to those Organ-at-risk (OAR). A guideline with UK Consensus on normal tissue dose constraints for stereotactic radiotherapy was published as reference (**Table 4**) [19].

6. Radiosurgery techniques and current devices

Dose selection is the basic but upmost significant step in planning of radiosurgery treatment. It is always a balance between the expected level of treatment success and complications risks at various doses so as to select the most optimal dose for the individual patient. The paired sigmoid dose–response curves illustrate the balance between increasing the desired response and increasing complications with higher radiation treatment doses, with the so-called therapeutic window is the area between the two curves (**Figure 3**). Another essential principles in radiosurgery planning are conformity and selectivity. Traditionally, stereotactic radiosurgery (SRS) refers to stereotactically guided delivery of focused radiation to a defined target volume in a single session. Most of the procedures are performed in stereotactic frame-based manner. Modern development of radiosurgery technique allows the fixation of patient's head on couch without the stereotactic frame i.e. frameless. Thus the concept of fractionated stereotactic radiosurgery (FSRS) evolved, or in better terminology, stereotactic radiotherapy (SRT).

Current choice of radiosurgery devices can be divided depends on the application of clinical beams. LINAC Radiosurgery makes use of either linear accelerators-based system or robot-assisted e.g. CyberKnife, while Gamma Knife Radiosurgery employs Cobalt (Co)-60 as the source (**Figure 4**). Both treatment of choices are effectively in treatment of intracranial meningiomas.

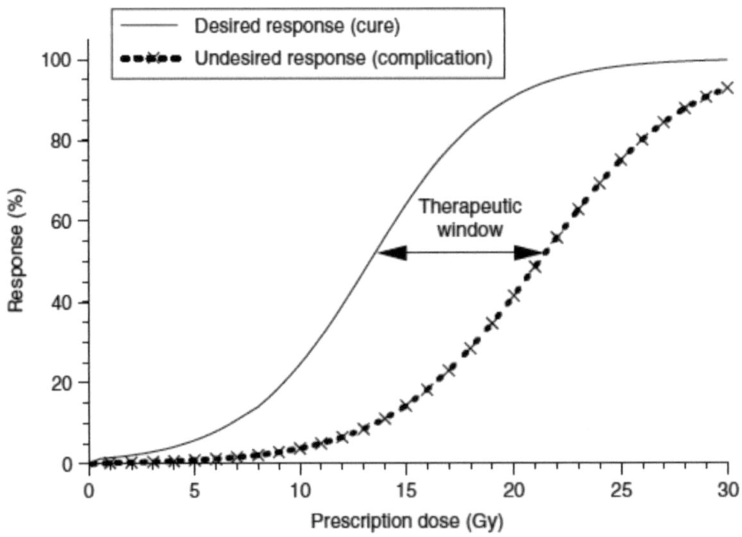

Figure 3.
Paired sigmoid dose–response curves for both desired response and complications.

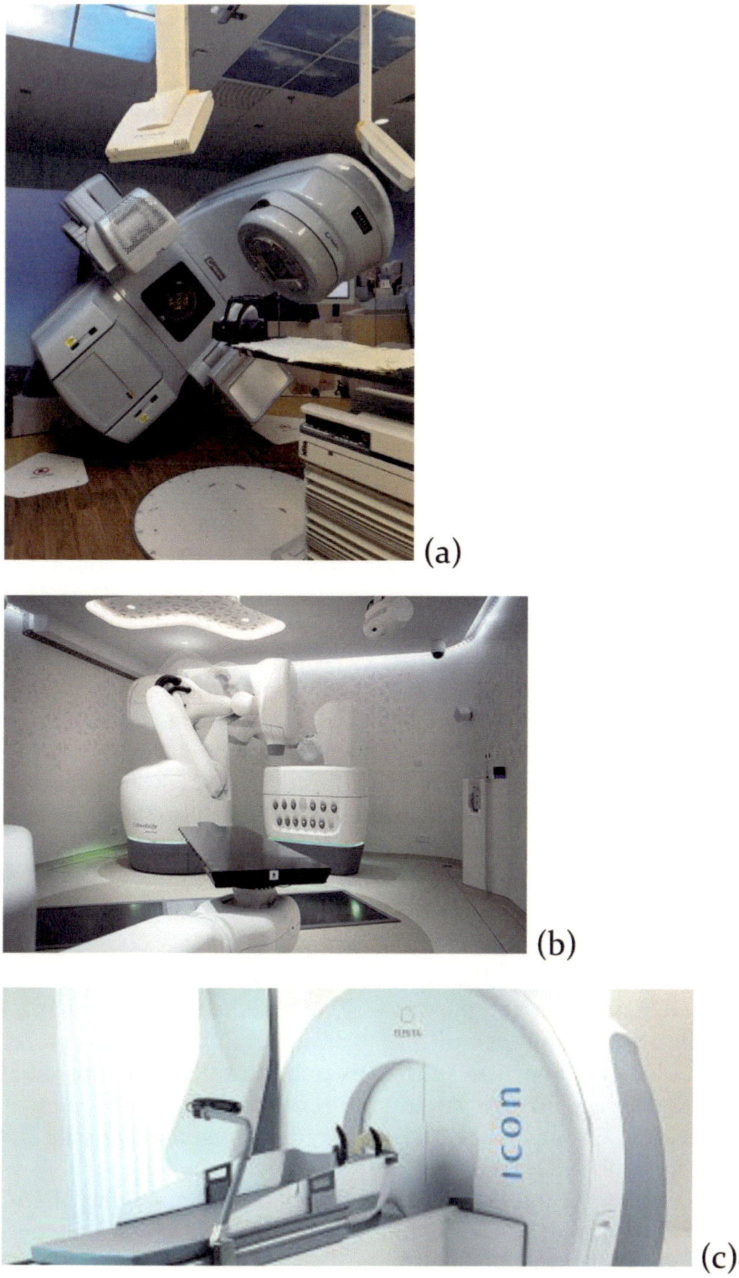

Figure 4.
Models of radiosurgery system in Hong Kong (a) LINAC in our centre (b) CyberKnife in private hospital (c) Gamma Knife Icon in private hospital.

7. Patient selection

The practice of radiosurgery is guided by the treatment purposes, the nature and extent of the lesion, proximity of the lesion to critical organs at risk and patient factors such as general condition, comorbidities and symptoms. In our centre, potential candidates for consideration of radiosurgery for treatment of meningiomas will all be discussed and reviewed in regular multi-disciplinary team meeting. The whole radiosurgery team includes neurosurgeon, clinical oncologist, radiation physicist and nurse as case manager. The following are considerable factors:

1. Patient factors – age, pre-morbid status, presenting symptoms or incidental finding, any past history of head and neck radiation

2. Tumor factors – size, number, location, relationship to organ-at-risk (OAR) e.g. optic nerve, optic chiasm, retina, brainstem, hippocampus, cochlea, any tumor growth during observation period [20]

In general, meningioma with diameter >3 cm with deteriorating clinical condition will be suggested to consider surgical excision instead of radiosurgery.

8. Treatment outcome

8.1 Gamma Knife vs. LINAC radiosurgery

Gamma Knife Radiosurgery was one of the most popular treatment modalities in centres worldwide. Professor Douglas Kondziolka in Pittsburgh had an early study on 946 patients between September 1987 and December 2004. The actuarial tumor control rates was 93% at 5 years and 10 years for benign types, and 83 +/−7% in 5 years and 72+/−10% for atypical and malignant types. Adverse radiation effect ranged from 5.7 to 16% [21]. Outcome of gamma knife radiosurgery of meningioma in 10 years were reviewed by Lippitz et al. 86 Swedish patients were included between March 1991 and May 2001. Totally 130 tumors were treated in 115 treatment sessions. Local tumor control was achieved in 87.8% with recurrence adjacent but outside the initial radiation field was found in 15.1% of patients. A significant lower rate of in-field local recurrences was seen in meningiomas treated with a prescription dose of >13.4 Gy (7.1% vs. 24%, p=0.02) [13]. Seo et al. had another review on 424 patient after Gamm Knife Radiosurgey from 1998 to 2010. The median tumor volume was 4.35 ml and the median marginal dose was 14 Gy. The actuarial tumor control rates were 91.7% at 5 years and 78.9% at 10 years [22]. Morever, Jang et al. showed overall tumor control rate of 95% with 15% peritumoral oedema in 628 pateints from January 2008 to November 2012, whom had received Gamma Knife Radiosurgery with maximal dosage 27.8 Gy and marginal dosage 13.9 Gy [17].

There are numbers of published papers from centres employing LINAC Radiosurgery in treatment of meningiomas with promising treatment outcome. UCLA group had a review of their early results in using LINAC system in treatment of 161 patients between May 1991 and July 2003. SRS with peripherial dose of 12–22 Gy (mean 15 Gy) was given to 26 lesions and SRT with dose ranged from 23 to 54 Gy (mean 48 Gy) was given to 7 cases. Tumor control rate was 92.3% in SRS group and 100% in SRT group, with 2 patients in SRS group suffered from worsening of neurological deficit [23]. Gallego et al. reported the results in using of LINAC Radiosurgery for treatment of 82 patients with cavernous sinus meningioma from 1992 to 2005. The mean volume of tumor was 17.96 ± 13.67 cm^3. Tumor volume reduced in 74.4% and remained stable in 14.6% [14]. Kaul et al. in Germany had retrospective review of 297 patients with LINAC Radiosurgery. The overall progression free survival was 92.3% at 3 years, 87% at 5 years and 84.1% at 10 years [16].

8.2 SRS vs. SRT

There is always debate on the indications or effectiveness of single fraction therapy in SRS or multiple-fraction therapy in SRT [15]. Huang et al. had a retrospective review of 228 patients with 245 tumors treated with radiosurgery between March 2006 and June 2017 using LINAC radiosurgery using Novalis system. 147 (64.5%) patients were SRS group with total dose of 12–16 Gy in one fraction as treatment protocol and 81 (35.5%) were SRT group with 7 Gy/fraction/day for three consecutive days to 21 Gy as total dose. The actuarial local control rate between two groups was not statistically significant during the total 10-year follow-up period (96.86% vs. 100%, $p=0.175$, in 2-year, 94.76% vs. 97.56%, $p=0.373$, in 5-year, 74.4% vs. 91.46%, $p=0.204$, in 10-year), and with comparable radiation-related side effects [24]. Wegner et al. from Pittsburgh also had a review on 56 patients with either SRS or SRT for meningioma treatment from 2008 to 2017. They concluded that fractionation had improved local control compared with single session (91% vs. 80% at 2 years, $p=0.009$) with minimal radiation-related toxicity [18].

Hypofractationated therapy by CyberKnife in meningioma treatment was reviewed by French group. Meniai-Merzouki et al. collected 126 patients with 136 meningiomas undergone treatment between December 2008 and June 2016 with median prescription dose of 25 Gy (12–40) in a 5 median fractions (3–10). They showed that the subgroup with more fractions (25–40 Gy in 5–10 fractions) had significant higher progression free survival that the subgroup with less fractions (21–23 Gy in 3 fractions), and only 2% of patients experienced radionecrosis at 24 months [25]. Di Franco et al. reviewed the treatment outcome of stereotactic radiosurgery and fractionated stereotactic radiotherapy with CyberKnife from January 2013 to April 2017. They achieved 100% local control for 28 patients at 12 months, 89% local control for 19 patients at 24 months and 9 patients at 36 months [26]. Smith et al. also reported 100% crude local control rate for large meningiomas with mean treatment volume 14.7 cm^3 (range 0.79–64.5 cm^3) with hypofractionated CyberKnife with dose of 22.5–30 Gy in five fractions [27]. Study of Oermann et al. in 38 patients treated with five-fraction CyberKnife showed similar response rate to SRS but have low peritumoral oedema around 13.2% [28]. Other centres employ fractionation in terms of 1–5 fractions. Bria had treated 73 patients with median volume of 5.54 cm^3. 60 patients had WHO grade I, 11 patients had WHO grade II and 2 patients had WHO grade III. Treatment median dose was 17.5 Gy with median of three fractions. The Actuarial local control at one year was 95% in WHO grade I, 71% in WHO grade II and 0% in WHO grade III. There was no acute significant toxicity and only one late toxicity noticed [29].

Fractionated treatment is also getting its popularity in centers using Gamma knife, particularly after the introduction of the sixth versions of Leksell Gamma Knife System, ICON®. In a retrospective review of 70 patients with large-volume meningiomas (>10 cm^3) that had undergone gamma knife treatment by Han et al., the single session group having 42 patients with median tumor volume 15.2 cm^3 (range 10.3–48.3 cm^3) and median prescription dose of 12 Gy (range 8–14 Gy) was compared with fractionated group having 28 patients with median tumor volume 21 cm^3 (range 10.2–54.7^3) and median prescription dose of 7.5 Gy in 2 fractions (range 5–8 Gy), 6 Gy in 3 fractions (range 5–6.5 Gy) and 4.5 Gy in 4 fractions. The fractionated group had higher progression free survival rate at 5 yars (92.9% vs. 88.1%) with lower complication rate (7.1% vs. 33.3%) compared with patients with single session treatment [30]. Another smaller series by Park et al. showed satisfactory tumor control after fractationated Gamma Knife radiosurgery with functional preservation for large skull base meningiomas in 23 patients with mean volume of tumors of 21.1+/−15.63 cm^3 (range 10.09–71.42) [31].

Meta-analysis study by Fatima et al. in 2019 had reviewed a total of 1736 patients from 12 retrospective studies. Treatment modalities included Gamma Knife surgery, linear accelerator and CyberKnife. Results showed SRT group had better radiographic tumor control, progression-free survival at 4–10 years, with significantly lower risk of clinical neurological deterioration during their follow-up (OR 2.07, 95% CI 1.06–4.06, p=0.03) and of immediate symptomatic oedema (OR 4.58, 95% CI 1.67–12.56, p=0.003) [32].

Regarding the radiation-induced oedema after radiosurgery, Milano et al. had reviewed 26 studies from 1998 to 2017. Symptomatic oedema was reported in 5–43% of patients among all oedema in 28–50%. The average time to oedema onset time ranged from around 3 to 9 months. Possible factors correlated with radiation-induced oedema included greater tumor margin and/or maximum dose, greater tumor size and/or volum, non-base of skull location particularly parasagittal, no prior resection for meningioma, and presence of pretreatment oedema [33].

9. Radiosurgery in special circumstances

9.1 Meningioma eligible to microsurgery

Microsurgery is the first choice if therapy is indicated and aims at radically removing the tumor if possible. However, the benefits of surgery have to be seriously balanced against the possible interventional related anesthetic risks. Also some patients, though having meningiomas eligible to surgery, refuse surgery due to personal reason. Ruge et al. analyzed 188 patients with 218 meningiomas that undergone LINAC radiosurgery with median tumor volume 4.2 cm^3 (0.1–22) and mean marginal radiation 13+/−3.1 Gy. The estimated 2-, 5-, 10- and 15-year regional recurrence rates were 1.5%, 3.0%, 6.6% and 6.6%, which provides reliable long-term local tumor control with low rates of mild morbidity [34].

9.2 Meningioma close to optical apparatus and skull base vital structures

Management of meningioma at anterior skull base close or adhered to optical apparatus is always challenging in radiosurgery considerations (**Figure 5**).

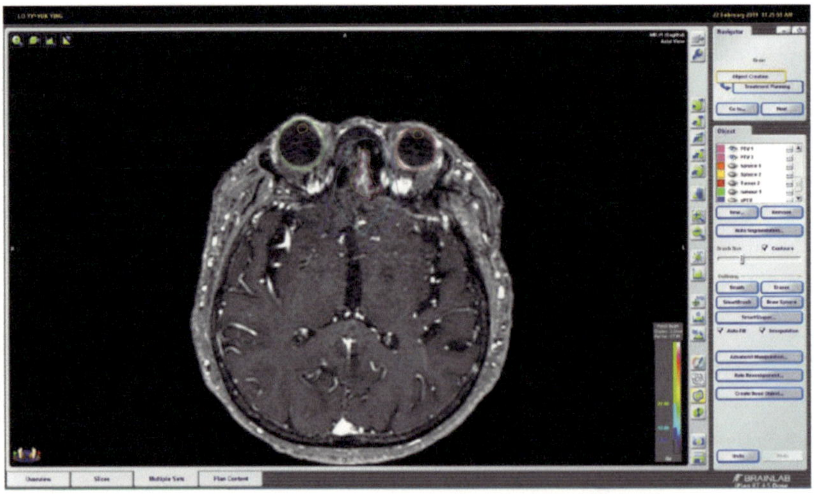

Figure 5.
Treatment of anterior cranial fossa meningioma near bilateral optic nerves using LINAC 27.5 Gy in 5 fractions in our centre.

Tumor control has to be balanced by risk of high-dose radiation exposure leading to optic neuritis and radiation-induced neuropathy. As mentioned, vision preservation can be achieved by confounding the maximum radiation exposure of optic pathway to 8–10 Gy per session. Su et al. in Taiwan treated 4 patients with large tumor volume by volume-staged Gamma Knife Radiosurgery. In stage I, the treatment was focused on the basal part of tumor (mean volume 13.2 cm^3, range 3.9–54.7 cm^3) with marginal dose of 13.5 Gy (range 12–15 Gy), followed by smaller upper portion of tumor close to the optical apparatus (mean volume 4.3, range 1.5–16.2 cm^3) with marginal dose of 9 Gy (range 9–10 Gy) in stage II. 34–46% tumor reduction was observed during the median follow-up period of 100.5 months with no new visual deterioration [35]. A study from Williams et al. on parasellar meningiomas treatment with Gamm Knife Radiosurgery had reviewed the tumor control together with any radiation induced neurological deficit. Totally 138 patients were reviewed from 1989 to 2006. The mean radiation volume was 7.5 cm^3 (range 0.2–54.8 cm^3). Radiographic progression free suvivial at 5 and 10 years were 95.4% and 69%. Only 4% of their patients had radiation related optic neuropathy [36].

Starke et al. had also similar promising findings in Gamma Knife Radiosurgery treatment for other skull base meningiomas. Around 10% of their cases had deterioration in neurological symptoms [37]. His group in another review specifically focus on posterior fossa cases in 152 patients. The radiographic progression free survival at 3, 5, and 10 years to b 98%, 96%, and 78% respectively. 9% of study patients showed deterioration in symptom. They concluded the predicative factors of new or worsening symptoms were clival or petrous-based location [38]. In Austria, Kreil et al. had a review of 200 patients with skull base meningimas with a follow up of 5–12 years. The tumor volume ranged from 0.38 to 89.8 cm^3 (median 6.5 cm^3), and the median dose was 12 Gy (7–25 Gy). They achieved actuarial progression free survival rate of 98.5% at 5 years and 97.2% at 10 years with only 1% radiation induced oedema and 4.5% neurological deterioration [39]. The promising tumor control with low new neurological deficit in Gamma Knife Radiosurgery can also be demonstrated in centres using LINAC system. Villavicencio et al. in Brigham and Women's Hospital had reviewed 56 patients with treatment for skull base meningiomas. The minimal peripheral dose ranged from 12 to 18.5 Gy (mean 15 Gy). The actuarial progression free rate was 95% in median follow-up of 26 months (range 6–66 months) [40].

In cases where skull base meningiomas had extension into the internal auditory meatus, the concern will be more towards the facial nerve function and hearing preservation after radiation. Pollock et al. had reviewed 16 patients from 1992 to 2002. The median tumor margin dose was 15 Gy. They achieved 63% tumor reduction in size at medial follow-up period of 36 months. No facial nerve palsy was reported, and 1 patient had worsened facial sensation. The actuarial incidences of hearing preservation was 93% at 1 year, 84% at 2 years and 42% at 5 years [41].

9.3 Cavernous sinus meningioma

Meningiomas at cavernous sinus are cases always have dilemma with clinical management due to its complex anatomy and its specific location in the antero-lateral skull base (**Figure 6**). Despite the advancement in microscopic and endoscopic surgical technique, still a complete radical excision with minimal anantomo-functional preservation remains very challenging. UCLA De Salles group had proposed a radiosurgery grading system for this specific group of tumor (**Table 5**) [42]. Pittsburgh group reviewed 79 patients with cavernous sinus meningioma between October 1987 and December 1995. The median marginal tumor dose was 15 Gy. The achieved actuarial tumor control rate was 95+/−2.8% at 5 years an 88.2+/−7% at 12 years with 12.7% patients experienced adverse radiation effects [43].

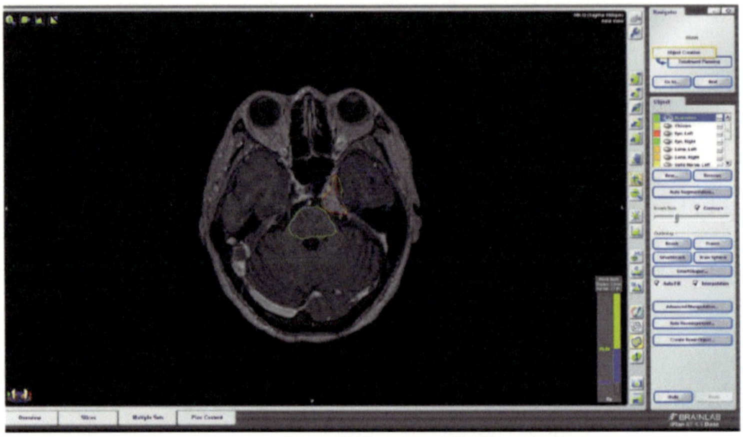

Figure 6.
Meningioma involving cavernous sinus and petrosal apex was treated by LINAC stereotactic radiotherapy using 25 Gy in 5 fractions in our centre.

Grade	Meningioma radiological aspect in MRI T1 contrast images
I	Confined to the cavernous sinus
II	Involvement of the petroclival region without brainstem compression
III	Extension to and compression of the optic nerve, chiasm or tract
IV	Involvement of the petroclival region with compression of brainstem
V	Extensive involvement of both cavernous sinus

Table 5.
Radiosurgery grading system for cavernous sinus meningiomas by UCLA.

Takanashi had reviewed 101 skull base meningioma patients with Gamma Knife Radiosurgery performed from 1991 to 2003. Among those cases, 38 cases are cavernous sinus in location with mean dose delivered to the tumor 14.5 to 15.2 Gy. The overall tumor control rate were 95.5% in the mean follow-up of 51.9 months (range 6–144 months) [44]. Fariselli et al. had proposed a multidisciplinary treatment algorithm involving microsurgery and stereotactic radiosurgery [45]:

1. Small and asymptomatic intracavernous meningiomas – for observation first, radiosurgery in case of progression

2. Larger meningiomas with lateral wall of cavernous sinus involvement – microsurgical resection

3. Large extra-intracavernous meningiomas – combined approach with resection of extracavernous part, followed by radiosurgery for residual tumor part

4. Pre-operative radiosurgery for tumor devascularization is still controversial

9.4 Large tumor volume

The consensus of tumor size in consideration of radiosurgery for meningioma is generally around 30–35 mm in diameter. Tumor volume greater than

8 cm^3 is believed to have poor outcome compared. Starke et al. retrospectively reviewed the Gamma Knife Radiosurgery outcome of 75 patients with mean follow-up of 6.5 years (range 0.5–21 years) whom had tumor volume more than 8 cm^3. The actuarial rates of progression-free survival were 90.3% at 3 years, 88.6% at 5 years and 77.2% at 10 years. Factors associated with tumor progression included [46]:

1. Presentation with any cranial nerve deficit from III to VI

2. History of radiotherapy

3. Tumor volume greater than 14 cm^3

10. Local experience

Our centre, the Queen Elizabeth Hospital in Hong Kong, have conducted a 10-year review of the patients who received LINAC-based SRS or SRT for intracranial meningioma from July, 2009 to June, 2019. We investigated the tumor control rate in the 1-, 2- and 5-years intervals. Tumor control was defined as a static or shrunken tumor. Functional outcome was determined by modified Rankin scale (mRS).

40 patients were included with 45 tumors irradiated. 42% of the tumors were parasagittal or parafalcine, followed by 20% petrous or petroclival and 18% convexity. 48% of the tumors were WHO grade I while 52% were WHO grade II. In 48% of the cases, Simpson I/II excision was achieved while in the remainder, Simpson III/IV was achieved. In 27% of the tumors, radiosurgery were done as primary treatment while 73% as postoperative adjuvant treatment.

In the recent 25 cases, we switched from frame-based to frameless radiosurgery, using the LINAC system. Mean radiation dose was 22.4Gy (SD: 7.2). Mean target volume was 5.0 (SD: 6.1) while mean treatment volume was 6.0 (SD: 6.8), with mean treatment-target ratio being 1.8 (SD: 1.0). Mean coverage was 96.3%. Mean conformity index was 1.7 (SD: 1.0).

Tumor control rate was achieved in 82%, 79% and 66% in 1-, 2- and 5-years intervals respectively. More than 80% patients enjoyed mRS 0–1 over the study period. SRS was associated with better tumor control in the 1- and 2-years interval compared with SRT. However, it was confounded by smaller target volume. Other teletherapy metrics were found to have no significant association with the outcome.

11% of the patients required reoperation, while 7% developed radionecrosis or radiation-induced edema. Multiple meningiomata was associated with poor tumor control in 5 years (20% vs. 82%, p=0.025). It may reflect the underlying pathology of the entire intracranial meninges, making local irradiation ineffective in overall intracranial control. Parasagittal or parafalcine locations predicted reoperation (21% vs. 0%, p=0.026). We observed that these tumors more likely recurred and caused symptoms which required surgical decompression. On the other hand, tumors inside the superior sagittal sinus were often not removed in operation. The residual tumors may progress, with nurture by the surrounding vasculature. Moreover, sometimes there is technical difficulty to plan effective radiation dose to cover the adequate dura origin in this location.

Overall, neither histology grading nor the extent of resection predicted tumor control rate when they were analyzed as ordinal scale in our study.

11. International recommendations

International Stereotactic Radiosurgery Society (ISRS) had a systemic review on stereotactic radiosurgery for intracranial noncavernous sinus benign meningioma in 2020. Totally 2844 relevant studies from January 1964 to April 2018 were reviewed. The 10-year local control rate ranged from 71–100%, and the 10-year progression-free-survival rate varied from 55–97%, based on prescription dose 12 Gy to 15 Gy. ISRS had summarized the following recommendations based on this review [47]:

11.1 Level II evidence

1. SRS may be proposed as a primary treatment modality for an asymptomatic or mildly symptomatic meningioma, and should be considered when a complete surgical excision cannot be achieved or is not amenable

2. After surgery, when a residual tumor is not evident or is minimal, a wait-and -scan approach appears to be reasonable with a regular radiological follow-up. At the time of recurrence or progression, SRS should be taken into consideration as a treatment modality. Some studies suggest that the recurrence/progression rate is lower when SRS is delivered as the primary treatment as compared to an adjuvant treatment and this remains to be confirmed

11.2 Level III evidence

1. Single-fraction SRS with a dose of 12 to 15 Gy appears to be sufficient to manage benign intracranial meningioma. A prescription dose of at least 14 Gy would be advisable

2. Hypofractionated stereotactic radiotherapy (HSRT) may be considered for the treatment of large or/and critically located meningioma. Optimal practice has yet to be defined, however, 25 Gy in 5 fractions is a common approach

3. SRS generally entails a low risk of neurological deterioration. Patients may experience a clinical improvement without tumor shrinkage

ISRS also had published a review of 49 full-text articles from January 1963 to December 2014. The 5-year progression-free survival (PFS) rates was 86–99% and 10-year PFS was 69–97%. The followings are recommendations for management of cavernous sinus (CS) meningioma in level III evidence [48]:

1. SRS/SRT is recommended as a primary/upfront treatment option for an asymptomatic, or mildly symptomatic CS meningioma.

2. Resection should be considered for the treatment of larger and symptomatic CS meningioma in patients both receptive to, and medically eligible, for open surgery

3. SRS/SRT delivered to a CS meningioma has a low risk of complications; most cranial nerve functions are preserved or improved due to tumor shrinkage, and carotid artery stenosis after SRS is rare

4. When no residual tumor is observed, or only a small tumor lining on dura of the CS exists postoperatively, serial neuroimaging studies is not unreasonable. At the time of recurrence or progression of residual tumor, SRS/SRT should be considered

5. In patients with a CS meningioma that has rapidly and substantially recurred after prior treatment, a subtotal surgical resection or biopsy may b considered. More aggressive features of the tumor (transformation of the tumor from WHO grade I to a higher grade) should be ruled out. These tumors have a predilection for progression and postoperative SRS/SRT with a higher dose should be strongly considered

6. The technique for SRS or SRT delivery will depend upon the tumor histology, tumor volume and proximity of the tumor to adjacent critical structures (e.g. the optic chiasm). SRS using single session marginal doses of 11 to 16 Gy offers a local tumor control rate of 90% or higher at 5 year post-SRS

National Comprehensive Cancer Network (NCCN) also had proposed guidelines for CNS tumors. Radiotherapy is recommended in the following clinical scenarios with Level 2A evidence [49]:

1. Small (<30 mm) asymptomatic tumors at presentation, if grade II and subtotally resected or grade III regardless of resection volume, and grade I when sub-totally resected with "potential" symptom

2. Large (>30 mm) asymptomatic tumors if grade III, and if grade II or incompletely resected grade I.

3. Following surgery for any grade III and should be considered for any grade II tumors or large (>30 mm) incompletely resected grade I.

4. Surgically inaccessible tumors or surgically contraindicated patients

12. Future directions

Planning of radiosurgery in meningiomas usually concentrated on the main tumor bulk as overall treatment volume. Lovo et al. recently try to include tumor dural tails of 143 patients with histologically confirmed or radiologically assumed WHO Grade I meningiomas in the radiosurgery treatment plans. All the final prescription isodose line in treatment plans were focused on tumor coverage and measurement of the dose received at maximum distance (MaxDis) of the dural tail and the midpoint distance (MPDis) from the prescription isodose line to the maximum dural tail distance. The dural tail of meningiomas were identified in at least three consecutive sections of the MRI T1-weighted sequence with contrast in 1 mm slice thickness. Tumor control was achieved in 96% of patients [50].

13. Conclusion

Intracranial meningiomas are one of the most common neoplasm in clinical practice. Management should be based on patient's factors and tumor factors. Multi-disciplinary approach in treatment modalities decision is essential to achieve the best treatment outcome. Use of Radiosurgery in terms of Gamma Knife, LINAC or CyberKnife, either in single fraction or multiple fractions, should be subjected to individual centre's preference and experience.

Author details

Tak Lap Poon* and Ka Wing See
Department of Neurosurgery, Queen Elizabeth Hospital, Hong Kong

*Address all correspondence to: poontaklap@yahoo.com.hk

References

[1] Buerki RA, Horbinski CM, Kruser T, Horowitz PM, James CD, Lukas RV. An overview of meningiomas. Future Oncol. 2018;14(21):2161-2177

[2] Louis DN, Perry A, Reifenberger G, Von Deimling A, Figarella-Branger D, Cavenee WK, Ohgaki H, Wiestler OD, Kleihues P, Ellison DW. The 2016 World Health Organization classification of tumors of the Central Nervous System: A summary. Acta Neuropathol 2016;131:803-820

[3] Minniti G, Amichetti M, Enrici RM. Radiotherapy and radiosurgery for benign skull base meningiomas. Radiation Oncology 2009;4:42

[4] Bloch O, Kaur G, Jian BJ. Stereotactic radiosurgery for benign meningiomas. J Neurooncol 2012;107:13-20

[5] Moraes FY, Chung C. Radiation to skull base meningiomas: Review of the literature on the approach to radiotherapy. Chin Clin Oncol 2017;6(Suppl 1):S3

[6] Ding D, Starke RM, Hantzmon J, Yen CP, Williams BJ, Sheehan JP. The role of radiosurgery in the management of WHO grade II and III intracranial meningiomas. Neurosurg Focus 2013;35(6):E16

[7] Vera E, Lorgulescu JB, Raper DMS, Madhavan K, Lally BE, Morcos J, Elhammady S, Sherman J, Komotar RJ. A review of stereotactic radiosurgery practice in the management of skull base meningiomas. J Neurol Surg B 2014;75:152-158

[8] Goldbrunner R, Minniti G, Preusser M, Jenkinson MD, Sallabanda K, Houdart E, Von Deimling A, Stavrinou P, Lefranc F, Lund-Johansen M, Moyal ECJ, Brandsma D, Henriksson R, Soffietti R, Weller M. EANO guidelines for the diagnosis and treatment of meningiomas. Lancet Oncol 2016;17:2383-2391

[9] Albert A, Lee A, Vijayakumar S, Kanakamedala M, Allbright R, Schreiber D. Adjuvant treatment of meningioma with stereotactic radiation surgery and hypofractionated stereotactic radiation surgery: Patterns of care and survival in a large, hospital database. Advances in Radiation Oncology 2018;3:280-287

[10] Demiral S, Dincoglan F, Sager O, Uysal B, Gamsiz H, Ozcan F, Dirican B, Beyzadeoglu. Contemporary management of meningiomas with radiosurgery. Int J Radiol Imaging Technol 2018;4:041

[11] Chang JH, Chang JW, Choi JY, Park YG, Chung SS. Complications after gamma knife radiosurgery for benign meningiomas. J Neurol Neurosurg Psychiatry 2003;74:226-230

[12] Flannery T, Poots J. Gamma knife radiosurgery for meningiomas. Prog Neurol Surg. Basel, Karger, 2019;34:91-99

[13] Lippitz BE, Bartek Jr J, Mathiesen T, Forander P. Ten-year follow-up after Gamma knife radiosurgery of meningioma and review of the literature. Acta Neurochirurgica 2020;162:2183-2196

[14] Gallego MP, Samblas J, Bustos JC, Diaz JAG, Gonzalez M, Sallabanda K. Long-term follow-up of 82 cavernous sinus meningiomas treated with radiosurgery. Journal of Cancer Therapy, 2014;5:1005-1011

[15] Elia AEH, Shih HA, Loeffler JS. Stereotactic radiation treatment for benign meningiomas. Neurosurg Focus 2007;23(4):E5

[16] Kaul D, Budach V, Wurm R, Gruen A, Graaf L, Habbel P, Badakhshi H. Linac-based stereotactic radiotherapy and radiosurgery in patients with meningioma. Radiation Oncology 2014;9:78

[17] Jang CK, Jung HH, Chang JH, Chang JW, Park YG, Chang WS. Long-term results of gamma knife radiosurgery for intracranial meningioma. Brain Tumor Res Treat 2015;3(2):103-107

[18] Wegner RE, Hasan S, Abel S, Anderson S, Fuhrer R, Williamson RW, Karlovits SM. Linear accelerator-based stereotactic radiotherapy for low-grade meningiomas: Improved local control with hypofractionation. Journal of Central Nervous System Disease 2019;11: 1-5.

[19] Hanna GG, Murry L, Patel R, Jain S, Aitken KL, Franks KN, Van As N, Tree A, Hatfield P, Harrow S, McDonald F, Ahmed M. Saran FH. Webster GJ, Khoo V, Landau D, Eaton DJ. Hawkins MA. UK consensus on normal tissue dose constraints for stereotactic radiotherapy. Clinical Oncology 2018;30:5-14

[20] Combs SE, Baumert BG, Bendszus M, Bozzao A, Brada M, Fariselli L, Fiorentino A, Ganswindt U, Grosu AL, Lagerwaard FL, Niyazi M, Nyholm T, Paddick In Weber DC, Belka C. ESRTO ACROP guideline for target volume delineation of skull base tumors. Radiotherapy and Oncology 20021;56:80-94

[21] Lee JYK, Kondziolka D, Flickinger JC, Lunsford LD. Radiosurgery for intracranial meningiomas. Prog Neurol Surg. Basel, Karger, 2007;20:142-149

[22] Seo Y, Kim DG, Kim JW, Han JH, Chung HT, Paek SH. Long-term outcomes after gamma knife radiosurgery for bening meningioma: A single institution's experience with 424 patients. Neurosrugery 2018;83: 1040-1049

[23] Torres RC, De Salles AAF, Frighetto L, Gravori T, Pedroso AG, Goss B, Medin P, Solberg TD, Ford JM, Selch M. Long-term follow-up using Linac radiosurgery and stereotactic radiotherapy as a minimally invasive treatment for intracranial meningiomas. Radiosurgery. Basel, Karger, 2004;5:115-123

[24] Huang SH, Wang CC, Wei KC, Chang CN, Chuang CC, Chen HC, Lin YJ, Chen KT, Pai PC, Hsu PW. Treatment of intracranial meningioma with single-session and fractionate radiosurgery: A propensity score matching study. Scientific Reports 2020;10:18500

[25] Meniai-Merzouki F, Bernier-Chastagner V, Geffrelot J, Tresch E, Lacornerie T, Coche-Dequeant B, Lartigu E, Pasquier D. Hypofractionated stereotactic radiotherapy for patients with intracranial meningiomas: Impact of radiotherapy regimen on local control. Scientific Report 2018;8:13666

[26] Di Franco R, Borzillo V, Ravo V, Falivene S, Romano FJ, Muto M, Cammarota F, Totaro G, Ametrano G, Rossetti S, Cavaliere C, D' Aniello C, Iovane G, Porricelli MA, Berretta M, Botti G, Starace L, La Salvia E, Facchini G, Muto P. Radiosurgery and stereotactic radiotherapy with cyberknife system for meningioma. The Neuroradiology Journal 2108;31(1):18-26

[27] Smith DE, Ghosh S, O'Leary M, Chu Colin, Brody D. Hypofractionated radiosurgery for meningiomas – A safer alternate for large tumors? Transl Cancer Res 2014;3(4):367-372

[28] Oermann EK, Bhandari R, Chen VJ, Lebec G, Gurka M, Lei S, Chen L, Suy S,

Azumi N, Berkowitz F, Kalhom C, McGrail K, Collins BT, Jean WC, Collins SP. Five fraction image-guided radiosurgery for primary and recurrent meningiomas. Frontiers in Oncology August 2013;3:Article 213

[29] Bria C, Wegner RE, Clump DA, Vargo JA, Mintz AH, Heron DE, Burton SA. Fractionated stereotactic radiosurgery for the treatment of meningiomas. Journal of Cancer Research and Therapeutics January–March 2011;7(1): 52-57

[30] Han MS, Jang WY, Moon KS, Lim SH, Kim IY, Jung TY, Jung S. Is fractionated gamma knife radiosurgery as safe and effective treatment approach for large volume (>10 cm^3) intracranial meningiomas? World Neurosurg 2017;99:477-483

[31] Park HR, Lee JM, Park KW, Kim KH, Jeong SS, Kim JW, Chung HT, Kim DG, Paek SH. Fractionated gamma knife radiosurgery as initial treatment for large skull base meningioma. Exp Neurobiol 2018;27(3):245-255

[32] Fatima N, Meola A, Pollom EL, Soltys SG, Chang SD. Stereotactic radiosurgery versus stereotactic radiotherapy in the management of intracranial meningiomas: A systematic review and meta-analysis. Neurosurg Focus 2019;46:E2

[33] Milano MT, Sharma M, Soltys SG, Sahgal A, Usuki KY, Saenz JMS, Grimm J, El Naqa Issam. Radiation-induced edema after single-fraction or multifraction stereotactic radiosurgery for meningiomas: A critical review. Int J Radiation Oncol Biol Phys, 2018;101(2)344-357

[34] Ruge MI, Tutunji J, Rueb D, Celik E, Baues C, Treuer H, Kocher M, Grau S. Stereotactic radiosurgery for treating meningiomas eligible for complete resection. Radiat Oncol 2021;16:22

[35] Su CF, Liu DW, Lee CC, Chiu TL. Volume-staged gamma knife surgery for the treatment of large skull base meningioma surrounding the optical apparatus: A snowman-shape design. Journal of the Chinese Medical Association 80 2017;697-704

[36] Williams BJ, Yen CP, Starke RM, Basina B, Nguyen J, Rainey J, Sherman JH, Schlesinger D, Shehan JP. Gamma knife surgery for parasellar meningiomas: Long-term results including complications, predictive factors, and progression-free survival. J Neurosurg 2011;144:1571-1577

[37] Starke RM, Williams BJ, Hiles C, Nguyen JH, Elsharkawy Y. Sheehan JP. Gamma knife surgery for skull base meningiomas. J Neurosurg 2012;116:588-597

[38] Starke RM, Nguyen JH, Rainey J, Williams BJ, Sherman JH, Savage J, Yen CP, Sheehan JP. Gamma knife surgery of meningiomas located in the posterior fossa: Factors predictive of outcome and remission. J Neurosurg 2011;114:1399-1409

[39] Kreil W, Luggin J, Fuchs I, Weigl V, Eustacchio, Papaofthymiou. Long term experience of gamma knife radiosurgery for bening skull base meningiomas. J Neurol Neurosurg Psychiatry 2005;76:1425-1430

[40] Villavicencio AT, Black PM, Shrieve DC, Fallon MP, Alexander E, Loeffler JS. Linac radiosurgery for skull base meningiomas. Acta Neurochir (Wien) 2001;143:1141-1152

[41] Pollock BE, Link MJ, Foote RL, Stafford SL, Brown PD, Schomberg PJ. Radiosurgery as primary management for meningiomas extending into the internal auditory canal. Stereotact Funct Neurosurg 2004;82:98-103

[42] De Salles AAF, Frighetto L, Grande CV, Solberg TD,

Cabatan-Awang C, Selch MT, Wallace R, Ford J. Radiosurgery and stereotactic radiation therapy of skull base meningiomas: Proposal of a grading system. Stereotact Funct Neurosurg 2001;76:218-229

[43] Lee HYK, Stippler M, Niranjan A, Kondziolka D, Flickinger JC, Lunsford LD. Gamma knife radiosurgery for cavernous sinus meningiomas. Radiosurgery, Basel, Karger, 2006;6:118-130

[44] Masami T, Fukuoka S, Hojyo A, Sasaki T, Nakagawara J, Nakamura H. Gamma knife radiosurgery for skull-base meningiomas. Prog Neurol Surg. Basel, Karger, 2009;22:96-111

[45] Fariselli L, Biroli A, Signorelli A, Broggi M, Marchetti M, Biroli F. The cavernous sinus meningioma' dilemma: Surgery or stereotactic radiosurgery. Reports of practical oncology and radiotherapy 2016;21:379-385

[46] Starke RM, Przybylowski CJ, Sugoto M, Fezeu F, Awad AJ, Ding D, Nguyen JH, Sheehan JP. Gamma knife radiosurgery of large skull base meningiomas. J Neurosurg 2015;122:363-372

[47] Marchetti M, Sahgal A, De Salles AAF, Levivier M, Ma L, Paddick I, Pollock BE, Regis J, Sheehan J, Suh JH, Yomo S, Fariselli L. Stereotactic radiosurgery for intracranial noncavernous sinus benign meningioma: International Stereotactic Radiosurgery Society systematic review, meta-analysis and practice guideline. Neurosurgery 2020;87:879-890

[48] Lee CC, Trifiletti DM, Sahgal A, De Salles A, Fariselli L, Hayashi M, Levivier M, Ma L, Alvarez RM, Paddick I, Regis J, Ryu S, Slotman B, Sheehan J. Stereotactic Radiosurgery for bening (World Health Organization Grade I) cavernous sinus meningiomas – International Stereotactic Radiosurgery Society (ISRS) practice guideline: A systematic review. Neurosurgery 2018;0:1-14

[49] NCCN guidelines: central nervous cancers. http://nccn.org/

[50] Lovo EE, Moreira A, Navarro PA, Barahona K, Campos F, Caceros V, Blanco A, Arguello-Mendez J, Arce L, Contreras WO. Multiplatform radiosurgery for intracranial meningiomas and dose to the dural tail. Cureus 2021;13(1):1-10

Chapter 5

Rare Brain Tumors with Infrequent Clinical Manifestations: Illustrative Cases

José Luis Navarro-Olvera, Armando Armas-Salazar, José Damián Carrillo-Ruiz, Jesús Q. Beltrán, Gustavo Parra-Romero and Gustavo Aguado-Carrillo

Abstract

This chapter describes the epidemiology, clinical and neuroimaging features, histological characteristics, surgical approach, outcomes, and prognostic factors of different cases of very rare intracranial tumors, associated with complex clinical syndromes. Highlighting the important aspects in the diagnosis and management that were considered relevant through the experience of our center. Here we included an intracranial Rosai-Dorfman disease manifested as an apparent multiple meningiomatosis, a choroid plexus papilloma clinically manifested as a hemifacial spasm originated by a compression of the facial colliculus, and a neuroenteric cyst associated with Klippel-Feil syndrome. This type of tumor presents a challenge to the neurosurgeon, originating various questions about its management. In this chapter, we present the experience we had with these pathologies to establish the most appropriate management decisions.

Keywords: rare intracranial tumors, multiple meningiomas, Rosai-Dorfman disease, Hemifacial spasm, choroid plexus papilloma, Klippel-Feil syndrome, neuroenteric cyst

1. Introduction

Brain tumors according to their location and growth rate can produce very typical clinical manifestations [1], in addition to the classic characteristics of imaging studies that provide the possibility of approaching the diagnosis of the specific type of tumor and guide to establish the treatment modality [2]. However, when the incidence of some of these tumors is very low and they present with very varied clinical manifestations, added to the radiological findings that do not provide too much information to approximate the diagnosis, these cases condition stricter study protocols where the undoubtedly diagnoses alters the treatment modality for each particular case [3]. For this reason, knowledge of the existence of some of these tumors should be the subject of study, to understand the difficulty in diagnosis and treatment, seeking to reduce errors in addressing these cases and improve the result.

2. Rosai-Dorfman disease manifested as an apparent multiple meningiomatosis

The first case presented in this chapter corresponds to an intracranial Rosai-Dorfman disease (RDD), which was manifested as an apparent multiple meningiomatosis that affected the anterior fossa, the sphenoidal plane, and the clivus. RDD is a non-Langerhans histiocytosis described in 1965 by Pierre P. Destombes and then characterized by J. Rosai and R. Dorfman [4, 5]. RDD has a prevalence of 1 in 200,000 and an incidence of 100 cases per year. It can occur at any age but is usually more common in adolescents [6]. The typical clinical manifestations of this disease are the presence of painless bilateral cervical lymphadenopathy added to the presence of fatigue, fever, and weight loss, associated with elevated erythrocyte sedimentation rate, anemia, fever, and hypergammaglobulinemia. Extranodal involvement occurs in less than 43% of cases, mostly in the skin, nasal cavity, and bone [7]. The central nervous system (CNS) is affected in less than 5% of cases, the isolated affection is possible, without systemic manifestations. There are approximately 200 reported cases of intracranial RDD [8, 9]. This case illustrates a patient with multiple intracranial lesions, where the symptoms and characteristics per image simulated the presence of multiple meningiomas, where the RDD finding was made until the moment of the histopathological study.

2.1 Case presentation

A 59-year-old male patient with a history of gradual right hearing loss that later presents the same symptoms in the contralateral ear. His current condition began 8 months ago with a high-intensity holo-cranial headache that predominated in the mornings accompanied by occasional dizziness. Three months before his hospital admission, he reported non-quantified weight loss, asthenia, and adynamia.

Two months before hospital admission, the patient reported decreased visual acuity and compromise of the temporal hemifields added to hyposmia. The reason for hospital admission in our institution was the presence of two generalized tonic–clonic seizures lasting more than one minute (less than five minutes), these seizures were characterized by the absence of aura, with a postictal period of 20 minutes. The second seizure required hospital admission for control. On physical examination, the cognitive functions were preserved, evaluation of the cranial nerves demonstrate hyposmia and bitemporal hemianopia. Fundoscopy showed edema of the papilla in the left eye and an atrophic papilla of the right eye. Regarding the complementary studies, the electroencephalogram showed abnormal bifrontal activity. Computed campimetry confirmed the bitemporal hemianopia, and regarding the neuroimaging studies, the computed tomography (CT)-scan showed three isodense with homogeneous enhancement lesions located in the midline in the floor of the anterior fossa in the cribriform plate, the sphenoidal plane with extension to the tuberculum sellae, and the middle and lower portion of clivus. The magnetic resonance imaging (MRI) revealed isointense lesions with peritumoral edema, with intense and homogeneous gadolinium-enhancement demonstrating a dural attachment (**Figure 1A–F**).

The diagnosis of multiple meningiomas was established, supported by the neuroimaging features and previous experience. The surgical plan was to resect the two main symptomatic lesions (olfactory groove and tuberculum sellae). The surgical approach was made through a bicoronal incision to perform a bifrontal craniotomy and a sub-frontal approach. The surgical approach allowed a complete resection of the lesions, after the olfactory groove lesion resection was possible to access the lesion of the tuberculum sellae. Debulking of the lesions was made

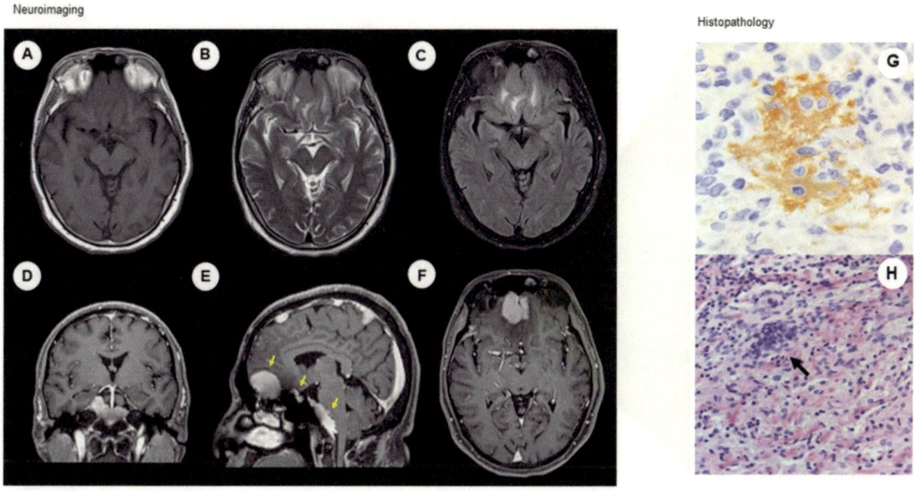

Figure 1.
Pre-operative brain magnetic resonance imaging (MRI) studies. Non-contrasted brain MRI shows an isointense olfactory groove lesion with perilesional edema in the T1-weighted (A), T2-weighted (B), and FLAIR (C). Contrasted brain MRI reveals three homogeneous enhancement lesions with dural attachment (yellow arrows in the sagittal section) in the floor of the anterior fossa in the crista Galli and cribriform plate, the sphenoidal plane with extension to the tuberculum sellae, and the middle and lower portion of clivus, observed in the coronal (D), sagittal (E), and axial sections (F). Histopathological analysis. G. Positive immunohistochemical profile for S100 protein. Furthermore, other immunochemical profiles show positive expression of CD68 (macrophages), CD20 (B lymphocytes), and CD2 (T lymphocytes), in which lymphagocytosis was observed. IgG and IgG4 positivity were also identified. A negative expression for CD30 and CD15 (reed Stenberg cells), and CD1A (Langerhans cells) was observed. H. H&E Stain: Mixed inflammatory infiltrate with plasma cells, lymphocytes, and macrophages, no evidence of meningothelial cells, emperipolesis was observed (black arrow).

with an ultrasonic aspirator, and according to meningioma surgery principles, it was decided to perform anterior fossa drilling to reduce the recurrence probability. The tumor lesions showed low vascularity and close contact with the optic chiasm (**Figure 2**). Immediately post-operative the patient remained without complications and was discharged five days after surgery, the CT scan performed 5 days after surgery showed complete resection of the lesions (olfactory groove and tuberculum sellae), with residual lesion of the middle and lower portion of clivus (**Figure 2F**). Due to the residual lesion, the patient was observed for the clinical oncology service to decide adjuvant management.

Histopathological findings established the diagnosis of RDD (**Figure 1G** and **H**). In the subsequent follow-up, extension studies were carried out, which were ruled out other infiltrates with a thoracic and abdomen-pelvic CT. The patient received treatment with prednisone and remain asymptomatic without clivus lesion growth at 8 months follow-up.

2.2 Case discussion

For the diagnostic process of RDD, it is important to consider the observations by imaging studies that usually mimic the characteristics of a meningioma, either as one or multiple extra-axial lesions with homogeneous contrast enhancement surrounded by vasogenic perilesional edema, they can arrive to present a dural tail and its location is very diverse [1]. Proton MRI spectroscopy improves the specificity of preoperative diagnoses in some patients; for example, in meningiomas, alanine is usually elevated in spectroscopy, with a peak at 1.48 ppm, in a patient with RDD disease, spectroscopy revealed an increased choline level [10]. In a review of 10 cases, a dural tail was found in all cases. Therefore, in data suggestive

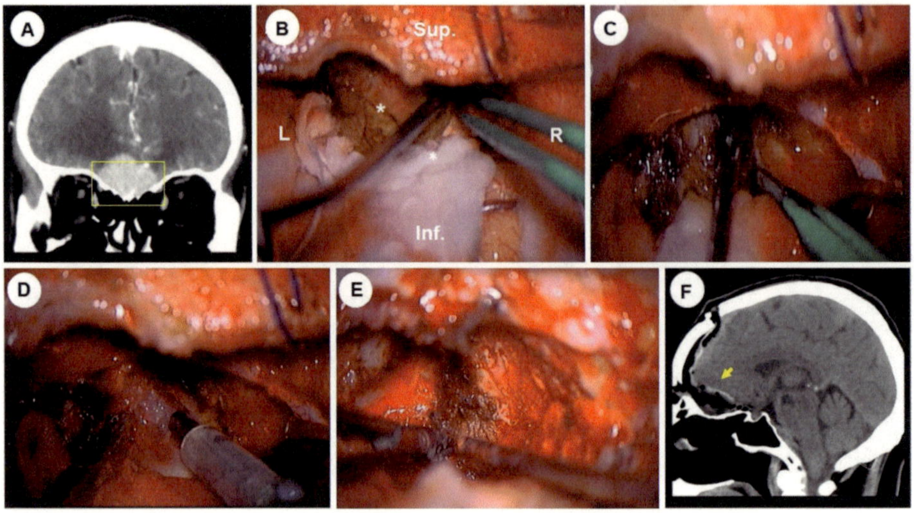

Figure 2.
(A) Preoperative enhanced coronal head CT-scan with an olfactory groove lesion (square). Surgical procedure: Approach to the anterior fossa lesion. Perimeter dissection of the anterior cranial fossa lesion (asterisk) is shown (B-C). Debulking with ultrasonic aspiration (D) and complete resection of olfactory groove (E) is demonstrated. (F) Sagittal section of postoperative CT with complete resection (arrow).

of meningioma obtained by neuroimaging studies, RDD is a differential diagnosis [11]. Zhu et al. [11] concluded that, unlike meningiomas, a typical hypointensity non-related to calcification on T2-weighted or fluid attenuation inversion recovery (FLAIR) images could suggest the RDD diagnosis.

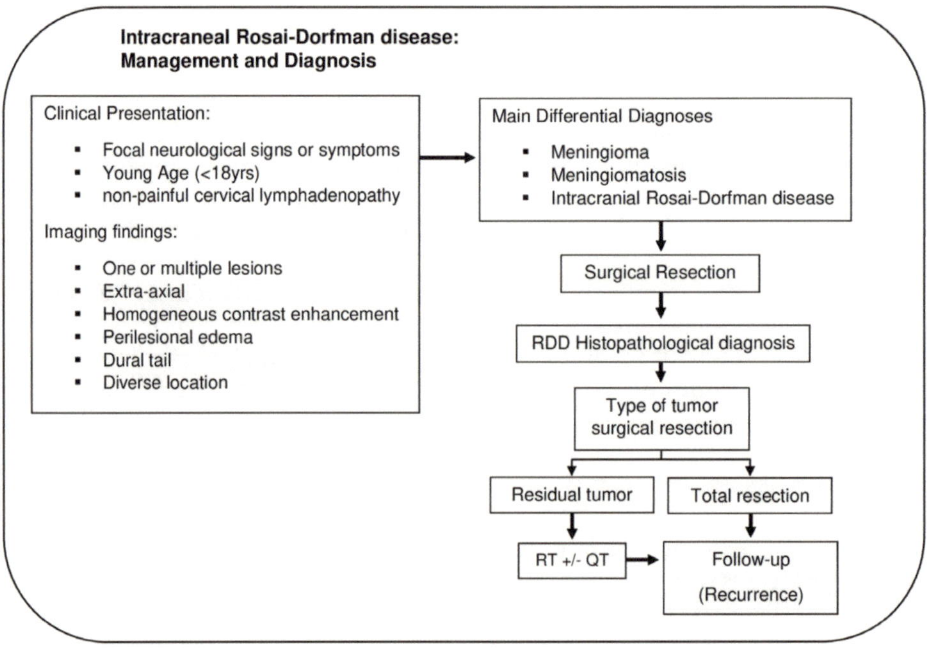

Figure 3.
Algorithm for management and diagnosis (clinical suspect) for intracranial Rosai-Dorfman disease. Clinical suspicion is obtained by clinical evaluation and imaging studies. The differential diagnosis is made with meningioma, corroborating it by the histopathological and immunohistochemical study. Relative to management, the presence of residual tumor after surgery suggests performing radiotherapy with or without chemotherapy. Strict monitoring after surgery is recommended due to the risk of recurrence.

Histopathological characteristics correspond to a large lymphohistiocytic infiltrate, with a large or vesicular nucleus, well-defined nuclear membranes and a single and prominent nucleolus. The main characteristic is the intracytoplasmic presence of lymphocytes and, to a lesser extent, intact erythrocytes, plasma cells, and neutrophils ("emperipolesis"), however, it may be absent in 30% of leptomeningeal lesions [7, 9]. Associated with histiocyte proliferation, a perivascular plasmacytic infiltrate can be observed. From the immunohistochemical point of view, they are characterized by presenting protein S100 +, CD68 +, CD11c +, MAC387 +, lysozyme +/−, being negative for CD1a, a positive marker in Langerhans cell histiocytosis [10, 12].

Illustrative case	Pearls and pitfalls
Intracranial Rosai-Dorfman Disease (RDD)	• The most affected population group are young people (<18 yrs), where the main clinical manifestation of is massive cervical lymphadenopathy. • RDD: Suggestive data of meningioma by neuroimaging studies • Brain MRI: hypointensity non-related to calcification on T2-weighted or FLAIR images could suggest the RDD diagnosis. • Total resection is the most recommended management. • Radiation therapy is indicated in case of residual disease. • Chemotherapy can be helpful in extensive (disseminated) disease. However, there is insufficient evidence on its efficacy in isolated disease. • A periodic follow-up (3–6 mos) with imaging studies should be carried out, in search of local recurrences or extensive disease.
Choroid plexus papilloma (Tumoral compression of the facial colliculus)	• Differentiation between primary and secondary HFS is elementary, imaging studies are fundamental, supported by electrodiagnostic studies. • In HFS not related to vascular compression, we recommend to intentionally search tumoral compression at the facial colliculus level at the floor of the fourth ventricle through an MRI scan with contrast. • Surgical approach: Telovelar approach to the fourth ventricle. • Intraoperative EMG register is an elemental tool to determine the impact of surgical treatment and resolution of symptoms.
Neuroenteric cyst (NEC) on posterior fossa	• Cystic lesion located in posterior fossa (90%). Differential diagnoses are mainly cystic lesions; arachnoid cysts, epidermoid cyst, dermoid cyst, neurocysticercosis, or metastases, cholesteatoma, ependymoma, schwannoma, hemangioblastoma, and pilocytic astrocytoma. • Diagnosis can be suspected in recurrent meningitis due to a fistula to the aerodigestive tract. • Slight diffusion restriction in Diffusion-weighted imaging (DWI) due to xanthogranulomatous changes or presence of melanin, hemosiderin, proteins, mucopolysaccharides and cholesterol. • Surgical treatment recommended for NEC is complete resection. If resection is partial, remnants adhered to neurovascular structures should be electrocoagulated to avoid reaccumulation. • Cystoperitoneal and ventriculoperitoneal shunts are second-line procedures recommended in recurrence with high difficulty for a new excision. • Minimum follow-up is recommended for 10 years, every 6 months at the first 2 years (complemented with CA 19–9 measurement on CSF).

RDD, Rosai-Dorfman disease; MRI, Magnetic resonance imaging; FLAIR, Fluid attenuation inversion recovery; HFS, Hemifacial spasm; EMG, Electromyography; NEC, Neuroenteric cyst; DWI, Diffusion-weighted imaging; CA 19-9, carbohydrate antigen 19-9; CSF, Cerebrospinal fluid.

Table 1.
Rare tumors: Pearls and pitfalls in diagnosis, surgical management, and prognosis.

Related to the management of this disease is primarily with surgery, seeking to eliminate the mass effect and the associated neurological sequelae. Total resection is the main objective, although a partial resection is allowed in case the lesions are in complex regions. The optimal management of residual disease remains unclear due to the rarity of the disease [13]. The use of radiotherapy has shown some efficacy of residual or recurrent disease, postoperative doses of 20 Gy in 10 fractions in 2 weeks after subtotal resection has shown a good effect in reducing symptoms and reducing the size of the lesions [14]. The use of chemotherapeutic agents such as alkaloids and anthracyclines, alkylating agents, and methotrexate have shown variable efficacy [15]. Rivera et al. [16] reported the use of the modified CHOP regimen in two cases of intracranial RDD observing a long-term remission [16].

Adeleye et al. [17] reported a series of 111 cases of RDD involving the CNS [17]. Of the population studied, 77% presented intracranial disease, which received various treatments with surgery, radiotherapy and chemotherapy. 37% of the study population had a long-term follow-up beyond one year (41% of these patients had no recurrence of the disease), where a relapse or growth of the most residual tumor was determined in 12%. Therefore, active monitoring after the surgery is prudent; however, it is not well established how often to follow up with imaging studies and when it would be prudent to classify the disease as remitted. Rivera et al. [18] reported the longest reported follow-up time (7 years) [18], of two patients with intracranial RDD with surgical resection and chemotherapeutic management with the modified CHOP scheme consisting of 8 cycles of cyclophosphamide (1 g), Vincristine (2 mg), doxorubicin (50 mg), and prednisone (50 mg) for 5 days every 3 weeks. Where it was observed that during follow-up there were no recurrences. Due to the low incidence of the disease, it is difficult to standardize diagnostic, therapeutic and prognosis. For this reason, we propose a simple algorithm for the diagnosis and management of intracranial RDD (**Figure 3**). **Table 1** describes the fundamental aspects in the management of this pathology.

3. Hemifacial spasm associated with compression of the facial colliculus by a choroid plexus papilloma

As a second case, we have an extremely rare cause of hemifacial spasm (HFS). HFS is an involuntary neuromuscular disorder in which it affects the facial musculature, which usually has as its primary cause a mechanical compression over the cisternal portion of the facial nerve in the root entry zone by an aberrant or ecstatic vessel in the 60–70% of the cases [19]. Etiology's different than vascular compression are called secondary causes, which correspond commonly to those pathologies that occupy the space in the cerebellopontine angle such as: aneurysms, arteriovenous malformations or tumor growths. Compression of the facial colliculus due to the presence of a tumor is an extremely rare cause, representing less than 0.6% of HFS cases [20]. What makes this case even more exceptional is that the tumor that was conditioning the compression of the facial colliculus was a choroid plexus papilloma (CPP), an uncommon benign intraventricular neuroepithelial tumor [21, 22].

3.1 Case presentation

A 43-year-old female who presents left severe HFS, associated with headaches, symptoms started 6 months before presentation at our service, characterized by the onset of periocular and expression muscles, increasing in intensity and frequency. The patient had the antecedent of one episode of left facial palsy 6 years ago with full

DOI: http://dx.doi.org/10.5772/intechopen.101062

recuperation 2 months later. The first management was with botulin toxin, showing a low response to initial treatment. Clinical examination at our functional neurosurgery service, found left HFS with labial commissure deviation, palpebral occlusion, and extension of the spasm to the neck. The patient did not refer pain and has no evidence of facial palsy. HSF presented every 2 min with a 15 seconds duration. Other cranial nerves did not show any alterations, and hearing was not affected. Clinical assessment was complemented with Brain MRI with gadolinium, showing a tumoral growth in the floor of the fourth ventricle that homogeneously captured gadolinium without infiltrating the floor of the fourth ventricle (**Figure 4A** and **B**). Preoperative and intraoperative electromyography (EMG) recordings were considered for the management. The preoperative register showed normal auditory and motor-evoked potentials. EMG was free from synchronic neuromyotonic discharges in muscles innervated by the left facial nerve, corresponding to the HFS clinically founded.

It was decided to perform surgery to remove the tumor growth of the superior colliculus to improve the clinical status of the HFS. A telovelar approach with intraoperative neurophysiology recordings of the facial nerve was performed. The surgical procedure was performed with the patient in the prone position and head fixation. An incision of 1 cm was made above the inion up to the C2 spinous process, the C1 posterior arch was recognized, and the tectorial membrane was dissected. Conventional suboccipital craniectomy was conducted. Dural opening in Y was realized before transverse sinus identification. Under the microscopic vision, the tela choridea was opened, and the tumor was identified. The tumor had a pearly appearance. After dissection complete resection was made. At the extraction of the tumor, there was a nervous hyperexcitability correction in intraoperative EMG recording

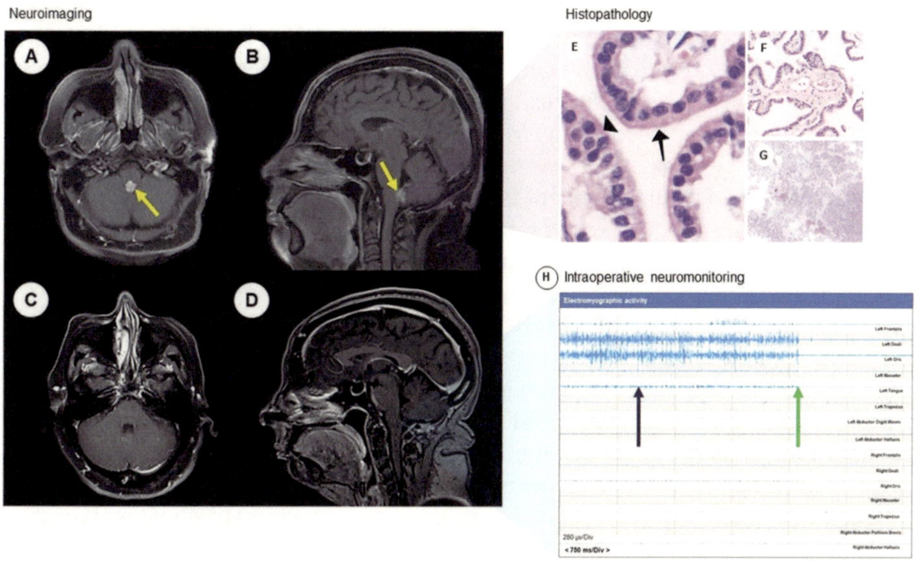

Figure 4.
Neuroimaging: Preoperative gadolinium-enhanced T1-weighted MRI showed that the right side of the fourth ventricle was occupied by a hyperintense tumor (arrows). (A) Axial view. (B) Sagittal view. T1-weighted sequences with gadolinium showing complete resection of the tumor. (C) Axial view. (D) Sagittal view. Histopathology: Choroid plexus papilloma. (E) HE x40: Cylindrical coating epithelium with flat apical domain and multiple microvilli (arrow). Cells have round-to-oval nuclei, moderate amount of acidophilous cytoplasm, and some focally pseudostratified (arrowhead) and oriented to the basal domain. (F) HE ×10: Lesion mimics the papillary architecture of a normal choroid plexus with thin fibrovascular stems and coated by a simple cylindrical epithelium. (G) HE ×4: Epithelial neoplasia. (H) Intraoperative neuromonitoring: Electromyographic activity shows synchronic neuromyotonic discharges in muscles innervated by the left facial nerve (blue arrow). Cessation of irritative activity over the left orbicularis oculi and orbicularis oris after en-bloc removal of the tumor (green arrow).

of the facial musculature (**Figure 4**). Motor-evoked potentials did not show alterations during the surgical intervention. Postoperative histopathology examination demonstrates CPP in the fourth ventricle (**Figure 4E–G**). The clinical outcome of the patient in the immediate postoperative period was a diminution in the intensity and frequency of spasms. At 12 months of follow-up, complete symptom resolution was observed without associated neurological deficits. Postoperative MRI at 1 year of follow-up showed complete resection of the tumor (**Figure 4C** and **D**).

3.2 Case discussion

HFS's most common pathophysiological mechanism corresponds in 60–70% of the cases to mechanical compression over the cisternal portion of the facial nerve in the root entry zone by an aberrant or ecstatic vessel in the 60–70% of the cases. Conversely, secondary common etiologies are pontocerebellar angle tumors, traumas, demyelination conditions, and infections. Therefore, the tumors in adults related to HFS are rare (0.3–2.5%), and the tumoral compression at the facial colliculus level, at the floor of the fourth ventricle is considered an exceptional etiology, being gliomas, subependymomas, ependymomas the neoplasia's reported [19]. The pathological mechanism of HFS is unclear. However, different theories suggest that the direct compression of the facial nerve in its cisternal portion by a vascular structure is the most related mechanism of injury, which leads to local demyelination. On the other hand, another hypothesis suggests a central/nuclear origin, that states change in the reorganization of functional connections within the facial nerve nucleus, generating irritative activity that produces abnormal discharges, precipitating HFS. A hypothesis that would be more related to the mechanism of HFS production in the presence of a tumor mass growing in the superior colliculus. This case supports the central theory of direct facial nucleus irritability, generating a hyperexcitability state that precipitates the discharges [23]. Microvascular decompression is the most frequent surgical treatment used for HFS. It is usually indicated when a vascular contact is found by MRI, which is usually effective management in more than 80% of cases [24]. However, because in this case a vascular contact was not found, the surgical management is different, focused on the complete resection of the tumor. Therefore, due to the uncertainty that may exist in the clinical outcome as it is an infrequent presentation, intraoperative monitoring is a very useful tool that helps to define the effectiveness that surgical intervention could have in symptomatic improvement, observing changes in symptoms, and synchronic neuromyotonic discharges during resection [25].

In conclusion, secondary HFS are infrequent conditions. Direct compression by tumors at the facial colliculus level associated with HFS is an exceptional case. Clinical findings do not allow differentiation between primary and secondary HFS, for this reason we recommend an adequate evaluation of the brain MRI, supported by electrodiagnostic studies. Tumoral compression at the facial colliculus level at the floor of the fourth ventricle is an exceptional etiology, and there is very few information in the medical literature about management and diagnosis. Therefore, about our experience, in **Table 1** we describe the fundamental aspects in the management of this pathology.

4. Neuroenteric cyst on posterior fossa associated with Klippel-Feil syndrome

Neuroenteric cysts (NEC) are rare benign (the malignant transformation is extremely rare) lesions of the spinal axis composed of heterotopic endodermal tissue generally located in the intradural extramedullary space in the lower cervical and upper thoracic spine, comprising 0.03% of intracranial lesions and 16% of cystic lesions of the CNS, they can found rarely intracranially, examples in the posterior fossa are ventral to the brainstem or in the cerebellopontine angle, and they present with hydrocephalus, headache, and cranial nerve deficits [26, 27]. The origin of these lesions is not completely understood, histologically are composed of cuboidal epithelium that resembles the gastrointestinal or respiratory tract. Therefore, are thought to arise from rostrally located vestigial remnants of the neuroenteric canal [28]. The consensus for treatment is complete surgical resection, when possible, partial resection should be avoided because of the high risk of recurrence. However, due to their rarity, there is a lack of information about management [29]. On the other hand, Klippel-Feil syndrome (KFS) is defined as the fusion of two or more cervical vertebrae, with a classic triad of limitation of cervical movements, short neck (brevicollis), and low hair implantation in 52% of patients [30]. Association between NEC and KFS has not been described.

4.1 Case presentation

A 21-year-old male patient began his current disease with a severe occipital headache of one month of evolution, the headache was aggravated by Valsalva maneuvers, occasionally associated with nausea and emesis. Physical examination showed brevicollis with restricted range of motion, low hair implantation (KFS). Moreover, examination shows papilledema, dysdiadochokinesia, and right dysmetria. Head CT exhibited a heterogeneous cystic lesion located on the posterior fossa, conditioning an obstructive hydrocephalus, for which an urgent ventriculoperitoneal shunt was placed (demonstrating clear cerebrospinal fluid). Sagittal section of a spine CT (**Figure 5A**) that demonstrates C1-C2 and C3-C4 anterior and posterior elements fusion, without thoracic, lumbar, or sacral alterations. Anteroposterior and lateral static and dynamic cervical spine radiographs and spine CT exposed lordosis rectification, flexion, and extension limitation. Brain MRI showed (**Figure 5B** and **C**) an infratentorial lesion, dorsal to the right cerebellar hemisphere, ovoid shape, with regular and defined borders, composed of a nodular portion in contact with pia mater, and multiple punctate flow absences, isointense on T1, heterogeneously hyperintense on T2 and FLAIR sequences, with diffusion restriction on its central portion and contrast enhancement, whose measurements were 17 × 14 × 15 mm in major axes, and spectroscopy displayed increased N-Acetyl-Aspartate and choline peaks (**Figure 5D**); another remaining cystic portion was hyperintense on T1, hypointense on T2, FLAIR, and apparent diffusion coefficient, without diffusion restriction or contrast enhancement, whose measurements were 46 × 49 × 46 mm. Due to data compatible with KFS, simple contrasted thoracoabdominal CT, echocardiography, and renal function tests were obtained; otorhinolaryngology assessment cursed without hearing alterations, and medical genetics confirmed the syndromic diagnosis.

A total complete surgical resection was decided. Subsequently, a midline suboccipital craniectomy was performed. The surgical procedure involves resection of the C1 posterior arch and tumor excision, obtaining a cystic lesion with a mural nodule at the inferolateral right torcular level, with leakage of greenish fluid (**Figure 5E**). Complete resection of the capsule was achieved, with a histopathological study that reported smooth, opaque, light gray color walls, with tortuous vessels, and peripheral solid, anfractuous, gray-green areas of firm consistency, clear brown content, and soft consistency compatible with NEC, positive to alcian blue and negative to periodic acid-Schiff stains (**Figure 5F**). The patient had a favorable clinical evolution, receiving medical discharge to home

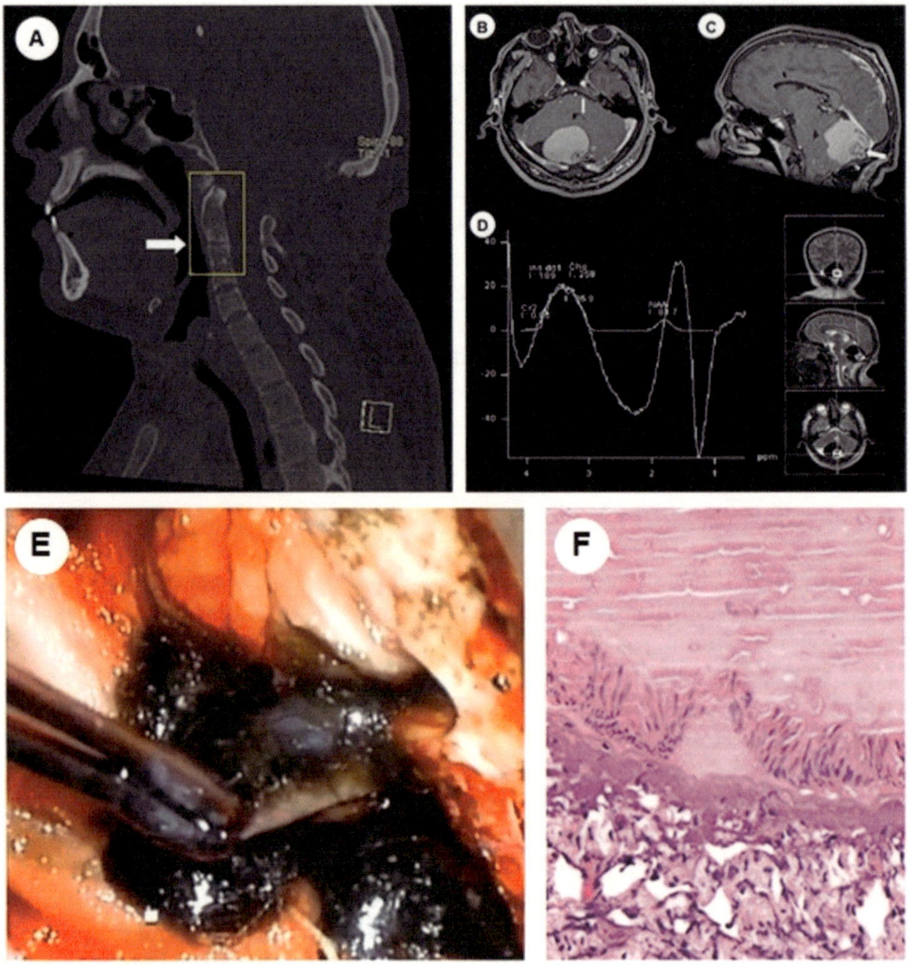

Figure 5.
(A) Cervical spine computed tomography (CT) with evidence of C1-C2 and C3-C4 anterior elements fusion (white arrow). Presurgical brain contrast-enhanced T1-weighted magnetic resonance imaging (MRI). (B) Axial section, there is evidence of an extra-axial lesion in the posterior fossa, which is contrast enhanced and displaces the cerebellum and brainstem ventrally, collapsing the fourth ventricle (white arrow). (C) MRI sagittal section. (D) Spectroscopy without choline (Cho) elevation according to the indicated voxel on T2-sequence hypointense lesion. Intraoperative images: (E) The tumor capsule with a good cleavage plane presents liquid content of oily material inside the capsule. (F) Histopathology image: HE (400X), demonstrate a cyst wall and proteinaceous content with some spaces for cholesterol crystals.

after 3 weeks, with adequate follow-up 9 months after surgery, identifying by MRI a residual nodular image adhered to the straight sinus.

4.2 Case discussion

NEC was described for the first time in 1928 and the first intracranial NEC was reported in 1962 [26], with more than one hundred cases reported since then [31]. Relative to the epidemiological characteristics of the patients, frequency is higher in men, and the age of presentation ranges from the neonatal period to 70 years. Regarding intracranial location, the initial findings are at the second or third decades of life. The predominant localization is on the posterior fossa (90%), specifically at prepontine and prebulbar cisterns, cisterna magna, cerebellopontine angle, fourth ventricle, and dorsal to the cerebellum. The etiopathogenesis is due to abnormal endodermal-ectodermal adhesion during gastrulation at embryological development, with the persistence of endodermal elements near the notochord in the neuroaxis, which would explain the association with spinal disorders (spina bifida, diastematomyelia, and vertebral body alterations). Supratentorial localizations are exceptional. Infratentorial lesions usually present headache, nausea, and cranial nerve alterations such as vertigo, hearing loss, tinnitus, hypoesthesia, or trigeminal neuralgia. Diagnosis can be suspected in recurrent meningitis due to a fistula to the aerodigestive tract that causes slow growth because of active secretion from epithelial cells. Accompanying disorders are intestinal malformations and cutaneous abnormalities. Clinical manifestations can be acute or insidious, with a course ranging from 4 months to 40 years [30, 32].

Regarding the characteristics observable by neuroimaging studies in the diagnosis of NEC, in head CT is hypodense lesions without contrast enhancement. However, density depends on protein concentration. MRI shows heterogeneous lesions (well-defined, extra-axial, rounded or lobulated cysts), hyperintense on T1, T2 and FLAIR, without contrast enhancement, with slight diffusion restriction in Diffusion-weighted imaging due to xanthogranulomatous changes or presence of melanin, hemosiderin, proteins, mucopolysaccharides and cholesterol. Differential diagnoses on the posterior fossa are mainly cystic lesions; arachnoid cysts, epidermoid cyst, dermoid cyst, neurocysticercosis, or metastases, cholesteatoma, ependymoma, schwannoma, hemangioblastoma, and pilocytic astrocytoma [33, 34]. During surgery macroscopically visualization corresponds to yellow, milky white, gray, or red cysts, with thin walls similar to arachnoid, and transparent, mucoid or xanthochromic liquid content, unusually blood, pus, calcifications, or keratinized debris adhering to the adjacent pia mater. Histopathological studies reveal benign lesions with simple, pseudostratified, columnar epithelium and collagenous fibrous connective tissue lined with gastrointestinal epithelium, with the presence of goblet cells [26]. In immunohistochemistry, they are positive for cytokeratin, epithelial membrane antigen, and carcinoembryonic antigen. Degeneration to adenocarcinoma is extremely unusual and only occurs in intracranial locations (9 patients reported) [27]. In these cases, carbohydrate antigen 19–9 (CA 19–9) is positive [26], elevated MIB-1 labeling index suggests malignancy [27]. No correlation between imaging findings and pathology has been found [35].

The surgical treatment recommended for NEC is complete resection. Wang et al. [35] described a technique that shows an improvement in prognosis and limits recurrence [35]. If resection is partial, remnants adhered to neurovascular structures should be electro-coagulated to avoid reaccumulation. Surgical approaches depend on the location and the optimal visualization of the lesion and adjacent structures to minimize the risk of neurological deficits [36]. Cystoperitoneal and ventriculoperitoneal shunts are second-line procedures recommended in recurrence with high difficulty for a new excision [28]. Postoperative complications are aseptic meningitis, abducens nerve palsy, pseudomeningocele, and cerebrospinal fluid fistula [36]. Although the prognosis is mostly favorable, one-third of patients experience a symptomatic recurrence in a period of 2 months to 32 years [36]. Minimum follow-up is recommended for 10 years, every 6 months at the first 2 years [35] and can be complemented with CA 19–9 measurement on cerebrospinal fluid to determine recurrence [37].

In this case report, we did not find a specific genetic alteration that explains the relationship between KFS and NEC. The commonly associated disorders in KFS are mostly spinal disorders how congenital scoliosis and spina bifida occulta, in some cases this disease is related to hearing alterations, genitourinary defects, cardiovascular anomalies, and other skeletal abnormalities [38]. The association between KFS and intracranial tumors is mainly related to teratomas, and dermoid cysts [39].

The diagnosis of KFS is usually incidental, the cervical spine X-rays show scoliosis, vertebral fusion, and instability, spinal CT with three-dimensional reconstruction is useful in surgical planning, and the spinal MRI is useful to detect neurologically (spinal compression, stenosis, and syringomyelia). Surgical treatment is based on the detection and management of associated systemic alterations, only 43% of patients will require decompression and spinal stabilization depending on risk patterns determined by Samartzis classification. Our patient did not require surgical management of this malformation due to the lack of clinical repercussion [40].

In conclusion, NEC prognosis is generally favorable, but a significant proportion of individuals undergoing partial resection experience recurrence. The association between KFS and NEC can be related to the persistence of embryological structures. The correct diagnostic approach must be carried out to choose the optimal surgical approach. Therefore, about our experience, in the points of **Table 1**, we describe the fundamental aspects in the management of this pathology.

5. Conclusion

Because these intracranial tumors are uncommon, studies that compare the benefits of various management strategies about outcomes and prognosis factors are lacking. Therefore, the level of evidence of management recommendations is low. However, we consider the knowledge of these entities important, so we determine the important characteristics in the diagnosis, management, and prognosis to establish a comprehensive review of these neoplasms.

Acronyms and abbreviations

CA 19-9	Carbohydrate antigen 19-9
CNS	Central nervous system
CPP	Choroid plexus papilloma
CT	Computed tomography
EMG	Electromyography
FLAIR	Fluid attenuation inversion recovery
HFS	Hemifacial spasm
KFS	Klippel-Feil syndrome
MRI	Magnetic resonance imaging
NEC	Neuroenteric cysts
RDD	Rosai-Dorfman disease

Author details

José Luis Navarro-Olvera[1*], Armando Armas-Salazar[1],
José Damián Carrillo-Ruiz[1,2,3], Jesús Q. Beltrán[1], Gustavo Parra-Romero[1]
and Gustavo Aguado-Carrillo[1]

1 Unit of Functional and Stereotactic Neurosurgery and Radiosurgery,
General Hospital of Mexico. "Dr. Eduardo Liceaga", Mexico City, Mexico

2 Faculty of Health Sciences, Anahuac University, Mexico City, Mexico

3 Research Direction, General Hospital of Mexico. "Dr. Eduardo Liceaga",
Mexico City, Mexico

*Address all correspondence to: luiginavarro97@hotmail.com

References

[1] Louis DN, Perry A, Reifenberger G, von Deimling A, Figarella-Branger D, Cavenee WK, et al. The 2016 World Health Organization classification of tumors of the central nervous system: A summary. Acta Neuropathologica. 2016;**131**(6):803-820. DOI: 10.1007/s00401-016-1545-1

[2] Ostrom QT, Gittleman H, Truitt G, Boscia A, Kruchko C, Barnholtz-Sloan JS. CBTRUS statistical report: Primary brain and other central nervous system tumors diagnosed in the United States in 2011-2015. Neuro-Oncology. 2018;**20**(suppl_4):iv1-iv86. DOI: 10.1093/neuonc/noy131

[3] Franceschi E, Frappaz D, Rudà R, Hau P, Preusser M, Houillier C, et al. EURACAN domain 10. Rare primary central nervous system tumors in adults: An overview. Frontiers in Oncology. 2020;**26**(10):996. DOI: 10.3389/fonc.2020.00996

[4] Rosai J, Dorfman RF. Sinus histiocytosis with massive lymphadenopathy. A newly recognized benign clinicopathological entity. Archives of Pathology. 1969;**87**(1):63-70 PMID: 5782438

[5] Destombes P. Adénites avec surcharge lipidique, de l'enfant ou de l'adulte jeune, observées aux Antilles et au Mali. (Quatre observations) [Adenitis with lipid excess, in children or young adults, seen in the Antilles and in Mali. (4 cases)]. Bull Soc Pathol Exot Filiales. 1965;**58**(6):1169-1175 French. PMID: 5899730

[6] Petzold A, Thom M, Powell M, Plant GT. Relapsing intracranial Rosai-Dorfman disease. Journal of Neurology, Neurosurgery, and Psychiatry. 2001;**71**(4):538-541. DOI: 10.1136/jnnp.71.4.538

[7] Abla O, Jacobsen E, Picarsic J, Krenova Z, Jaffe R, Emile JF, et al. Consensus recommendations for the diagnosis and clinical management of Rosai-Dorfman-Destombes disease. Blood. 2018;**131**(26):2877-2890. DOI: 10.1182/blood-2018-03-839753

[8] Huang BY, Zong M, Zong WJ, Sun YH, Zhang H, Zhang HB. Intracranial Rosai-Dorfman disease. Journal of Clinical Neuroscience. 2016;**32**:133-136. DOI: 10.1016/j.jocn.2015.12.046

[9] Jiang Y, Jiang S. Intracranial Meningeal Rosai-Dorfman Disease Mimicking multiple Meningiomas: 3 Case reports and a literature review. World Neurosurgery. 2018;**120**:382-390. DOI: 10.1016/j.wneu.2018.09.060

[10] Symss NP, Cugati G, Vasudevan MC, Ramamurthi R, Pande A. Intracranial Rosai Dorfman Disease: Report of three cases and literature review. Asian J Neurosurg. 2010;**5**(2):19-30 PMID: 22028755

[11] Zhu H, Qiu LH, Dou YF, Wu JS, Zhong P, Jiang CC, et al. Imaging characteristics of Rosai-Dorfman disease in the central nervous system. European Journal of Radiology. 2012;**81**(6):1265-1272. DOI: 10.1016/j.ejrad.2011.03.006

[12] Russo N, Giangaspero F, Beccaglia MR, Santoro A. Intracranial dural histiocytosis. British Journal of Neurosurgery. 2009;**23**(4):449-454. DOI: 10.1080/02688690902756173

[13] Boissaud-Cooke MA, Bhatt K, Hilton DA, Muquit S. Isolated intracranial Rosai-Dorfman disease: Case report and review of the literature. World Neurosurgery. 2020;**137**:239-242. DOI: 10.1016/j.wneu.2020.01.229

[14] Petzold A, Thom M, Powell M, Plant GT. Relapsing intracranial Rosai-Dorfman disease. Journal of Neurology, Neurosurgery, and Psychiatry.

2001;**71**(4):538-541. DOI: 10.1136/jnnp.71.4.538

[15] Joshi SS, Joshi S, Muzumdar G, Turel KE, Shah RM, Ammbulkar I, et al. Cranio-spinal Rosai Dorfman disease: Case series and literature review. British Journal of Neurosurgery. 2019;**33**(2): 176-183. DOI: 10.1080/02688697.2017.1329517

[16] Rivera D, Pérez-Castillo M, Fernández B, Stoeter P. Long-term follow-up in two cases of intracranial Rosai-Dorfman Disease complicated by incomplete resection and recurrence. Surgical Neurology International. 2014;**28**(5):30. DOI: 10.4103/2152-7806.128003

[17] Adeleye AO, Amir G, Fraifeld S, Shoshan Y, Umansky F, Spektor S. Diagnosis and management of Rosai-Dorfman disease involving the central nervous system. Neurological Research. 2010;**32**(6):572-578. DOI: 10.1179/016164109X12608733393836

[18] Rivera D, Pérez-Castillo M, Fernández B, Stoeter P. Long-term follow-up in two cases of intracranial Rosai-Dorfman Disease complicated by incomplete resection and recurrence. Surgical Neurology International. 2014;**28**(5):30. DOI: 10.4103/2152-7806.128003

[19] Yaltho TC, Jankovic J. The many faces of hemifacial spasm: Differential diagnosis of unilateral facial spasms. Movement Disorders. 2011;**26**(9):1582-1592. DOI: 10.1002/mds.23692

[20] Elgamal EA, Coakham HB. Hemifacial spasm caused by pontine glioma: Case report and review of the literature. Neurosurgical Review. 2005;**28**(4):330-332. DOI: 10.1007/s10143-005-0392-7

[21] Sethi D, Arora R, Garg K, Tanwar P. Choroid plexus papilloma. Asian Journal of Neurosurgery. 2017;**12**(1):139-141. DOI: 10.4103/1793-5482.153501

[22] Navarro-Olvera JL, Covaleda-Rodriguez JC, Diaz-Martinez JA, Aguado-Carrillo G, Carrillo-Ruiz JD, Velasco-Campos F. Hemifacial spasm associated with compression of the facial colliculus by a choroid plexus papilloma of the fourth ventricle. Stereotactic and Functional Neurosurgery. 2020;**98**(3):145-149. DOI: 10.1159/000507060

[23] Liu J, Liu P, Zuo Y, Xu X, Liu H, Du R, et al. Hemifacial spasm as rare clinical presentation of vestibular Schwannomas. World Neurosurgery. 2018;**116**:e889-e894. DOI: 10.1016/j.wneu.2018.05.124

[24] Piatt JH Jr, Wilkins RH. Treatment of tic douloureux and hemifacial spasm by posterior fossa exploration: Therapeutic implications of various neurovascular relationships. Neurosurgery. 1984;**14**(4):462-471. DOI: 10.1227/00006123-198404000-00012

[25] Sindou M, Mercier P. Microvascular decompression for hemifacial spasm: Surgical techniques and intraoperative monitoring. Neuro-Chirurgie. 2018;**64**(2):133-143. DOI: 10.1016/j.neuchi.2018.04.003

[26] Gauden AJ, Khurana VG, Tsui AE, Kaye AH. Intracranial neuroenteric cysts: A concise review including an illustrative patient. Journal of Clinical Neuroscience. 2012;**19**(3):352-359. DOI: 10.1016/j.jocn.2011.10.005

[27] Fujisawa N, Oya S, Higashi M, Matsui T. Malignant transformation of a neurenteric cyst in the posterior Fossa presenting with intracranial metastasis: A case report and literature review. NMC Case Report Journal. 2015;**2**(4): 123-127. DOI: 10.2176/nmccrj.2014-0416

[28] Chen CT, Lee CY, Lee ST, Chang CN, Wei KC, Wu CT. Neurenteric cysts: Risk factors and management of recurrence. Acta Neurochirurgica.

2016;**158**(7):1325-1331. DOI: 10.1007/s00701-016-2828-y

[29] Breshears JD, Rutkowski MJ, McDermott MW, Cha S, Tihan T, Theodosopoulos PV. Surgical management of intracranial neuroenteric cysts: The UCSF experience. Journal of Neurological Surgery Part B. Skull Base. 2015;**76**(6):475-479. DOI: 10.1055/s-0035-1554906

[30] Frikha R. Klippel-Feil syndrome: A review of the literature. Clinical Dysmorphology. 2020;**29**(1):35-37. DOI: 10.1097/MCD.0000000000000301

[31] Kim JH, Wang KC, Phi JH, Park SH, Cheon JE, Kim SK. Intracranial neurenteric cyst arising at the suprasellar cistern with extension to middle cranial fossa. Child's Nervous System. 2018;**34**(12):2491-2495. DOI: 10.1007/s00381-018-3892-9

[32] Tracy MR, Dormans JP, Kusumi K. Klippel-Feil syndrome: Clinical features and current understanding of etiology. Clinical Orthopaedics and Related Research. 2004;**424**:183-190 PMID: 15241163

[33] Watanabe N, Akasaki Y, Fujigasaki J, Mori R, Aizawa D, Ikeuchi S, et al. Imaging alterations due to squamous metaplasia in intracranial neurenteric cysts: A report of two cases. The Neuroradiology Journal. 2016;**29**(3):187-192. DOI: 10.1177/1971400916638356

[34] Yamamoto J, Shimajiri S, Akiba D, Nakano Y, Nishizawa S. Intracranial neurenteric cyst with an enhanced mural nodule and melanin pigmentation: Radiologic-pathologic correlation. World Neurosurgery. 2017;**97**:758.e11-758.e19. DOI: 10.1016/j.wneu.2016.09.126

[35] Wang X, Song G, Chen G, Guo H, Li M, Liang J, et al. Single-center clinical characteristics and treatment experience of Foramen Magnum neurenteric cyst: Report of 6 cases and brief review of the literature. World Neurosurgery. 2018;**112**:e608-e616. DOI: 10.1016/j.wneu.2018.01.097

[36] Shimanskiy VN, Shevchenko KV, Poshataev VK, Odamanov DA, Karnaukhov VV, Shishkina LV, et al. Intrakranial'naia neĭroéntericheskaia kista: opyt Instituta neĭrokhirurgii im. akad. N.N. Burdenko, v XXI veke [Intracranial neurenteric cysts: experience of the Burdenko Neurosurgical Institute in the XXIth century]. Zhurnal Voprosy Neĭrokhirurgii Imeni N. N. Burdenko. 2017;**81**(6):16-25. Russian. DOI: 10.17116/neiro201781616-24

[37] Prasad GL, Sharma BS, Mahapatra AK. Ventral foramen magnum neurenteric cysts: A case series and review of literature. Neurosurgical Review. 2016;**39**(4):535-544. DOI: 10.1007/s10143-015-0687-2

[38] Pavone V, Praticò A, Caltabiano R, Barbagallo G, Falsaperla R, Pavone P, et al. Cervical neurenteric cyst and Klippel-Feil syndrome: An abrupt onset of myelopathic signs in a young patient. Journal of Pediatric Surgery Case Reports. 2017;**24**:12-16

[39] Can A, Dos Santos Rubio EJ, Jasperse B, Verdijk RM, Harhangi BS. Spinal neurenteric cyst in association with Klippel-Feil syndrome: Case report and literature review. World Neurosurgery. 2015;**84**(2):592.e9-592.14. DOI: 10.1016/j.wneu.2015.03.015

[40] Nouri A, Martin AR, Tetreault L, Nater A, Kato S, Nakashima H, et al. MRI analysis of the combined prospectively collected AOSpine North America and international data: The prevalence and spectrum of pathologies in a global Cohort of patients with degenerative cervical Myelopathy. Spine (Phila Pa 1976). 2017;**42**(14):1058-1067. DOI: 10.1097/BRS.0000000000001981

Chapter 6

Awake Surgery for Brain Tumors

Julio Plata-Bello, Helga Fariña-Jerónimo and Yaiza Pérez-Martín

Abstract

Surgery is one of the most important steps in most of brain tumors management. In this regard, the extent of resection has been considered as an important prognostic factor. However, the resection may be limited by the presence of functional brain tissue around or in the tumor. Preventing functional damage during brain surgery is essential to keep a good postoperative performance status and for facing the successive steps in brain tumor management (i.e., radio- and/or chemotherapy). This chapter will describe all the procedures around an awake surgery for a brain tumor: from presurgical preparation to postoperative treatments and follow-up. It will not focus only on surgical approaches, but also on the specific aspect of the disciplines that are involved in this procedure.

Keywords: brain tumor, awake surgery, intraoperative neuromonitoring

1. Introduction

Principles of brain tumor surgery consist of the achievement of maximal resection by preserving the function. In this regard, different tools have been developed in the last decades, which help neurosurgeons to achieve that goal. Presurgical functional and anatomical studies, neuronavigation, fluorescence-guided surgery, and intraoperative neurophysiological monitoring (IONM) have become a standard in neuro-oncological surgery.

IONM has not only demonstrated being useful in preserving the function, but also its use is associated with an increase in the extent of resection and an improvement in the quality of life. IONM includes different techniques, and among them, direct cortical and subcortical stimulations in an awake patient are considered as the gold standard for the identification and preservation of functional areas. The information provided by direct cortical and subcortical stimulation in an awake patient cannot be completely substituted by any presurgical imaging or functional study. Therefore, bearing in mind that different complex functions should be preserved to maintain or improve, not only the neurological status, but also the quality of life in each patient, awake surgery for brain tumors is a widespread technique.

This chapter performs a narrative review about awake surgery in brain tumors, addressing the whole procedure (from patient selection to postsurgical rehabilitation) and adding the author's point of view derived from their own experience.

2. Indications of an awake surgery in brain tumor patients

Awake craniotomy is indicated in any patient with a supratentorial intra-axial lesion adjacent or in eloquent areas, that is, regions with functional importance for the patient, among which, we highlight the motor and language areas. However, there are other functions, relevant and frequently underestimated in patients who are undergoing surgical treatment, such as working memory, attention, mentalizing, semantics [1]. In fact, monitoring during the surgical procedure must be adapted not only to the lesion location, but also to preserve all relevant functions that ensure a good quality of life.

The lesions that are usually operated by awake craniotomy are mainly low- and high-grade gliomas, since in these cases an attempt is made to achieve the maximum tumor resection with the least possible neurological damage (overall survival is related to the extent of tumor resection). However, it is also used in patients with refractory epilepsy, deep brain stimulation, and vascular injury surgery, especially arteriovenous malformations [2].

Regarding glial lesions, there is controversy in the indication of awake surgery in tumor recurrences, but there are several studies that confirm that glioma recurrence surgery does not provide neuropsychological sequelae, since no significant differences are detected in the pre- and post-surgical neuropsychological status of the patient in his/her first- and second-surgery [1].

Until a few years ago, patients with right hemisphere lesions were usually operated under general anesthesia, except if it was necessary to monitor sensorimotor function and motor evoked potentials or somatosensory evoked potentials were not available. However, to maintain the quality of life of brain tumor patients, it is also necessary to preserve other functions (visuospatial function, executive functions such as memory, attention, judgment). For this reason, nowadays the benefit of an awake craniotomy is considered for all patients with a supratentorial glial lesion, regardless of their location (dominant or non-dominant hemisphere).

Therefore, the awake surgery aims to maximize the extent of resection (EOR) but mainly preserve (but not restricted to) the following functions:

Sensorimotor function. It is considered when the lesion is located within or adjacent to the perirrollandic cortex, the supplementary motor area, or the corticospinal tract. Direct electrostimulation (DES) has elucidated the complexity and breadth of motor function. The corticospinal tracts present a somatotopic organization, like the supplementary motor network, responsible for stopping or accelerating movement when stimulated in awake patients [3]. Furthermore, there is evidence of bilateral motor responses caused by unilateral subcortical stimulation, which indicates the existence of a wide and complex bilateral cortico-subcortical network that connects premotor areas, basal ganglia, and spinal cord to control bimanual coordination, language, movement, and cognition [4].

Likewise, the use of DES has demonstrated motor interference when stimulating sensitive tracts, probably related to transient inhibition of fibers, indicating the existence of a wide fronto-thalamic-parietal network involved in sensorimotor control [3].

Visual area. Direct stimulation of optical radiation can cause a temporary visual field deficit (homonymous hemianopia) if the stimulation is of the fibers that connect with the calcarine fissure, or visual hallucinations if the stimulation is of the fibers that connect with the association visual cortex, involved in visual processing [3].

Language. Since the introduction of direct intraoperative cortical and subcortical stimulation, Broca-Wernicke's model ("localizationist model") has been re-evaluated, providing a new model based on the existence of multiple interconnected direct and indirect cortico-subcortical networks involved in phonological, articulatory, syntactic, and semantic processes [5]. Theoretically, there is a dual-flow language model: a ventral pathway (semantics) and a dorsal pathway (phonological and articulatory processes). The dorsal pathway is projected toward the parietal and inferior frontal lobe, involving the superior longitudinal fasciculus (DES) and the arcuate fasciculus (AF) as white matter pathways [6]. During the picture-naming task, the DES of the inferior parietal lobe and inferior frontal gyrus is associated with the appearance of phonological paraphasias, while cortical stimulation of the ventral premotor cortex, supramarginal gyrus, and posterior portion of the superior temporal gyrus generates articulatory mistakes. Likewise, AF stimulation causes conduction aphasia and SLF has been implicated in working phonological memory, essential for learning new words and syntactic processing. In the ventral or semantic pathway, one has to consider the role of the inferior fronto-occipital fascicle (IFOF) and an indirect circuit composed of the inferior longitudinal fascicle (ILF), temporal pole, and the uncinate fasciculus (UF). IFOF stimulation during the picture-naming task leads to semantic paraphasias [7] and can also produce verbal perseveration, suggesting a role in semantic control [8]. The indirect circuit (ILF and UF) participates in verbal semantic processing and the posterior portion of the ILF is important for visual recognition and reading [9].

Others. Depending on the patient's profile, the cortico-subcortical mapping can be adapted to preserve specific functions that may be associated with the self-perceived quality of life. For example, multi-language mapping and the ability to voluntarily switch languages, mathematical calculation in teachers, music processing and interpretation in musicians, visuospatial perception in dancers, or bimanual coordination in pianists.

2.1 Contraindications

The only absolute contraindication for awake craniotomy is the patient's denial of it. Relative contraindications include the following: neurological causes (severe dysphasia, drowsiness, confusional state, or cognitive disorders that limit patient collaboration); claustrophobia; psychiatric instability; tumor characteristics (large size producing midline displacement >2 cm or highly vascularized lesions); difficulties to control the airway (uncontrollable cough, morbid obesity, obstructive apnea); and medical conditions that associate with high surgical risk and contraindicate any type of neurosurgical intervention. Age is not considered a contraindication for awake craniotomy (ages recorded in the last 10 years range from 9 to 90 years) [1].

2.2 Advantages and disadvantages

The main objective of glioma surgery is to improve overall survival and quality of life by maximizing tumor resection and it is known that awake surgery, with direct cortical and subcortical electrostimulation, allows locating and protecting the relevant functions for each patient. Thus, greater and safer resection can be achieved, by reducing postoperative sequelae and improving the prognosis.

Awake surgery has been demonstrated to reduce morbidity and mortality, with better control of postsurgical seizures and a higher postsurgical Karnofsky performance status (KPS). All of this leads to a shorter hospital stay and lower healthcare costs.

The main disadvantage that may be associated with awake surgery is the emotional stress for the patient (10–40% of patients experienced anxiety perioperatively) and up to 30% reported pain during the procedure [10].

3. Presurgical preparation for an awake surgery

3.1 Neuropsychological evaluation

Awake surgery for brain tumors aims to extend the life of the patient, preserve their capabilities, functionality, and quality of life through real-time intra-surgical monitoring of sensorimotor, visuospatial, language, executive, and behavioral functions [11]. For this reason, pre- and intrasurgical work requires careful preparation in which different professionals are involved: neurosurgeon, anesthesiologist, neuropsychologist. Regarding the work of neuropsychology, the importance of its role in awake brain surgeries has been already highlighted in international protocols [12].

The presurgical neuropsychological evaluation allows to know the psychological, cognitive, and functional state of the person. A presurgical neuropsychological evaluation should include the following aspects:

Personal aspects: Decision-making capacity, previous experiences (especially with cancer), disposition of social and family resources, coping strategies, personality type, substance abuse, patient expectations in relation to surgery, and their disease or stress level.

Emotional aspects: It will especially affect the presence of anxiety. Anxiety may be related to the patient's own characteristics but also to the uncertainty associated with the disease and/or the procedure, fear, or the lack of perception of control. This is a factor that can affect attention/concentration capacity and leads to emission mistakes and generates difficulties in establishing the baseline and surgical intervention. Depressive symptoms should also be evaluated. These symptoms may be related to the tumor pathology itself, the difficult adaptation process, or other characteristics or circumstances of the patient. In any case, the preparation of a depressed patient will always require a higher level of attention from the staff.

As Boele et al. highlighted, a wide range of brain tumor patients present psychotic symptoms or hallucinations that should also be explored before surgery as well as a decrease in the level of arousal, irritability, or agitation [13].

Cognitive factors: The evaluation of these aspects will allow the establishment of a baseline and increase the chances of success during the intervention. Some cognitive functions have been described as basic for the correct participation of a patient in awake surgery [14]. A complete neuropsychological evaluation allows to examine normal or impaired performance and determine the strengths and weaknesses that a patient has, as well as the implications that their cognitive deficits have so that they can reintegrate, in the best way, in the activities of their daily life or at the same time. In any case, a minimum evaluation protocol should include the analysis of the following: attentional processes, language in all its aspects, amnestic processes, executive functions, and perceptual abilities. A **fluent language** to express oneself and be able to communicate cognitive and physical alterations and discomfort during surgery; **verbal comprehension** for cooperation and following instructions; **memory** to guarantee the storage of information and instructions to follow during the surgery; care for the performance of intraoperative activities and **visual skills** in case of picture-naming tasks is needed.

Most studies show that language is the cognitive domain that has been most evaluated in awake surgery. However, in recent years various tests have already been used to map other cognitive functions, such as visuospatial functions, calculation, emotions, facial recognition, or executive functions. This fact, together with the great diversity of psychological variables that must be evaluated, makes it necessary to have a neuropsychology professional within the multidisciplinary team involved in the management of awake brain surgery candidate patient. In our team, the neuropsychologist is the expert who not only supports the patient in this surgical situation but is also the professional who must determine if the affectation observed during the mapping is due to electrostimulation or if it is caused by other causes, such as problems to concentrate or psychological factors.

3.2 Task selection and adaptation

The selection of tasks for intraoperative monitoring is done during the presurgical phase considering the location of the lesion, the age, and the educational-cultural level of the patient and cognitive abilities. To minimize the risk of false positives, only those items in which the patient performs flawlessly will be selected.

Using language domain as an example of function monitored during an awake surgery, the most common tasks used are naming objects, counting, naming verbs, naming famous people, reading sequences, naming colors, naming days of the week or months of the year, or repetition. These tasks can be associated with other motor control tasks such as the movement of an arm or tapping tasks or previous tasks such as promoting spontaneous language through a conversation about the patient's life (with information that has been obtained in the presurgical evaluation), or if the patient is comfortable or feels pain or cold, etc.

Regarding language monitoring, one must bear in mind:

Language without semantic content: Automatic speech tasks require motor planning and articulatory processing. To evaluate this type of language, the patient is encouraged to recall the numbers from 1 to 20 or to say the months of the year. This type of tasks uses overlearned sequences of words. Repetition of phonemes quickly (e.g., Fa-Ma-Ba) or word/nonword repetition can also be used.

Lexico-semantic processes: The most frequently used task is the presentation of drawings or pictures of objects for naming. In several studies, an introductory phrase has been added (this is a ...). Following Ojemann and Mateer, adding the introductory phrase allows us to distinguish between an anomic error and a speech arrest, but a failure could be the result of an orthographic mistake or an inability to read. Another frequently used task is action-naming [15]. A drawing, image, or video of a person performing an action are presented to the patient and the patient must name the action in the infinitive. The famous face naming requires the same processes as object naming, adding facial recognition and access to biographical information. Auditory object naming is used too. In this case, the patient hears a description of the object and its use, and then it must be named.

The pyramids and palms test is frequently used in intrasurgical monitoring. The patient must choose between two stimuli that are associated with an image presented at the top of the screen. This test allows to know the capacity of access to the semantic information of the pictures and the words and associate this information.

Grammatical processes: Naming actions (already described previously) have been used frequently. Other tasks are reading sentences slowly or complete sentences, in which one word is missing (to allows assess different grammatical), sentence repetition, writing sentences.

3.3 Evaluation of presurgical imaging studies

When the decision to perform an awake surgery must be taken, one can use the information provided by a set of tools that allow us to decide the degree of eloquence for a specific function. The location of the lesion or the clinical information is not enough to evaluate the relationship between the lesion and its functional boundaries.

However, in this point, it is essential to define more precisely what we understand as an "eloquent area." This concept has significantly evolved in the last decades, from considering eloquent areas only those involved in motor control and language, to considering other regions involved in sensorial and cognitive processing. The evolution of this concept is also associated with the better understanding of brain function that has currently been achieved. The "localizationist" vision has again been abandoned and substituted by an hodotopic view, where connectivity between one brain regions to another becomes relevant to the development of a function [16]. Furthermore, the hodotopic model includes a dynamic representation of functional systems (i.e., that change with time), fitting better with the current knowledge in brain plasticity. Therefore, an "eloquent area" can be considered as the gray matter and white matter pathways that are essential for the development of a specific function that, in the personal context of each patient, must be preserved. Each "eloquent area" can change its location with time, thanks to brain plasticity mechanisms that are activated in disease situations.

The identification of eloquent areas before a surgical procedure for a brain tumor may help in different ways:

1. To identify the anatomical relationship between the tumor and eloquent areas.

2. To decide which tasks are the most appropriate to activate eloquent areas involved in a specific function.

3. To establish an anatomic and functional map of gray matter regions and white matter pathways that is useful for the planification of the surgery.

4. To evidence the existence of functional migration to nonexpected location secondary to the plasticity mechanisms.

One of the tools that have demonstrated to be useful in achieving these aims is magnetic resonance imaging (MRI) [17]. The use of this technique is widely extended, and it constitutes an essential part of the diagnostic protocol of a brain lesion. Apart from the images acquired for diagnosis, additional sequences and procedures can be performed to obtain functional information. More specifically, the use of functional magnetic resonance imaging (fMRI) and diffusion tensor imaging (DTI) allows us to identify cortical regions and white matter tracts, respectively, that are involved in specific functions [18].

Functional MRI is based on the detection of changes in magnetization secondary to the levels of oxyhemoglobin, which increases in brain regions whose neurons increase their activity to be able to perform a specific task. fMRI has been demonstrated to be useful in the identification of the somato-motor regions using simple motor tasks with high sensitivity and specificity. However, the reported values of sensitivity and specificity for the identification of language processing areas are much lower. This difference is more pronounced during the evaluation of the sensitive component of this complex task. Furthermore, there is also a lack of evidence about the use of fMRI to map the regions involved in other cognitive tasks in patients with a brain tumor, although a significant amount of literature has described the relationship between the activities in specific regions with a specific function, but they are all in the research environment. In this regard, the development of new language tasks or paradigms to be used in fMRI studies might improve the reliability of the information provided by this technique. In the same way, cognitive tasks adapted to fMRI should be tested in brain tumor patients, to identify their usefulness in presurgical brain mapping.

Regarding the selection of fMRI tasks for presurgical mapping, one must bear in mind that there is a significant restriction of movement inside the scanner; thus, the selected task must not be associated with the excessive movement. Furthermore, we consider that the fMRI task should be as similar as possible to the task that is going to be performed during the surgical procedure.

The combination of fMRI with DTI would give us much information that may be useful to predict the cortical regions that will be positive during stimulation as well as the white matter tracts that are associated with the tumor. All this information will help us to decide which tasks will be used during the procedure; to decide the location and the size of the craniotomy; to predict the entry point to perform the corticectomy; and to give a precise information to the patient and relatives about the risks and prognosis.

3.4 Training and preparation of the patient

Once an awake craniotomy is considered for a patient, a multidisciplinary team should discuss about the feasibility of performing this procedure in this patient. The multidisciplinary team includes, necessarily, anesthesiologists, neuropsychologists/speech therapists, and neurosurgeons. Additionally, this team could also include radiologists and clinical psychologists. These professionals would finally decide if the patient is a good candidate for an awake surgery and they will plan the training of the patients for the procedure.

Keeping awake during the whole or part of a surgical procedure that involves the brain is an additional stress not only for the patient but also for the surgical team. This stress would be associated with the beliefs or expectations that may have the patient in terms of pain, immobility, or the experiencing of intraoperative complex situations. Regarding the surgical team, the lack of familiarity with the procedure may hinder the anticipation of possible complications that may appear during the surgery.

Bearing all this in mind, to achieve a successful procedure, it is essential that both the patient and the surgical team have to be instructed and trained before the surgery.

Regarding the surgical team, the ideal would be to designate a specific team for this kind of surgery. A group of anesthesiologists, surgeons, and nurses, after adequate training, should accumulate experience in such procedures, avoiding global changes in the members of the team, but allowing the occasional participation of new members to acquire experience.

On the other hand, regarding the training of the patient, we consider that he/she must know and understand the purpose of each step of the procedure. The patient must understand why an awake surgery is planned and what are its aims. After that, the patient must be explained in detail how the procedure will be taken place, from the arrival to the surgical area, to the admission in the postsurgical area. Apart from all the explanations, it is adequate to perform a specific training that should include the tasks that have been selected for the surgery, the positioning, and the layout of the operating room. In this sense, it is advisable that this training is performed in simulation conditions, mimicking the conditions that the patient will find during the surgery.

In our center, the training of the selected tasks is performed by the same neuropsychologist who has evaluated the patient and who is going to be during the surgery. This reinforces the link between the patient and the professional and contributes in reducing the anxiety and stress related to the procedure. Furthermore, the neuropsychologist can use the training sessions to adapt the tasks to the situation and features of the patient. This may lead to a more efficient procedure, thus lesser surgical times. The simulation of the procedure (positioning and operating room distribution) is performed in a room with a stretcher and with furniture that mimics those, we found in an operating room. The patient is explained about the positioning and is indicated about the interlocutors during the surgery. This may help to know the people with whom the patient must communicate with. The number of training sessions is adjusted by the functional and cognitive status of each patient. We usually recommend at least two training sessions for tasks and two for simulating the procedure.

3.5 Surgery planning

The plan of the surgery should consider different aspects:

a. The aim of the surgery (resection vs. biopsy).

Most of the awake surgeries are performed to maximize the extent of tumor resection, but, in some cases, an awake surgery may be indicated for a biopsy. This is the case of lesions located in or near eloquent regions and/or the patient may not be in good condition for a long surgery. In those cases, less time will be required for the surgery and probably only direct cortical stimulation will be performed.

b. The clinical status of the patient (including cognitive evaluation).

As it was previously explained, a complete cognitive evaluation is mandatory in any patient considered for awake surgery. This evaluation added to the clinical assessment will draw a precise picture of the clinical situation of the patient, determining the functional and cognitive state of the patient. In our experience, patients, who present any neurological or cognitive deficit, usually present shorter periods of adequate attention and collaboration in performing the selected tasks, independently of precise anesthetic management. In other words, patients with functional or cognitive dysfunction usually show fatigue symptoms before the patients without the neurological impairment. This must be considered in the planification of the procedure, trying to shorten the presurgical period (vascular accesses, material preparation, patient positioning, surgical field preparation), and the surgical approach (cutaneous phase and craniotomy). Bearing this in mind, the first DCS will be performed in a brief period and, if the surgery course is adequately developed, the subcortical stimulation may also start sooner. This can limit the negative effect of fatigue in the development of awake surgery.

c. Structural and functional findings of presurgical studies.

DTI for tractography and fMRI studies have both a significant role in surgical planning. DTI studies are useful to identify the white matter pathways around or in the tumor, while the fMRI allows identifying cortical regions that are functionally involved in specific tasks. Both imaging techniques may help us to decide the size and location of the craniotomy, as well as the place of the corticectomy. They also allow us to predict the result of the direct cortical and subcortical stimulation.

Regarding these considerations, an awake procedure should fulfill the following premises:

- The procedure must be safe.
- The patient must not feel pain or discomfort.
- The patient must not feel anxiety or fear.
- The procedure must be efficient regarding time.

4. Anesthetic considerations in awake surgery

The role of the anesthesiologist during awake brain surgery is to ensure that the patient can actively and comfortably participate in tasks during DCS in a comfortable way. As we previously indicated, the first thing when considering awake surgery is to make a correct patient selection through a prior clinical and neuropsychological evaluation. It is essential to assess the airway and inquire about sleep apnea, cognitive impairment, psychiatric disorders, and to know the neurological deficits that the patient presents before the surgery.

4.1 Anesthetic modalities for performing awake brain tumor surgery

There are three anesthetic modalities that may be considered for an awake surgery: asleep-awake-asleep, conscious sedation, and completely awake.

4.1.1 Asleep-awake-asleep

It consists of general anesthesia in the initial phase, waking up the patient during stimulation/mapping and subsequently, reintroducing general anesthesia for closure. During the general anesthesia phase, the ideal is to achieve airway control with a laryngeal mask (it offers advantages over the placement of a tracheal tube as it is easier to place, avoids head extension, and associates less risk of coughing with vomiting).

Generally, this anesthetic modality is achieved with the use of propofol and remifentanil, since they are short-acting drugs and allow sedation with rapid awakening (5–20 min). The great advantage of propofol is its rapid recovery and a titratable sedative effect, which helps to avoid excessive and unnecessary sedation, but also reduces intracranial pressure and has anti-seizure and anti-emetic properties [19]. In the case of propofol, the infusion should be stopped 15 minutes before the onset of cortical stimulation in adults, 20 minutes before in children [2], and should be restarted for dura closure. It is usually given in combination with a low dose of remifentanil.

The advantages of this modality are better airway control and adequate deep sedation with greater comfort for the patient in the initial phases. In fact, this is the modality that best adjusts to prolonged procedures (>5 h). However, the drawbacks include the complexity involved in repositioning the device in the airway for closure and that general anesthesia increases the risk of hypoventilation, nausea, and agitation during brain mapping [2, 20].

4.1.2 Conscious sedation

It consists of the administration of sedation during the first stage of the awake craniotomy without airway control (patient breathes spontaneously) [20]. A combination of propofol and remifentanil has been the standard for sedation, but it has been associated with a higher risk of respiratory depression. Dexmedetomidine, a selective alpha2 agonist with sedative, anxiolytic, analgesic, and opioid-sparing properties, has recently been shown to provide easily reversible sedation without associated ventilation depression risk [21]. Likewise, compared with the propofol-remifentanil combination, it reduces the incidence of vomiting and coughing, increasing patient comfort during surgery, and facilitating surgical resection by reducing cerebral blood flow [2]. The advantages and disadvantages of this anesthetic modality are registered in **Table 1**.

	Asleep-awake-asleep	Conscious sedation	Awake
Advantages	Good airway control	No adverse effects of sedation	Less adverse effects tan AAA
	Greater comfort for the patient	Better communication with the patient	Greater comfort in adjusting the patient's position
	Preferable for prolonged procedures (> 5 h)	Less postoperative pain	
Disadvantages	Complexity for device repositioning in the airway.	Not recommended for long-term procedures	Not recommended for long-term procedures
	Increased risk of vomiting, agitation, hypoventilation	Worse airway control	Worse airway control
		Requires more collaboration from the patient	Requires more collaboration from the patient

Table 1.
Advantages and disadvantages of each anesthetic modality for awake brain surgery.

4.1.3 Awake

This modality is the least commonly used. It consists of using local anesthesia and avoiding sedation in any of the stages of surgery with the idea of avoiding the inconveniences of general anesthesia/sedation. It raises the option of avoiding pain, through the infiltration of the scalp and selective blocking of the trigeminal sensory branches [2]. In addition to reducing postoperative pain, it has the great advantage of being able to optimize patient position and improve considerably communication with the patient by avoiding sedative medication [20, 22]. In these cases, some protocols propose the use of hypnosis to produce a dissociative state [23, 24]. The advantages and disadvantages of this anesthetic modality are registered in **Table 1**.

4.2 Anesthetic monitoring during the procedure. Complications

Premedication is not standardized. Corticosteroids are often used to reduce the mass effect of the tumor lesion and nausea. The risk of seizures is higher than standard surgery due to DCS; thus, anticonvulsant therapy is also usually administered prophylactically, although there is not enough literature evidence to support this indication.

In addition to premedication, it is essential to carry out rigorous anesthetic monitoring during the procedure. This monitoring should include electrocardiogram, invasive blood pressure measurement, pulse oximetry, respiratory rate, capnography, temperature, urinary catheterization, and BIS encephalographic recording.

Although it is usually a safe procedure in experienced professionals, some intraoperative complications related to the anesthetic procedure may occur: seizures (3–30%), high blood pressure (17–24%), desaturation/hypoventilation (7–16%), nausea and vomiting (0–9%), and brain swelling (7–14%) [25]. However, the conversion to a general anesthesia procedure only occurs in less than 2% of surgeries and there is no relationship between failure rate and the type of anesthetic modality [26].

5. Development of awake brain tumor surgery

5.1 Surgical field preparation

Awake surgery involves several specialists (neurophysiologists, neuropsychologists, surgeons, anesthesiologists, nurses) that must stay together in the operating room; thus, an adequate distribution of the space is essential. First, the position of the patient must ensure not only its comfort but also access to the surgical field; an access to the airway and vascular catheters; and the possibility to perform the corresponding tasks during the procedure. As in any operation, care must be taken to avoid nerve, vascular, ischemic, and musculo-ligamentous injuries related to compression or traction.

Regarding positioning, the most common position for temporal, insular, and low frontoparietal lesions is the patient lying supine with slight lateralization toward the contralateral side of the lesion with cephalic support (Mayfield®, Integra), with the contralateral arm extended and the ipsilateral resting on the body. If the lesion is in the frontal or parietal lobes, it is also possible to use a semi-sitting supine position.

After confirming that the patient is comfortable, the surgical field is prepared. The first step is to remove the hair that interferes with the opening and closure of the skin incision, preferably with an electric razor, followed by washing with antiseptic shampoo. Then, the skin is cleaned with antiseptic (povidone Iodine or chlorhexidine) for three times. Subsequently, the drapes are placed to isolate the surgical field, preferably using a sterile and transparent paper that is placed toward the basal side; in this way, we allow the surgeon to have visual access to the content that is being shown to the patient in any moment.

5.2 Local anesthesia and regional block

Regardless of the anesthetic modality, local anesthesia must also be used. Bupivacaine, mepivacaine, levo-bupivacine, and lidocaine are the local anesthetics most frequently used in skull surgery. Lidocaine is very useful for dura mater infiltration, but it increases the risk of seizures. The use of an anesthetic with a vasoconstrictor reduces the risk of bleeding, ensures a prolonged duration, and reduces the risk of toxicity (once infiltrated, it is necessary to wait 15 minutes to rule out acute toxicity). The total amount of local anesthetic use during the procedure will be determined by the patient's weight, comorbidities, and the concentration of the anesthetic.

Bearing in mind the locations for local anesthesia, the infiltration of the head support anchor points and infiltration of the skin incision is recommended. If we want to achieve a selective blockade (more effective for pain control during the procedure), the following locations should be also infiltrated:

- Supraorbital and supratrochlear nerves (branch of the frontal nerve).
- Zygomatic-temporal nerve (terminal branch of the zygomatic nerve).
- Temporal auricle and great occipital nerve (posterior branch of C2).
- Occipital minor (anterior branches of C2–C3).

In long-term procedures, the appearance of pain in the temporal area and its relationship with the manipulation of the dura mater are common. In these cases, additional infiltration of the zygomatic-temporal branch is recommended.

5.3 Brain mapping

Direct cortical and subcortical stimulation is used to identify the cortical regions and tracts involved in the functions we are interested in. This stimulation produces depolarization of a specific region, leading to a neuronal excitation by current diffusion, both anti- and orthodromic. The stimulation can be performed using bipolar or monopolar probes. Bipolar stimulation is performed using a pair of 2-mm-tip stimulators with 5 mm of separation between tips. This is considered a more precise method for stimulation than monopolar (2–3 mm single-tip stimulator). However, when a more precise sensorimotor mapping is going to be performed, monopolar stimulation is preferred, because the use of bipolar probes may result in ambiguous spatial distribution.

The stimulation is initiated from 1.5 to 2 mA and progressively increases 0.5 mA to achieve 6 mA of stimulation current when no response is observed. The generator supplies a constant current with biphasic quadratic waves of 1.25 ms in 4-second trains at 60 Hz. Subcortical stimulation must be done each 2 mm of resected tumor near eloquent areas.

Regions considered with positive stimulation are those where a disruption during the performance of the task is observed during the stimulation. Those regions will be identified by using a kind of marker. The positive region covered approximately 1 cm^2 around the position of the tip of the stimulator.

Apart from the direct stimulation, in most of the centers that awake surgeries with direct stimulation are performed, electrocorticography is usually performed for the detection of after-discharge potentials, which are a subclinical indicator of epileptic activity.

During brain mapping, we do not usually use mannitol or hypertonic saline to avoid brain shift and changes in the elastance of the brain that may influence the results of mapping or make the dissection of the lesion more difficult. Furthermore, if subarachnoid dissections must be done, we perform it once the lesion is functionally disconnected from subcortical pathways because the excessive release of cephalo-spinal fluid may also influence the results of mapping.

5.4 Concomitant use of other tools to maximize the degree of resection

Brain mapping during an awake procedure can also be combined with other techniques or tools that are useful in brain tumor resection. Image-guided surgery, using neuronavigation or real-time imaging systems (intraoperative MRI or ultrasound), is perfectly compatible with awake surgery. On the other hand, the use of fluorescent compounds (5 aminolevulinic acid, fluorescein, or indocyanine green), which allows to identify the areas of tumor invasion or regions where the blood-brain barrier is disrupted, can also be used during awake surgeries. In any case, the limitations of the resection will always be defined by the functional boundaries established by the direct cortical and subcortical stimulation during task performance.

5.5 Continuous evaluation of patient's feedback

It is essential to maintain continuous communication with the patient during the surgery. The key to succeeding in an awake surgery lies in adequate preparation of the patient; adequate control of sedation levels; the correct use of analgesia; and ensuring a comfortable position for the patient. Therefore, continuous monitoring of all these aspects contributes to achieve good results in awake surgery for brain tumor.

6. Postsurgical follow-up after an awake surgery

6.1 Cognitive follow-up

Apart from the regular clinical-radiological assessment after the surgery, a neuropsychological evaluation is particularly important in patients who have been operated awake.

Cognitive deficits are one of the most frequent symptoms in patients with brain tumors, mainly in attention, memory, language, and executive functions. These deficits may not only be present before surgery but can also appear after it because of the tumor itself or due to the surgical procedure. Cognitive dysfunction negatively impacts the quality of life of patients and their reincorporation into their daily functioning. Therefore, it is necessary to plan an intervention adapted to the circumstances of each patient.

Neuropsychological rehabilitation combines the application of cognitive intervention strategies and compensatory systems. These targeted strategies reduce emotional problems and promote socio-labor integration. According to scientific evidence, effective intervention methods are those that combine metacognitive and emotional regulation strategies and generalization of their effects on daily life [27, 28]. These interventions combine psychoeducational programs (providing information on cognitive functioning and their consequences in daily life, from both the patients and their families) with direct or compensatory training of the affected functions and environmental strategies (focused on restructuring the patient's environment to meet the new demands of daily activity).

6.2 Optimization of postsurgical rehabilitation in the context of adjuvant treatments

After any brain surgery, even when it has not been associated with any complication, a recovery period for normal brain function is needed. Sometimes, the improvement in the neurological function appears immediately after the surgery because the de-lesion was producing a mass effect or dysfunction in the surrounding regions. However, it is relatively common that, after surgery, brain tumor patients (mainly those whose lesion is in or near eloquent regions, as those who present an indication for an awake procedure) show a worsening in some neurological functions, even when the mapping technique and the surgery have been adequately performed. In fact, a worsening in language function has been reported in 14–50% of patients, but 78–100% of patients have recovered a normal function at 1 month. Furthermore, postsurgical transitory cognitive dysfunction in 55% of patients treated with an awake procedure has been reported. This worsening is associated with the increase of edema related to surgical handling, as well as the presence of blood resting in the tumor cavity. In our experience, this worsening is normally higher in patients with high- than low-grade gliomas.

In any case, after the surgery, a recovery period must be considered in all patients, which may include the indication of simple tasks to facilitate the spontaneous recovery process or an organized rehabilitation program. This therapy would try to accelerate and/or modify brain plasticity mechanisms to make them more efficient. However, the recovery period after brain surgery may be truncated or limit their effectiveness due to the use of other oncological adjuvant treatments. More specifically, the early use of radiotherapy in low- and high-grade gliomas or brain metastasis may slow the normal process of recovery down by damaging and limiting the development of brain plasticity mechanisms. From a tumoral biology point of view, the best moment for applying radiotherapy is in the first 4–6 weeks after the surgery. Plasticity mechanisms can develop until 8–12 weeks after surgery; thus, radiotherapy may constitute a limitation in the recovery capacity of neuro-oncological patients. This aspect may be considered in future studies because if the surgical aim is to achieve the maximal extent of resection but preserving the function, adjuvant treatments should not undermine what surgery has achieved. In this regard, we consider that radiotherapy should be delayed as much as possible, without limiting its effectiveness related to tumor biology. On the other hand, the rehabilitation program should start as soon as possible after the surgery, in an intensive and integrative manner. This will allow us to take advantage of the "plasticity window" after the surgery. In any case, it would be useful to identify serological or imaging neural plasticity biomarkers for a better follow-up, to decide the best moment to start the rest of the oncological treatments.

7. Conclusions

Awake surgery for a brain tumor is a safe procedure that should be considered in all patients with a brain tumor whose neurological function may be compromised during the surgical procedure, especially in those cases in which the function that must be preserved cannot be monitored under general anesthesia. The implication of a multidisciplinary team, a presurgical training period, and a standardized surgical protocol are essentials for the success of the procedure. Finally, adequate recovery periods, attending to brain plasticity mechanisms, must be considered in each patient by appropriately scheduling the rest of adjuvant treatments.

Author details

Julio Plata-Bello*, Helga Fariña-Jerónimo and Yaiza Pérez-Martín
Neurosurgery Department, Hospital Universitario de Canarias, Tenerife, Spain

*Address all correspondence to: jplata5@hotmail.com

References

[1] Tomasino B, Ius T, Skrap M. Gliomas. In: Brain Mapping: Real-Time Neuropsychological Testing Experience during Low-Grade Tumor Resection. Exon Publications; 2021

[2] Ghazanwy M, Chakrabarti R, Tewari A, Sinha A. Awake craniotomy: A qualitative review and future challenges. Saudi Journal of Anaesthesia. 2014;**8**(4):529-539

[3] Duffau H. Stimulation mapping of myelinated tracts in awake patients. Brain Plast (Amsterdam, Netherlands). 2016;**2**(1):99-113

[4] Catani M, Dell'acqua F, Vergani F, Malik F, Hodge H, Roy P, et al. Short frontal lobe connections of the human brain. Cortex. 2012;**48**(2):273-291

[5] Duffau H. The huge plastic potential of adult brain and the role of connectomics: New insights provided by serial mappings in glioma surgery. Cortex. 2014;**58**:325-337

[6] Martino J, De Witt Hamer PC, Berger MS, Lawton MT, Arnold CM, de Lucas EM, et al. Analysis of the subcomponents and cortical terminations of the perisylvian superior longitudinal fasciculus: A fiber dissection and DTI tractography study. Brain Structure & Function. 2013;**218**(1):105-121

[7] Tate MC, Herbet G, Moritz-Gasser S, Tate JE, Duffau H. Probabilistic map of critical functional regions of the human cerebral cortex: Broca's area revisited. Brain. 2014;**137**(Pt 10):2773-2782

[8] Khan OH, Herbet G, Moritz-Gasser S, Duffau H. The role of left inferior fronto-occipital fascicle in verbal perseveration: A brain electrostimulation mapping study. Brain Topography. 2014 May;**27**(3):403-411

[9] Zemmoura I, Herbet G, Moritz-Gasser S, Duffau H. New insights into the neural network mediating reading processes provided by cortico-subcortical electrical mapping. Human Brain Mapping. 2015;**36**(6):2215-2230

[10] Beez T, Boge K, Wager M, Whittle I, Fontaine D, Spena G, et al. Tolerance of awake surgery for glioma: A prospective European Low Grade Glioma Network multicenter study. Acta Neurochirurgica. 2013;**155**(7):1301-1308

[11] Duffau H. Mapping the connectome in awake surgery for gliomas: An update. Journal of Neurosurgical Sciences. 2017;**61**(6):612-630

[12] Ruis C, Wajer IH, Robe P, van Zandvoort M. Anxiety in the preoperative phase of awake brain tumor surgery. Clinical Neurology and Neurosurgery. 2017;**157**:7-10

[13] Boele FW, Rooney AG, Grant R, Klein M. Psychiatric symptoms in glioma patients: From diagnosis to management. Neuropsychiatric Disease and Treatment. 2015;**11**:1413-1420

[14] Becker J. Establishing Valid Neuropsychological Assessments in Patients with Gliomas Undergoing Awake Surgery. Doctoral Thesis. Christian-Albrechts-Universität zu Kiel; 2016. Available from: https://macau.uni-kiel.de/receive/diss_mods_00020713

[15] Ojemann G, Mateer C. Human language cortex: Localization of memory, syntax, and sequential motor-phoneme identification systems. Science. 1979;**205**(4413):1401-1403

[16] Duffau H. New philosophy, clinical pearls, and methods for intraoperative cognition mapping and monitoring "à la carte" in brain tumor patients. Neurosurgery. 2021;**88**(5):919-930

[17] Whiting BB, Lee BS, Mahadev V, Borghei-Razavi H, Ahuja S, Jia X, et al.

Combined use of minimal access craniotomy, intraoperative magnetic resonance imaging, and awake functional mapping for the resection of gliomas in 61 patients. Journal of Neurosurgery. 2019;**25**:1-9

[18] Voets NL, Pretorius P, Birch MD, Apostolopoulos V, Stacey R, Plaha P. Diffusion tractography for awake craniotomy: Accuracy and factors affecting specificity. Journal of Neuro-Oncology. 2021;**153**(3):547-557

[19] Marik PE. Propofol: Therapeutic indications and side-effects. Current Pharmaceutical Design. 2004;**10**(29): 3639-3649

[20] Sewell D, Smith M. Awake craniotomy: Anesthetic considerations based on outcome evidence. Current Opinion in Anaesthesiology. 2019;**32**(5): 546-552

[21] Bekker A, Sturaitis MK. Dexmedetomidine for neurological surgery. Neurosurgery. 2005; **57**(Suppl. 1):1-10

[22] Geze S, Yilmaz AA, Tuzuner F. The effect of scalp block and local infiltration on the haemodynamic and stress response to skull-pin placement for craniotomy. European Journal of Anaesthesiology. 2009;**26**(4):298-303

[23] Frati A, Pesce A, Palmieri M, Iasanzaniro M, Familiari P, Angelini A, et al. Hypnosis-aided awake surgery for the management of intrinsic brain tumors versus standard awake-asleep-awake protocol: A preliminary, promising experience. World Neurosurgery. 2019;**121**:e882-e891

[24] Zemmoura I, Fournier E, El-Hage W, Jolly V, Destrieux C, Velut S. Hypnosis for awake surgery of low-grade gliomas: Description of the method and psychological assessment. Neurosurgery. 2016;**78**(1):53-61

[25] Eseonu CI, ReFaey K, Garcia O, John A, Quiñones-Hinojosa A, Tripathi P. Awake craniotomy anesthesia: A comparison of the monitored anesthesia care and asleep-awake-asleep techniques. World Neurosurgery. 2017;**104**:679-686

[26] Stevanovic A, Rossaint R, Veldeman M, Bilotta F, Coburn M. Anaesthesia management for awake craniotomy: Systematic review and meta-analysis. PLoS One. 2016;**11**(5): e0156448

[27] Langenbahn DM, Ashman T, Cantor J, Trott C. An evidence-based review of cognitive rehabilitation in medical conditions affecting cognitive function. Archives of Physical Medicine and Rehabilitation. 2013;**94**(2):271-286

[28] Cicerone KD, Langenbahn DM, Braden C, Malec JF, Kalmar K, Fraas M, et al. Evidence-based cognitive rehabilitation: Updated review of the literature from 2003 through 2008. Archives of Physical Medicine and Rehabilitation. 2011;**92**(4):519-530

Chapter 7

Immunotherapy against Gliomas

Mathew Sebastian, Bayli DiVita Dean and Catherine T. Flores

Abstract

Immunotherapy has been demonstrably effective against various cancers, particularly those in the hematopoietic system and those with a high tumor-specific antigenic burden. Unfortunately, the development of immunotherapeutic strategies has proven more challenging against central nervous system (CNS) malignancies due to several unique characteristics of brain tumors that pose extraordinary barriers. To date, there is a lack of phase III trials demonstrating improved progression-free survival (PFS) and/or overall survival (OS) using immunotherapies in brain cancers. However, a better mechanistic understanding of current resistance to immunotherapies along with data from novel innovative techniques to overcome these barriers has been encouraging. This chapter gives an overview of current immunotherapies in the development of brain cancers. We will evaluate the present studies available in the clinical setting and any of their potential findings. The chapter will also discuss pertinent preclinical strategies whose translation for human use would potentially prove efficacious or provide invaluable scientific discovery.

Keywords: immunotherapy, brain cancer, immune system, malignancy

1. Introduction

Primary malignant brain tumors remain one of the most lethal and clinically challenging of all cancers. Despite comprising only an estimated 1.3% of all new cancer cases, brain tumors represent one of the highest causes of cancer mortality with 18,600 (3.1%) deaths predicted in 2021 [1]. Glioblastoma (GBM) is one of the most common and aggressive of the primary malignant adult brain tumors with a median survival of less than 21 months despite standard of care which includes surgical resection, targeted radiation therapy, high-dose chemotherapy, and tumor-treating fields [2–8].

Cancer immunotherapies have emerged as new therapeutic mainstays in a variety of cancers [9–14]. However, the unique characteristics of brain tumors pose extraordinary barriers that, thus far, have foiled efforts and the success of immunotherapeutic approaches. These characteristics include high tumor heterogeneity and relatively few coding mutations [15, 16], an immunosuppressive microenvironment [17–23], a relative lack of immune effector cell types [19, 24], and relative isolation from systemic circulation because of the blood-brain barrier [25–29]. This chapter will discuss some of the current immunotherapy types with emphasis on the prominent clinical trials for each and the limitations observed.

However, despite a lack of phase III trials demonstrating improved progression-free survival (PFS) and/or overall survival (OS) in many of these immunotherapies, incremental progress continues to be made in brain malignancies in both the clinical and preclinical settings. Novel immunotherapeutic strategies and combinations are currently being tested in the preclinical setting. This chapter will also discuss novel preclinical strategies to enhance immunotherapies, including modified chimeric antigen receptor (CAR) T cells, small molecular inhibitors that target immunologic pathways, and combinatorial checkpoint approaches.

2. Current immunotherapies

2.1 Cancer vaccines

Cancer vaccines involve exogenous administration of tumor antigens that can stimulate an adaptive immune system against tumor cells. The basic requirements for cancer vaccines include the delivery of tumor-specific antigens to antigen-presenting cells (APCs) such as dendritic cells (DCs), DC activation, activation of both T cell subsets and infiltration into the tumor microenvironment to exert durable responses [30]. Vaccine strategies have been employed against primary brain tumor targets using a variety of antigen substrates, including peptides, full-length proteins, RNA, and DNA in various formulations including antigens alone, antigens in combination with various local or systemic adjuvants, or dendritic cell vaccines. Though vaccination strategies have demonstrated a survival benefit in early phase clinical trials, there have yet to be any phase III clinical trials in patients with GBM demonstrating survival benefit. However, vaccination strategies continue to hold great promise with the rationale and hope that they would stimulate effective tumor-specific immunity, target tumor cells but not normal brain, and provide immunological memory against tumor recurrence [31].

2.1.1 Single peptide vaccines

Multiple single peptide vaccines have been generated to target a variety of tumor antigens including mutated isocitrate dehydrogenase 1 (IDH-R132H), survivin, Wilms Tumor 1 (WT1), and epidermal growth factor receptor variant III (EGFRvIII). Peptide vaccinations are highly specific and provide the benefit of reduced off-target effects, preventing autoimmune toxicities.

Mutated IDH1 defines a molecular subtype of diffuse glioma. A phase I trial of an IDH1(R132H)-specific peptide vaccine was conducted in 33 patients with newly diagnosed WHO grade 3 and 4 astrocytomas [32]. This study met its primary safety endpoint and demonstrated a three-year progression-free rate of 63% and a three-year death-free rate of 84% [33]. This study assessed intratumoral inflammatory reactions associated with the use of vaccines by the presence of pseudoprogression. Intriguingly, this study found high frequencies of pseudoprogression, 37.5% in the treatment group compared to 16.7% in a molecularly matched control cohort, indicating intratumoral inflammatory reactions. In one patient with pseudoprogression, the analysis found that a cluster of T cells was dominated by a single IDH1(R132H)-reactive T cell receptor.

Survivin is an anti-apoptotic protein expressed in malignant gliomas. One early phase study assessed the survivin peptide vaccine in nine patients with survivin-positive malignant gliomas and found it to be safe and tolerable [34]. The treatment group had a median PFS of 17.6 weeks and a median OS of 86.6 weeks compared to an analysis of phase II chemotherapy trials of patients with recurrent glioma with a PFS of 10 weeks and OS of 30 weeks [35]. A phase II trial was initiated with the survivin peptide vaccine in 63 participants with newly diagnosed glioblastoma [36]. In 2020, a trial update found 96.8% of patients did not experience disease progression within 6 months with a 93.5% survival rate a year after diagnosis [37]. This is an ongoing study.

Wilms Tumor 1 (WT1) is a pleiotropic transcription factor with functional roles in GBM that range from driving cellular proliferation [38] to inhibiting apoptosis [38, 39]. An uncontrolled nonrandomized phase II trial of WT1 peptide vaccination for patients with recurrent WT1-positive GBM was conducted with 21 patients. This study demonstrated that the vaccination was safe and produced a clinical response with a median PFS period of 20.0 weeks, median overall survival after initial vaccination of 36.7 weeks, and a 6 month PFS of 33.3% [40]. The median PFS and median OS found in this study were said to be comparable to various combination regimens of chemotherapy and/or radiotherapy.

Epidermal growth factor receptor (EGFR) amplification is enriched in the classical subset of GBM and is seen in 57.4% of primary GBM patients [41, 42]. Epidermal growth factor receptor variant III (EGFRvIII) regulates EGFR activity by inducing the expression of EGFR ligands [43]. A phase II trial assessed the immunogenicity of an EGFRvIII-targeted peptide vaccine [44]. The 6-month PFS after vaccination was 67% (versus 59% in the historical cohort) with a median overall survival of 26.0 months (versus 15.0 months in the matched control group) [45]. However, no benefit was observed in a randomized phase III trial [46]. Further analysis found significant loss of EGFRvIII expression in a subset of patients with tumor tissue available at recurrence in both those that received the vaccine and in those receiving standard-of-care chemoradiation [47].

To date, single peptide vaccines have yet to lead to clinical benefit in phase III trials in brain cancers. The EGFRvIII work hints that the selection of a single molecular target as a peptide vaccine might be inadequate to overcome the considerable challenges of tumor antigen down-regulation and tumor heterogeneity. Thus, targeting multiple targets could lead to robust durable responses. Thus, studies investigating multi-peptide vaccines, with several tumor antigen targets, have now been initiated.

2.1.2 Multipeptide vaccines

To identify multiple tumor-associated peptides for immunotherapy, a study set out to assess the potential of using HLA-associated tumor peptidomes as a source of tumor-associated antigens to be used in immunotherapy [48]. The components found gave rise to the multipeptide vaccine IMA950. A phase I/II set out to assess IMA950 and its 11 tumor-associated peptides which include brevican (BCAN); chondroitin sulfate proteoglycan 4 (CSPG4); fatty acid-binding protein 7, brain (FABP7); insulin-like growth factor 2 messenger mRNA-binding protein 3 (IGF2BP3), neuroligin 4, X-linked (NLGN4X); neuronal cell adhesion molecule (NRCAM), protein tyrosine phosphatase, receptor-type, z polypeptide 1 (PTPRZ1); tenascin C (TNC); Met proto-oncogene (MET); baculoviral IAP repeat-containing 5 (BIRC5); and hepatitis B virus core antigen [48]. In this study, IMA950 was adjuvanted with poly-ICLC (polyinosinic-polycytidylic acid stabilized with polylysine and carboxymethylcellulose) [49]. The multi-peptide vaccine was used in 19 patients, 16 with GBM and 3 with grade III astrocytoma. Results showed a median overall survival of 19 and 17 months for the whole cohort and GBM patients-only, respectively, with a PFS of 68% at 6 months for the whole cohort and 69% for GBM patients only when calculated from the study entry [50]. There was no mention of a historical control group used as a comparator in this study. Due to the findings in this study, a follow-up trial is actively recruiting patients with recurrent GBM to test IMA950/poly-ICLC alone or in combination with pembrolizumab, a checkpoint inhibitor that will be discussed later [51].

Another multi-peptide vaccine was generated based on observations of three tumor-associated antigens that were observed to be highly expressed in pediatric gliomas. This vaccine targets the peptide epitopes of EPH receptor A2 (EphA2; a tyrosine kinase), interleukin-13 receptor alpha 2 (IL-13Rα2), and survivin. This study was conducted in 26 pediatric patients with diffuse brainstem gliomas (BSG) or high-grade gliomas (HGG) [52]. Results showed a median survival of 13.3 months from diagnosis in the overall cohort with a median survival of 12.7 months in the BSG group and a median survival of 25.1 months in the HGG group. Though no historical control group was discussed in this phase I study, the authors mentioned that for children with BSGs, current therapies at the time failed to increase median overall survival beyond 9–12 months [53].

Though these studies are showing promising results, the lack of clear indication of efficacy and eventual tumor progression in these phase I-III trials may be attributed to the multiple obstacles in place by brain cancers including the high degree of heterogeneity of antigenic expression, an outgrowth of subclones not expressing the antigens, lack of major histocompatibility complex molecules and/or an immunosuppressive tumor microenvironment.

2.1.3 Dendritic cell (DC) vaccines

The aforementioned peptide cancer vaccines require uptake and activation of endogenous antigen-presenting cells (APCs) such as DCs. These DCs then present antigens to tumor-specific T cells leading to T cell activation. To circumvent the reliance of endogenous DC antigen loading and activation, some studies utilize DC vaccines and load DCs *ex vivo* with a variety of tumor antigens including autologous tumor lysates, tumor-associated peptides, and tumor-associated viral antigens. DC vaccines have a variety of advantageous characteristics making them an ideal choice for antitumor vaccines. They are considered to be the professional APC and most effective in sensitizing naïve T cells to specific antigens. They also are able to cross-prime, allowing them to present exogenous antigens for presentation on major histocompatibility complex (MHC) class I molecules, activating cytotoxic T lymphocytes.

A phase I trial of the DC vaccine DCVax-L was completed which loads autologous DCs with tumor lysate from newly diagnosed or recurrent GBM participants [54]. In this trial that enrolled 23 patients, the 1-year survival rate was 91% with a median OS of 31.4 months from the time of initial surgical diagnosis. The authors compared this median OS to the median OS of 18.6 months found in a large study of GBM patients who underwent tumor resection and chemoradiotherapy [55]. However, the study noted that it was unclear whether the extended survival of participants is a direct result of the vaccine effects or good responses to follow-up therapies after failing the vaccine [56]. DCVax-L has since gone on to a large phase III clinical trial with 331 participants with the primary endpoint of PFS and the secondary endpoint of OS [57]. Preliminary results of the study reveal a median OS of 23.1 months from surgery in the overall intention-to-treat population (ITT) and 34.7 months from surgery in patients with a methylated O^6-methylguanine-DNA-methyltransferase (MGMT) gene promoter. The authors compared the median OS in the ITT population to a median OS of 15–17 months from surgical intervention typically achieved with a standard of care in past studies. The PFS was not evaluated in this interim analysis. In this blinded interim survival analysis, the authors found that patients were living longer than expected and that this warrants further follow-up and analyses [58].

ICT-107 is another DC vaccine loaded with synthetic tumor-associated peptides of antigens commonly overexpressed in CD133-positive cancer stem cells that includes Erbb2 (HER2), second tyrosinase-related protein (TRP-2), glycoprotein 100 (gp100), melanoma-associated antigen 1 (MAGE-1), IL-13Rα2, and absent in melanoma 2 (AIM-2). In a phase I trial of 21 participants who were HLA-A1 or HLA-A2-positive and with newly diagnosed GBM (n = 17), recurrent GBM (n = 3), or with a brain stem glioma (n = 1), the median PFS was 16.9 months with a median OS of 38.4 months. These results suggest a correlation with prolonged OS and PFS though no comparator group or historic controls were mentioned [59]. The same group then conducted a phase II randomized, double-blind, placebo-controlled study using ICT-107 in 124 participants with newly diagnosed GBM following resection and radiotherapy with concomitant temozolomide [60]. The primary endpoint of median OS was not increased but a significant increase in the PFS by 2.2 months was observed in the intent-to-treat population treated with ICT-07 (11.2 months versus 9 months) [61]. A phase III trial was halted due to insufficient financial resources [62].

Another pair of studies made use of the immunodominant cytomegalovirus (CMV) antigen phosphoprotein 65 (pp65) in their DC vaccines. This antigen is expressed in GBM but not in normal brains [63]. The first was a randomized blinded phase I clinical trial in 12 patients with newly diagnosed GBM who received pre-conditioning in the form of tetanus/diptheria toxoid (a potent recall antigen) or unpulsed mature DCs before bilateral vaccinations with DCs pulsed with CMV pp65 RNA [64]. Td pre-conditioning led to a significant increase in both median PFS and median OS compared to the DC alone cohort which had a median PFS and OS of 10.8 and 18.5 months (consistent with patients treated with standard of care) [65]. A later study from the same group evaluated DCs pulsed with CMV pp65 RNA along with dose-intensified temozolomide (TMZ) and adjuvant GM-CSF [64]. Here they observed a median PFS of 25.3 months and a median OS of 41.1 months in the treatment group compared to 8.0 months and 19.2 months in historical controls, respectively [66]. A phase II randomized, blinded, placebo-controlled trial of DCs pulsed with CMV pp65 and Td is underway with a target of 120 patients [67]. Another phase II trial utilizing DCs pulsed with CMV pp65 was recently completed with results pending which is assessing whether basiliximab, a monoclonal anti-CD25 antibody, may inhibit the functional and quantitative recovery of T-regulatory cells after TMZ-induced lymphopenia in newly diagnosed GBM [68].

The potential for DC vaccines is vast in their ability to generate antitumor immunity however, to date, they have provided suboptimal and overall unsatisfactory clinical benefits in large trials. Work now includes methods to improve *in vitro* APC generation [69, 70], improve DC vaccine activity with additional treatments [65], and increase inflammation at the vaccine site [56, 66, 71]. It is now thought that the next major advances in DC vaccines will come from their combination with other immunotherapies such as checkpoint inhibitors [20].

2.2 Immune checkpoint inhibitors

The principal breakthrough in cancer treatment over the last 15 years is the introduction of immune checkpoint inhibitors (ICIs) blocking the immune checkpoints programmed death 1 (PD-1), programmed death-ligand 1 (PD-L1), and cytotoxic lymphocyte antigen 4 (CTLA-4). Immune checkpoints are negative regulators of T-cell immune function and are central for the modulation of physiological immune responses and the maintenance of self-tolerance. T cells are created in the thymus where they undergo positive and negative selection and undergo apoptosis if they fail to recognize self-MHC or bind too strongly to MHC with self-peptides. This process is called central tolerance [72]. T cells that appropriately respond to MHC molecules are then sent into the circulation where they eventually interact with APCs displaying mutated self-proteins (in cancers) or foreign antigens (in infection) [73]. However, central tolerance is sometimes incomplete and some T cells escape and become autoreactive. To prevent autoreactivity, there are multiple inhibitory checkpoint pathways that regulate the activation of T cells at multiple levels during an immune process called peripheral tolerance [74].

Central to cancer immunotherapy is that tumor cells can take advantage of peripheral tolerance and hijack these checkpoint mechanisms, inhibiting T cells from attacking. The arrival of checkpoint inhibitors in 2011 introduced a new mechanism to treat cancer and revolutionized cancer management in a variety of solid tumors [75–78]. There are now several FDA-approved monoclonal antibodies against solid tumors including ipilimumab targeting CTLA-4, pembrolizumab, and nivolumab targeting PD-1, and atezolizumab and durvalumab targeting PD-L1. However, despite numerous articles describing preclinical efficacy of checkpoints in central nervous system (CNS) tumors, activity against brain metastases from melanoma and non-small-cell lung cancer [79, 80], and multiple studies describing increased PD-L1 expression in GBM [81, 82], no FDA approval has occurred for immune checkpoints in GBM. Here, we will discuss some of the phase III trials that have occurred with immune checkpoint inhibitors, what has been learned, and where the research is going.

2.2.1 Phase III trials

One randomized phase III study assessed the effect of nivolumab versus bevacizumab (anti-vascular endothelial growth factor A) in 439 patients with recurrent glioblastoma [83]. The study found no statistical difference between the median OS of nivolumab monotherapy (9.8 months) and bevacizumab (10.0 months) [84]. Interestingly, this study observed that corticosteroid use at baseline seemed to be associated with worse outcomes in the nivolumab group. This may be due to the direct effects of corticosteroids on T cell function which may abrogate activation or priming of the immune system.

Additionally, a phase III study compared nivolumab versus temozolomide in newly diagnosed patients with unmethylated MGMT GBM [85]. In 2019, Bristol-Myers Squibb announced that the study did not meet its primary endpoint, which assessed overall survival [86].

Another randomized phase III single-blind study set out to compare TMZ plus radiation therapy combined with nivolumab or placebo in newly diagnosed patients with MGMT-methylated glioblastoma [87]. In 2019, Bristol-Myers Squibb provided an update that the nivolumab group did not meet one of its primary endpoints, progression-free survival, but that the data monitoring committee recommended continuing the trial to allow the other primary endpoint, overall survival, to mature [88]. The final results are pending.

It remains to be seen whether the lack of demonstrated efficacy of checkpoint therapeutic efficacy is due to difficulty getting to the tumor site or the tumor itself. Though it has been shown that T cells can traffick to the CNS, the relatively immune-privileged CNS may prove to be a limitation if checkpoint inhibition must enter into these tumors to be effective [20]. However, at least one study demonstrated clinically meaningful intracranial efficacy with ipilimumab combined with nivolumab in patients with melanoma with untreated brain metastasis, suggesting that immune checkpoint strategies can target tumors located intracranially [80]. Lack of effective checkpoint strategies in primary CNS tumors could be due to a variety of challenges that interplay with one another. First, glioblastomas generally are considered cold tumors, lacking intratumoral inflammatory cells though this is also considered to be heterogenous. Lack of efficacy could also be due to the relatively low mutational burden since it has been consistently shown that malignancies with a high burden of clonal neoantigens have a higher response rate to checkpoint inhibition [89]. Also, the high degree of heterogeneity found within gliomas, makes specific immunological targeting difficult. Lastly, the observed systemic T cell dysfunction and sequestration imposed by an intracranial tumor remain another domineering challenge as this singly does away with the requirement of a viable T cell compartment for immune checkpoints to act on [90].

Though multiple challenges must be overcome for immune checkpoint inhibitors to overcome glioblastoma specifically, a better understanding of treatment resistance in addition to many promising synergistic combinatorial approaches will provide important incremental advances to efficacy. Finally, as seen in other solid tumors, resistance to immune checkpoint blockade leads to upregulation of a host of alternative inhibitory immune checkpoint molecules that are currently also being targeted in ongoing clinical trials. These new inhibitory immune checkpoint targets potentially offer increased therapeutic targets to be used as single agents or in combination with other immunotherapies [91].

2.3 Adoptive cellular therapy (ACT) immunotherapy

Immunotherapy can be considered active or passive. The difference between each centers on how they modulate the immune system. Active immunotherapy, such as the aforementioned vaccines, relies on the process of endogenous immune cells activation, producing a durable response and generation of immunological memory. Passive immunotherapy, however, produces an immediate response due to the administration of cytokines, antibodies, or immune cells. A form of passive immunotherapy is adoptive cellular therapy (ACT) which specifically allows for the *ex vivo* generation and expansion of autologous immune cells that can then be given back to patients. This section will first discuss the non-specific adoptive cellular therapies such as lymphokine-activated killer (LAK) cells and natural killer (NK) cells followed by adoptive T cell therapies.

2.3.1 Lymphokine-activated killer (LAK) cells

LAK cells were thought to be a promising candidate for adoptive cellular therapies due to their ease of generation (culturing peripheral blood lymphocytes in the presence of IL-2), rapid expansion, the long shelf life *in vitro*, and tumor lysing capabilities [92]. These characteristics and favorable results in other cancers led to a phase I/II clinical trial in adult patients with recurrent or progressive supratentorial malignant glioma who were candidates for reoperative surgery. In this study, 19 eligible patients underwent craniotomy with debulking and placement of LAK cells and IL-2 in a reservoir inserted in the tumor resection cavity. Compared to an institutional historical control group of GBM after reoperation with a median OS of 28 weeks, LAK-treated patients had a median OS of 53 weeks. After treatment, the 1-year survival was 53% compared to less than 6% in a control contemporary chemotherapy group after reoperation suggesting improved long-term survival [93].

Another phase I/II trial was initiated in 40 patients with GBM who had autologous LAK cells placed in the tumor cavity. Findings from this study showed a median survival from the original diagnosis of 17.5 months compared to 13.6 months in a contemporary age-matched group [94]. The same group conducted a phase II trial with LAK cell treatment in 33 GBM patients who had not experienced clinical or radiographic evidence of progressive disease during or shortly after completion of initial therapy which showed a median survival from diagnosis of 20.5 months with a 1-year survival of 75%. The authors stated that 20.5 months median survival is 88% longer than the 12-month survival associated with GBM and 33% longer than the 15-month median survival observed in the clinical trials that established the benefit of temozolomide therapy [95].

Overall, the use of LAK has since fallen out of favor [20, 96]. In phase III randomized trial of IL-2 with or without LAK in the treatment of patients with advanced renal cell carcinoma (RCC), the addition of LAK did not improve the response rate against RCC [97]. It is thought the efficacy of LAK cell ACT is due to the amplification of a subset of therapeutic cells found in the peripheral blood that are reactive against tumors [96]. Thus, the use of tumor-infiltrating lymphocytes (TILs; discussed later), which are more specific to the target tumor, might have better potential.

2.3.2 Natural killer (NK) cells

The NK cell ACT field is rapidly expanding in both biological understanding of NK cells, including their distinct immune checkpoints [98, 99] in addition to clinical development of NK cell ACT. These cytotoxic cells are part of the innate immune system and have many advantageous characteristics which include rapid *ex vivo* activation and expansion without the use of autologous tumor cells and are not MHC restricted [100]. It is recognized that NK cells target other cells types based on a lack of MHC-I expression [101]. Glioblastoma is known to employ immune evasion tactics including downregulation of MHC-I [102–104] which may make it amenable to ACTs using NK cells.

An early preliminary trial was conducted in nine patients with recurrent malignant gliomas using autologous NK cells injected into the tumor cavity, using a reservoir system, and intravenously. This study found that NK cell therapy was safe with some clinical benefit demonstrating three patients with partial response (50% decrease in tumor volume), two with a minor response (25% decrease in tumor volume), seven with progressive disease (increase of 25% in tumor volume), and four with no change [100].

Currently, there is at least three phase I trials in the process utilizing NK cells in high-grade gliomas [105–107].

2.3.3 Tumor-infiltrating lymphocytes (TILs)

As mentioned before, ACT allows for *ex vivo* generation and expansion. During expansion, several modifications and enhancements can occur to confer advantageous characteristics in antitumor activity. T cells can be positively selected based on specificity to tumor antigens and increased effector function. Or, they can also be transduced to express specific tumor-associated T cell receptors (TCRs) that, though MHC-restricted and MHC-dependent, can target intracellular antigens. Alternatively, T cells can be modified to express chimeric antigen receptors (CARs) for specific tumor cell surface proteins.

As the name implies, tumor-infiltrating lymphocytes are thought to have undergone *in vivo* recognition of their cognate antigen and migration into the tumor. Thus, the administration of autologous TILs have produced durable objective responses in patients with advanced melanoma [108]. However, TILs are less feasible in GBM owing to the difficulty in isolating and expanding them [109] and T cell exhaustion while within the tumor microenvironment [110]. A more feasible approach is the aforementioned targeting of the ubiquitously expressed human CMV antigen pp65 in GBM tissue [111]. This approach was conducted in an early phase clinical trial and was able to successfully expand CMV-specific T cells from 13 out of 19 patients of which 11 received all four T-cell infusions and found that the median overall survival of these patients since the first recurrence was 403 days. The overall median OS in this study was >57 weeks (a range of 19–345 weeks) and a median PFS of >35 weeks (a range between 15.4–254 weeks). No comparator group or historic controls were mentioned in this early phase trial. Interestingly, molecular profiling of CMV-specific T cells from the patients revealed distinct gene expression signatures which correlated with their clinical response [111]. Another phase I randomized study was initiated in 22 CMV-seropositive, newly diagnosed GBM patients. This study assessed CMV pp65-specific T cells that were generated *ex vivo* with autologous CMV pp65 RNA-transfected DCs with or without a CMV-DC vaccination [112]. Though this study was not powered to detect differences between cohorts with regard to PFS and OS, the study found an association between higher IFNγ^+, TNFα^+, and CCL3$^+$ polyfunctional, CMV-specific CD8$^+$ T cells and OS [113].

2.3.4 Chimeric antigen receptors T cells (CAR T cells)

A major recent advancement in adoptive cellular therapies has been the development of chimeric antigen receptors as a means for T cells to bypass MHC restriction, and dependence and have specificity for a cell surface antigen. CAR T cell therapy recently received approval targeting CD19 in B cell leukemia and lymphoma [114]. CAR T cells are genetically modified to express an extracellular single-chain variable fragment that specifically recognizes a tumor cell's surface antigen. The extracellular binding fragment is bound to intracellular signaling domains and/or co-stimulatory domains that allow for T cell activation when the fragment is bound to its cognate antigen. CAR T cells have the advantage of recognizing target antigens independent of HLA and also disregarding tumor cell immunoevasion by MHC expression reduction.

A phase I safety study was conducted using autologous CAR T cells targeting EGFRvIII in 10 recurrent EGFRvIII$^+$ GBM patients [115]. The median OS was 251 days (~8 months; PFS could not be calculated due to the confounding factor of neurosurgical intervention in most of the patients). No specific historical controls were mentioned though the authors stated that GBM patients with significant residual disease after surgery have an average survival that is around ~6 months. The group demonstrated that EGFRvIII specific CAR T cells were found in the brain tumor and exerted antigen-directed activity. They also found that most of the patients had decreased expression of EGFRvIII in tumors resected after CAR T therapy [116].

Another member of the family of EGFR-related receptor tyrosine kinase is HER2. HER2 is commonly overexpressed in high-grade gliomas [117–120]. A phase I dose-escalation study was initiated to assess the safety and antitumor efficacy of autologous HER2-specific CAR T cells in 17 patients with progressive recurrent GBM [121]. This study found that though HER2-specific CAR T cells did not expand, they were detected in peripheral blood for up to 12 months. They found that eight patients had clinical benefit from either partial response or stable disease. The median OS was 11.1 months from the first CAR T cell infusion and 24.5 months from diagnosis with an 18-month OS of 29.4% [122]. As a comparator, this study mentions achieving similar outcomes as another study that used bevacizumab and lomustine where the median OS was 12 months with an 18-month OS of 20% [123].

Similar to the aforementioned peptide and DC vaccines, there are CAR T approaches targeting IL-13Rα2 due to its expression in a majority of adult and pediatric GBM tumors but not in normal brains [124, 125]. One group demonstrated that administration of IL-13Rα2-specific CAR T cells was feasible and showed evidence for transient anti-glioma responses in two out of three patients with recurrent GBM [126, 127]. The same group has initiated an ongoing phase I study utilizing IL-13Rα2-specific CAR T cell administration into the resected tumor cavity and the ventricular system in patients with recurrent or refractory malignant glioma [128]. A case report derived from this phase I study observed regression of all CNS tumors along with concomitant increases in cytokines and immune cells in the cerebrospinal fluid. Subsequent relapse was later found to be due to IL-13Rα2-negative tumors [129].

These studies demonstrate the barriers found in targeting single antigens in a highly heterogenous tumor. Newer approaches for enhanced CAR T therapy efficacy will require targeting multiple antigens, a combinatorial approach with other immunotherapies, or the development of CAR T cell designs that induce significant epitope spreading [20]. Aside from antigen target constructs, current work in CAR T therapy looks toward maximizing and maintaining the activity of the administered CAR T cells to overcome barriers in the solid tumor microenvironment [130]. As mentioned with cancer vaccines, the benefit will likely occur with the combination of CAR T therapy and immune checkpoint blockade. Another strategy is to express chemokine receptors in CAR T cells to improve their tumor-directed trafficking (discussed below) or, conversely, express blocking chemokines and receptors expressed by tumor cells to inhibit recruitment of inhibitory immune cells. Another strategy is disrupting the tumor vasculature with anti-VEGFR CAR T therapy. Strategies are also looking into the combination of depleting immune-inhibitory cells to then allow for CAR T therapies to maintain durable responses. Though CAR T therapy remains a promising therapy for GBM, further work is needed to lead to clinical benefit.

3. Novel preclinical strategies

3.1 Targeting glioma stem cells (GSCs)

Glioma stem cells (GSCs) are a subpopulation of glioma cells with stem-like properties. These cells are thought to promote tumor initiation, chemo- and radio-resistance, and tumor invasiveness. GSCs were first defined by their expression of prominin 1 or CD133, however, it was later discovered that CD133-negative cells were also capable of causing tumor initiation. In addition, several different models of GSC initiation have been proposed.

Vora *et al.* generated three different therapeutic modalities to target $CD133^+$ GSCs and tested their efficacy using human GBM models. The first modality, a CD133-binding IgG, was found to be ineffective at causing a significant reduction in proliferation *in vitro* and *in vivo* tumor burden. The second modality, a dual-antigen T cell engager or DATE, specific for CD133 and CD3, caused significant tumor-killing both *in vitro* and *in vivo*. Finally, the CD133-specific CAR T cells provided profound T cell proliferation and secretion of the anti-tumor cytokines IFNγ and TNFα upon co-culture with various human GBM cells. In addition, when mice were intracranially injected with human GBM cells followed by subsequent intracranial injection of CD133-specific CAR T cells, a significant reduction in tumor burden and prolonged survival was observed relative to control-treated mice. Importantly, they found administration of CD133-specific CAR T cells did not significantly impair hematopoiesis [131].

An additional novel method of targeting GSCs is through the use of NK cells. These cells are cytotoxic lymphocytes capable of killing target tumor cells. GSCs have been shown to express activating ligands of NK cells, such as CD155 and B7-H6. In addition, NK cells were shown to be able to lyse GSCs *in vitro* upon co-culture with target GSCs. Contrarily, GSCs were found to promote NK cell dysfunction that was determined to be contact-dependent. Mechanistically, the NK cell dysfunction was found to be mediated via TGFβ-1 released by GSCs and upon treatment with a TGFβ inhibitor, the dysfunction could be significantly diminished. When evaluated in an *in vivo* model of human GSC, the combination of allogeneic NK cells and a TGFβ inhibitor provided superior survival relative to any control groups. These results suggest combinatorial NK cell therapy and TGFβ inhibitor may provide promising anti-tumor responses [132].

3.2 Modified CAR T cells

CAR T cells combine the single-chain variable fragment (scFV) of monoclonal antibodies with the internal component of the T cell receptor. There are three main generations of CAR T cells—first-generation CAR T cells include an scFV as well as CD3ζ endodomain. The second generation built upon this by adding a costimulatory molecule such as CD28 or 4-1-BB to promote expansion. Finally, third-generation CAR T cells consist of an scFV, CD3ζ, as well as two or more costimulatory molecules. CAR T cells, especially third-generation CAR T cells, have had great success in patients with B cell malignancies [133].

However, single-agent CAR T cells have had limited success in patients with CNS malignancies. This is likely due to several factors, including a high degree of heterogeneity in the tumor microenvironment (TME), loss of antigen during tumor progression, exhaustion of the CARs within the TME, and finally upregulation of immunosuppressive molecules that inhibit CAR T cell killing [134].

Bielamowicz *et al.* utilized human GBM cells to identify three antigens expressed on human glioma cells: HER2, IL-13Rα2, and EphA2. Single-agent CAR T cells, bispecific CAR T cells targeting IL-13Ra2 and EphA2, as well as trivalent CAR T cells specific for all three antigens were developed and tumor-killing was first assessed *in vitro*. Upon coculture with target human glioma cells, secretion of IL-2 and IFNγ were significantly higher upon treatment with trivalent CAR T cells relative to nontransduced T cell controls. In addition, the specific lysis of target cells was significantly greater when co-cultured with trivalent CAR T cells relative to controls. Efficacy was also evaluated using intracranially injected human glioma cells followed by intracranial injection of single CAR T (targeting IL-13Rα2), bivalent CAR T (targeting EphA2 and IL-13Rα2), trivalent CAR T cells (targeting HER2, IL-13Rα2, and EphA2), or nontransduced T cell controls. The authors found the trivalent CAR T cells provided superior anti-tumor efficacy relative to controls [135].

Several other modified CARs have shown increased efficacy relative to their first-generation counterparts. Krenciute *et al.* modified IL-13Rα2-specific CAR T cells to secrete IL-15, a cytokine that promotes activation, proliferation, and cancer cell lysis. Relative to IL-13Rα2 CAR T cells that did not secrete IL-15 (first-generation), these second-generation CAR T cells showed increased lysis of target tumor cells and increased proliferation *in vitro*. In addition, when evaluated *in vivo*, mice treated with the second-generation CAR T cells had significantly increased PFS and OS relative to those treated with the first-generation CAR T cells. The authors found mice that succumbed to the tumor after treatment CAR T cell therapy downregulated the expression of IL-13Rα2 [136].

In the context of neuroblastoma, disialoganglioside (GD2) represents a promising tumor-associated target for CAR T cell therapy. GD2 has been shown to promote malignant phenotypes such as proliferation, migration, and invasion [137]. In a phase I clinical trial, GD2-specific CAR T cells were evaluated in neuroblastoma patients in combination with cyclophosphamide and fludarabine as well as the checkpoint inhibitor, anti-PD-1 [138]. Although the therapy was found to be safe, only modest anti-tumor responses were observed [139]. To improve upon the efficacy of these CAR T cells, Moghimi *et al.* modified GD2-specific CAR T cells to express B7H3 and found enhanced anti-tumor responses both *in vitro* and *in vivo* relative to untreated controls. They go on to determine the enhanced efficacy is likely due to improved metabolic function [140].

Another promising CAR T cell target for brain tumors is CD70. In terms of normal immunology, CD70 is a co-stimulatory molecule expressed in activated immune cells. However, Jin *et al.* found CD70 to be overexpressed in tumor samples isolated from IDH wild-type low-grade glioma and GBM patients [141]. Using a model of high-grade glioma, modified CD70 CAR T cells that express CXCR1 or CXCR2 improved T cell migration to the tumor site. In addition, survival of tumor-bearing mice was improved when treated with CXCR1 or CXCR2 modified CD70 CAR T cells relative to unmodified CD70 CAR T cells [142]. Collectively, these results suggest modified CAR T cells may hold promising anti-tumor responses relative to their first-generation counterparts.

A huge limitation of CAR T cells is the eventual expression of exhaustion molecules, leading to a lack of anti-tumor efficacy. Weber *et al.* recently utilized transient periods of rest using a small molecule as well as dasatinib, a tyrosine kinase inhibitor that inhibits T cell signaling. The authors utilized GD2.CD28ζ CAR T cells in a model of human osteosarcoma. The use of rest in pre-exhausted CAR T cells redirected their fate from a state of exhaustion toward a memory-like state. Furthermore, in T cells that already acquired markers of exhaustion, the use of rest reversed the exhaustion phenotype and caused epigenetic remodeling similar to non-exhausted controls. CAR T cells subjected to intermittent rest through alternating CAR expression or dasatinib-treatment demonstrated superior anti-tumor effects. These findings have profound translational implications to improve therapeutic response using CAR T cells [143].

3.3 Small molecule inhibitor

Myeloid-derived suppressor cells (MDSCs) have been shown to be expanded in the periphery of GBM patients [144]. MDSCs within the TME have been shown to contribute to tumor immunosuppression via the secretion of immunosuppressive molecules such as arginase 1 and inducible nitric oxide synthase (iNOS). Alban *et al.* expanded upon these findings and found the monocytic subset of MDSCs (mMDSCs) express high levels of CD74 and its ligand, macrophage migration inhibitor factor (MIF). They used MN-166, a small molecule inhibitor of phosphodiesterase capable of penetrating the blood-brain barrier to inhibit the CD74/MIF interaction on myeloid cells and therefore prevent mMDSC formation. They found MN-166-treated MDSCs prevented MDSC-mediated T cell suppression. In addition, increased intratumoral $CD8^+$ T cells were found when tumor-bearing mice were treated with MN-166. Despite no difference in survival being observed, the authors suggest this therapy could combine well with activating immunotherapies [145].

Signal transducer and activator of transcription 3 (STAT3) is a transcription factor shown to be upregulated in GBM and is correlated with decreased survival. Wightman *et al.* have shown treatment of GBM cells with IL-6 increased phosphorylation and overall STAT3 expression. The authors used bazedoxifene, a selective estrogen receptor modulator, to inhibit IL-6-mediated STAT3 activation. Importantly, they show treatment of GBM cells with bazedoxifene decreases markers of GSCs, such as SRY-box transcription factor 2 (SOX2) and octamer-binding transcription factor 4 (OCT4). In addition, they demonstrate treatment of tumor-bearing mice with bazedoxifene significantly prolongs survival relative to vehicle-control treated mice [146].

3.4 Gene therapy

Alghamri *et al.* recently published a thorough investigation of mutant versus wild-type IDH (wtIDH) gliomas in both murine and human models. Focusing on the murine data, the authors found wild-type IDH gliomas possessed more suppressive CD11b$^+$Ly6G$^+$ granulocytic MDSCs (gMDSCs) as well as increased PD-L1, iNOS, and Arg1 relative to gMDSCs derived from mutant IDH (mIDH) glioma bearing mice. Furthermore, murine mIDH glioma neurospheres were found to secrete significantly more G-CSF relative to their wtIDH counterparts. This increased secretion was determined to be caused by enrichment of H3K4me3 in the *Csf3* gene, which encodes G-CSF. Finally, when the immune-stimulatory gene therapy herpes simplex virus 1—thymidine kinase/Feline McDonough sarcoma (Fms)—like tyrosine kinase 3 ligand (TK/Flt3L) was used in combination with recombinant G-CSF (rG-CSF) in a wtIDH mouse model, a significant survival benefit was observed relative to TK/Ft3L or rG-CSF alone [147].

3.5 Combination checkpoint inhibition

Tumor-treating fields (TTFs) work as a non-invasive anti-cancer therapy via alternating electric fields. As stated earlier, TTFs are already FDA-approved for GBM in combination with temozolomide. Voloshin *et al.* expanded upon these findings and found TTFs elicited tumor cell death in murine models of lung and colon cancer. In addition, the authors found TTFs could induce maturation of bone marrow-derived DCs. Furthermore, using an orthotopic model of murine lung cancer, the combination of TTFs and the ICI, anti-PD-1, was found to reduce growth relative to control-treated mice. This anti-tumor effect was found to be mediated by the expansion of macrophages, DCs, and CD8$^+$ T cells within the TME. In addition, when subcutaneous colon cancer-bearing mice were treated with anti-PD-1, TTFs, or the combination, a reduction in tumor growth was observed in combination-treated mice relative to controls. Combination-treated mice were found to have a decrease in intratumoral DCs and macrophages but increased CD3$^+$CD4$^+$ and CD3$^+$CD8$^+$ T cells. These results suggest the combination of an ICI such as anti-PD-1 and TTFs could enhance anti-tumor responses in the context of brain tumors [148].

As stated earlier, ICI as monotherapies has had limited success in patients with CNS-derived malignancies. Therefore, several groups are evaluating combinatorial ICI approaches to enhance anti-tumor effects. Flores *et al.* found the combination of lineage-negative hematopoietic stem and progenitor cells (HSPCs) and the ICI, anti-PD-1 provided significantly prolonged survival relative to HSPC or anti-PD-1 monotherapy. The authors found the enhanced survival is likely due to increased secretion of IFNγ by T cells in the TME. In addition, they found the CCR2$^+$ HSPCs were the population responsible for providing the enhanced anti-tumor efficacy. Interestingly, they observed that utilizing CCR2$^+$ HSPCs in the context of an adoptive cellular therapy (ACT) platform, which combines tumor RNA-pulsed DCs, tumor-reactive T cells, and radiotherapy, significantly enhanced survival relative to ACT using bulk lineage-negative HSPCs. These results suggest these CCR2$^+$ HSPCs cells may be combined with various types of immunotherapies to enhance anti-tumor efficacy [149].

Alternatively, Flores-Toro *et al.* identified an expansion of CCR2$^+$ myeloid cells within the TME using two models of intracranial glioma. The authors used a small molecule inhibitor of CCR2, CCX872, in combination with the ICI, anti-PD-1 to enhance survival using a murine model of high-grade glioma as well as a GSC model. They went on to determine this mechanism of anti-tumor efficacy was likely due to a combination of reduced recruitment of Ly6C$^+$ myeloid cells to the TME, an increase in intratumoral $CD4^+$, $CD8^+$, $CD3^+$ $IFN\gamma^+$ cells, and a reduction in $CD8^+$ $TIM3^+$ PD-1^+ T cells relative to vehicle control-treated mice [150].

Finally, Sabbagh *et al.* used novel combinatorial immunotherapy approach to enhance anti-tumor efficacy. They utilized low-intensity pulsed ultrasound (LIPU) to open the BBB for better penetration of various therapeutics. Although LIPU as monotherapy did not provide a robust anti-tumor response, when combined with anti-PD-1, enhanced median survival was observed relative to IgG control-treated mice. In addition, the authors used EGFRvIII-specific CAR T cells in combination with LIPU and found increased trafficking of administered CAR T cells to the TME as well as enhanced survival relative to CAR T cells alone. These results suggest utilizing combinatorial immunotherapeutic approaches with LIPU may lead to enhanced anti-tumor efficacy [151].

4. Conclusions

Malignant brain tumors pose a unique and difficult set of challenges including high tumor heterogeneity and tumor antigen loss, low mutation burden, an immunosuppressive microenvironment, systemic T cell dysfunction, and relative isolation from systemic circulation due to the blood-brain barrier. These overwhelming obstacles have, thus far, limited immunotherapy efficacy. Despite these hurdles, immunotherapies are making incremental advances to overcome these challenges simultaneously [152, 153]. New developments are occurring in the peptide vaccine platforms by the conjugation with toll-like receptor agonists which can enhance activation of DCs to elicit tuned immune responses [154–156]. Studies are also moving forward to focus on targeting multiple antigens simultaneously to combat tumor antigen loss in CAR T therapy [157]. Other groups are working on addressing the immunosuppressive tumor microenvironment and T cell exhaustion with several studies underway in a variety of cancers that combine vaccines and immune checkpoint inhibitors [158]. In the CAR T therapy arena, groups are overcoming T cell exhaustion by knocking out the checkpoint molecules [159, 160], endowing CAR T cells with the capabilities of secreting anti-PD-L1 antibodies [161], and linking the PD-1 extracellular domain to the CD28 intracellular domain to lead to an activation signal instead of inhibition [162, 163]. Other groups are working on overcoming the blood-brain barrier challenge by using laser interstitial thermal therapy or the aforementioned low-intensity pulsed ultrasound to cause local disruption and permeability which may increase trafficking of therapies to the tumor site [151, 164, 165]. These approaches utilizing various combinations and novel technologies may provide solutions to the aforementioned obstacles.

In summary, the next advances in immunotherapies for CNS malignancies will come from enhanced foundational understanding of immune cells and the tumor microenvironment, better mechanistic understandings of current immunotherapy resistance, increased rational combinations of current immunotherapies with complementary mechanisms of action, and novel immunotherapeutic approaches. Together, the above-mentioned clinical studies and novel preclinical work provide an optimistic future in cancer with much-needed improvement in patient survival.

Acknowledgements

This work was supported by the University of Florida Clinical and Translational Science Institute, which is supported in part by the NIH National Center for Advancing Translational Sciences under the award TL1TR001428. NIH funding was also received through the National Cancer Institute (F30CA232641 to MS) (T32CA257923 to BDD) and the National Institute of Neurological Disorders and Stroke (R01NS112315 and R01NS111033 to CF). Additionally, this work was supported by Alex's Lemonade Stand Foundation and the University of Florida MD-PhD Training Program.

Conflict of interest

CF holds interest in iOncologi, Inc., a biotechnology company focused on immuno-oncology. Other authors declare no conflicts of interest.

Notes/thanks/other declarations

We thank all of the patients and their families who participated in the referenced studies that made this work possible and allows us to move the needle forward on patient outcomes.

Author details

Mathew Sebastian, Bayli DiVita Dean and Catherine T. Flores*
Preston A. Wells Jr. Center for Brain Tumor Therapy, Lillian S. Wells Department of Neurosurgery, University of Florida College of Medicine, Gainesville, FL, USA

*Address all correspondence to: cfdrake@ufl.edu

References

[1] Cancer Stat Facts: Brain and Other Nervous System Cancer. 2021. Available from: https://seer.cancer.gov/statfacts/html/brain.html

[2] Gilbert MR, Dignam JJ, Armstrong TS, Wefel JS, Blumenthal DT, Vogelbaum MA, et al. A randomized trial of bevacizumab for newly diagnosed glioblastoma. The New England Journal of Medicine. 2014;**370**(8):699-708

[3] Hegi ME, Diserens AC, Gorlia T, Hamou MF, de Tribolet N, Weller M, et al. MGMT gene silencing and benefit from temozolomide in glioblastoma. The New England Journal of Medicine. 2005;**352**(10):997-1003

[4] Imperato JP, Paleologos NA, Vick NA. Effects of treatment on long-term survivors with malignant astrocytomas. Annals of Neurology. 1990;**28**(6):818-822

[5] Stummer W, Pichlmeier U, Meinel T, Wiestler OD, Zanella F, Reulen HJ, et al. Fluorescence-guided surgery with 5-aminolevulinic acid for resection of malignant glioma: A randomised controlled multicentre phase III trial. The Lancet Oncology. 2006;**7**(5):392-401

[6] Stupp R, Mason WP, van den Bent MJ, Weller M, Fisher B, Taphoorn MJ, et al. Radiotherapy plus concomitant and adjuvant temozolomide for glioblastoma. The New England Journal of Medicine. 2005;**352**(10):987-996

[7] Stupp R, Taillibert S, Kanner A, Read W, Steinberg D, Lhermitte B, et al. Effect of tumor-treating fields plus maintenance temozolomide vs maintenance temozolomide alone on survival in patients with glioblastoma: A randomized clinical trial. Journal of the American Medical Association. 2017;**318**(23):2306-2316

[8] Walker MD, Green SB, Byar DP, Alexander E Jr, Batzdorf U, Brooks WH, et al. Randomized comparisons of radiotherapy and nitrosoureas for the treatment of malignant glioma after surgery. The New England Journal of Medicine. 1980;**303**(23):1323-1329

[9] Esfahani K, Roudaia L, Buhlaiga N, Del Rincon SV, Papneja N, Miller WH Jr. A review of cancer immunotherapy: From the past, to the present, to the future. Current Oncology. 2020;**27**(Suppl 2):S87-S97

[10] Kelly PN. The cancer immunotherapy revolution. Science. 2018;**359**(6382):1344-1345

[11] Palucka K, Banchereau J. Cancer immunotherapy via dendritic cells. Nature Reviews. Cancer. 2012;**12**(4):265-277

[12] Sharpe AH. Introduction to checkpoint inhibitors and cancer immunotherapy. Immunological Reviews. 2017;**276**(1):5-8

[13] Waldman AD, Fritz JM, Lenardo MJ. A guide to cancer immunotherapy: From T cell basic science to clinical practice. Nature Reviews. Immunology. 2020;**20**(11):651-668

[14] Yang Y. Cancer immunotherapy: Harnessing the immune system to battle cancer. The Journal of Clinical Investigation. 2015;**125**(9):3335-3337

[15] Patel AP, Tirosh I, Trombetta JJ, Shalek AK, Gillespie SM, Wakimoto H, et al. Single-cell RNA-seq highlights intratumoral heterogeneity in primary glioblastoma. Science. 2014;**344**(6190):1396-1401

[16] Vogelstein B, Papadopoulos N, Velculescu VE, Zhou S, Diaz LA Jr, Kinzler KW. Cancer genome landscapes. Science. 2013;**339**(6127):1546-1558

[17] Gong D, Shi W, Yi SJ, Chen H, Groffen J, Heisterkamp N. TGFbeta signaling plays a critical role in promoting alternative macrophage activation. BMC Immunology. 2012;**13**:31

[18] Perng P, Lim M. Immunosuppressive mechanisms of malignant gliomas: Parallels at non-CNS sites. Frontiers in Oncology. 2015;**5**:1

[19] Quail DF, Joyce JA. The microenvironmental landscape of brain tumors. Cancer Cell. 2017;**31**(3):326-341

[20] Sampson JH, Gunn MD, Fecci PE, Ashley DM. Brain immunology and immunotherapy in brain tumours. Nature Reviews. Cancer. 2020;**20**(1):12-25

[21] Uyttenhove C, Pilotte L, Theate I, Stroobant V, Colau D, Parmentier N, et al. Evidence for a tumoral immune resistance mechanism based on tryptophan degradation by indoleamine 2,3-dioxygenase. Nature Medicine. 2003;**9**(10):1269-1274

[22] Wainwright DA, Balyasnikova IV, Chang AL, Ahmed AU, Moon KS, Auffinger B, et al. IDO expression in brain tumors increases the recruitment of regulatory T cells and negatively impacts survival. Clinical Cancer Research. 2012;**18**(22):6110-6121

[23] Zhang I, Alizadeh D, Liang J, Zhang L, Gao H, Song Y, et al. Characterization of arginase expression in glioma-associated microglia and macrophages. PLoS One. 2016;**11**(12):e0165118

[24] Gajewski TF, Schreiber H, Fu YX. Innate and adaptive immune cells in the tumor microenvironment. Nature Immunology. 2013;**14**(10):1014-1022

[25] Bechmann I, Galea I, Perry VH. What is the blood-brain barrier (not)? Trends in Immunology. 2007;**28**(1):5-11

[26] Cserr HF, Knopf PM. Cervical lymphatics, the blood-brain barrier and the immunoreactivity of the brain: A new view. Immunology Today. 1992;**13**(12):507-512

[27] Huber JD, Egleton RD, Davis TP. Molecular physiology and pathophysiology of tight junctions in the blood-brain barrier. Trends in Neurosciences. 2001;**24**(12):719-725

[28] Kipnis J. Multifaceted interactions between adaptive immunity and the central nervous system. Science. 2016;**353**(6301):766-771

[29] Tietz S, Engelhardt B. Brain barriers: Crosstalk between complex tight junctions and adherens junctions. The Journal of Cell Biology. 2015;**209**(4):493-506

[30] Saxena M, van der Burg SH, Melief CJM, Bhardwaj N. Therapeutic cancer vaccines. Nature Reviews Cancer. 2021;**21**(6):360-378

[31] Hoang-Minh LB, Mitchell DA. Immunotherapy for brain tumors. Current Treatment Options in Oncology. 2018;**19**(11):60

[32] Phase I Trial of IDH1 Peptide Vaccine in IDH1R132H-mutated Grade III-IV Gliomas (NOA-16). US National Library of Medicine; 2015 [cited 2021]. Available from: https://clinicaltrials.gov/ct2/show/NCT02454634

[33] Platten M, Bunse L, Wick A, Bunse T, Le Cornet L, Harting I, et al. A vaccine targeting mutant IDH1 in newly diagnosed glioma. Nature. 2021; **592**(7854):463-468

[34] Vaccine Therapy and Sargramostim in Treating Patients With Malignant Glioma. US National Library of Medicine; 2010. Available from: https://clinicaltrials.gov/ct2/show/NCT01250470

[35] Fenstermaker RA, Ciesielski MJ, Qiu J, Yang N, Frank CL, Lee KP, et al. Clinical study of a survivin long peptide

vaccine (SurVaxM) in patients with recurrent malignant glioma. Cancer Immunology, Immunotherapy. 2016;**65**(11):1339-1352

[36] Study of Pembrolizumab Plus SurVaxM for Glioblastoma at First Recurrence. US National Library of Medicine; 2019. Available from: https://clinicaltrials.gov/ct2/show/NCT04013672

[37] Ahluwalia MS, Peereboom DM, Ciolfi M, Schilero C, Hobbs B, Ciesielski MJ, et al. Phase II study of pembrolizumab plus SurVaxM for glioblastoma at first recurrence. Journal of Clinical Oncology. 2020; **38**(Suppl 15):TPS2581-TPS

[38] Kijima N, Hosen N, Kagawa N, Hashimoto N, Kinoshita M, Oji Y, et al. Wilms' tumor 1 is involved in tumorigenicity of glioblastoma by regulating cell proliferation and apoptosis. Anticancer Research. 2014;**34**(1a):61-67

[39] Tatsumi N, Oji Y, Tsuji N, Tsuda A, Higashio M, Aoyagi S, et al. Wilms' tumor gene WT1-shRNA as a potent apoptosis-inducing agent for solid tumors. International Journal of Oncology. 2008;**32**(3):701-711

[40] Izumoto S, Tsuboi A, Oka Y, Suzuki T, Hashiba T, Kagawa N, et al. Phase II clinical trial of Wilms tumor 1 peptide vaccination for patients with recurrent glioblastoma multiforme. Journal of Neurosurgery. 2008;**108**(5): 963-971

[41] Jawhari S, Ratinaud MH, Verdier M. Glioblastoma, hypoxia and autophagy: A survival-prone 'menage-a-trois'. Cell Death & Disease. 2016;7:1

[42] Brennan CW, Verhaak RGW, McKenna A, Campos B, Noushmehr H, Salama SR, et al. The somatic genomic landscape of glioblastoma. Cell. 2013;**155**:462. Erratum in:2014;157(3):753

[43] Ramnarain DB, Park S, Lee DY, Hatanpaa KJ, Scoggin SO, Otu H, et al. Differential gene expression analysis reveals generation of an autocrine loop by a mutant epidermal growth factor receptor in glioma cells. Cancer Research. 2006;**66**(2):867-874

[44] Vaccine Therapy in Treating Patients With Newly Diagnosed Glioblastoma Multiforme (ACTIVATe). US National Library of Medicine; 2008 [cited 2021]. Available from: https://clinicaltrials.gov/ct2/show/NCT00643097

[45] Sampson JH, Heimberger AB, Archer GE, Aldape KD, Friedman AH, Friedman HS, et al. Immunologic escape after prolonged progression-free survival with epidermal growth factor receptor variant III peptide vaccination in patients with newly diagnosed glioblastoma. Journal of Clinical Oncology. 2010;**28**(31):4722-4729

[46] Phase III Study of Rindopepimut/GM-CSF in Patients With Newly Diagnosed Glioblastoma (ACT IV). US National Library of Medicine; 2011 [cited 2021]. Available from: https://clinicaltrials.gov/ct2/show/NCT01480479

[47] Weller M, Butowski N, Tran DD, Recht LD, Lim M, Hirte H, et al. Rindopepimut with temozolomide for patients with newly diagnosed, EGFRvIII-expressing glioblastoma (ACT IV): A randomised, double-blind, international phase 3 trial. The Lancet Oncology. 2017;**18**(10):1373-1385

[48] Dutoit V, Herold-Mende C, Hilf N, Schoor O, Beckhove P, Bucher J, et al. Exploiting the glioblastoma peptidome to discover novel tumour-associated antigens for immunotherapy. Brain. 2012;**135**:1042-1054

[49] Phase I/II Trial of IMA950 Multi-peptide Vaccine Plus Poly-ICLC in Glioblastoma. US National Library of

Medicine; 2013 [cited 2021]. Available from: https://clinicaltrials.gov/ct2/show/NCT01920191

[50] Migliorini D, Dutoit V, Allard M, Grandjean Hallez N, Marinari E, Widmer V, et al. Phase I/II trial testing safety and immunogenicity of the multipeptide IMA950/poly-ICLC vaccine in newly diagnosed adult malignant astrocytoma patients. Neuro-Oncology. 2019;**21**(7):923-933

[51] Pembrolizumab in Association With the IMA950/Poly-ICLC for Relapsing Glioblastoma (IMA950-106). US National Library of Medicine; 2018 [cited 2021]. Available from: https://clinicaltrials.gov/ct2/show/NCT03665545

[52] A Pilot Study of Glioma Associated Antigen Vaccines in Conjunction With Poly-ICLC in Pediatric Gliomas. US National Library of Medicine; 2010 [cited 2021]. Available from: https://clinicaltrials.gov/ct2/show/NCT01130077

[53] Pollack IF, Jakacki RI, Butterfield LH, Hamilton RL, Panigrahy A, Potter DM, et al. Antigen-specific immune responses and clinical outcome after vaccination with glioma-associated antigen peptides and polyinosinic-polycytidylic acid stabilized by lysine and carboxymethylcellulose in children with newly diagnosed malignant brainstem and nonbrainstem gliomas. Journal of Clinical Oncology. 2014;**32**(19):2050-2058

[54] Vaccine Therapy in Treating Patients With Malignant Glioma. US National Library of Medicine; 2003 [cited 2021]. Available from: https://clinicaltrials.gov/ct2/show/NCT00068510

[55] Stupp R, Hegi ME, Mason WP, van den Bent MJ, Taphoorn MJ, Janzer RC, et al. Effects of radiotherapy with concomitant and adjuvant temozolomide versus radiotherapy alone on survival in glioblastoma in a randomised phase III study: 5-year analysis of the EORTC-NCIC trial. The Lancet Oncology. 2009;**10**(5):459-466

[56] Prins RM, Soto H, Konkankit V, Odesa SK, Eskin A, Yong WH, et al. Gene expression profile correlates with T-cell infiltration and relative survival in glioblastoma patients vaccinated with dendritic cell immunotherapy. Clinical Cancer Research. 2011;**17**(6):1603-1615

[57] Study of a Drug [DCVax®-L] to Treat Newly Diagnosed GBM Brain Cancer (GBM). US National Library of Medicine; 2002 [cited 2021]. Available from: https://clinicaltrials.gov/ct2/show/NCT00045968

[58] Liau LM, Ashkan K, Tran DD, Campian JL, Trusheim JE, Cobbs CS, et al. First results on survival from a large phase 3 clinical trial of an autologous dendritic cell vaccine in newly diagnosed glioblastoma. Journal of Translational Medicine. 2018;**16**:142

[59] Yu JS, Phuphanich S, Wheeler C, Rudnick J, Mazer M, Wang HQ, et al. Phase I trial of a multi-epitope pulsed dendritic cell vaccine targeting cancer stem cells in patients with newly diagnosed glioblastoma. Journal of Immunotherapy. 2012;**35**(9):747-748

[60] A Study of ICT-107 Immunotherapy in Glioblastoma Multiforme (GBM). US National Library of Medicine; 2011 [cited 2021]. Available from: https://clinicaltrials.gov/ct2/show/NCT01280552

[61] Wen PY, Reardon DA, Armstrong TS, Phuphanich S, Aiken RD, Landolfi JC, et al. A randomized double-blind placebo-controlled phase II trial of dendritic cell vaccine ICT-107 in newly diagnosed patients with glioblastoma. Clinical Cancer Research. 2019;**25**(19):5799-5807

[62] Phase 3 Randomized, Double-blind, Controlled Study of ICT-107 in Glioblastoma. US National Library of

Medicine; 2015 [cited 2021]. Available from: https://clinicaltrials.gov/ct2/show/NCT02546102

[63] Rahman M, Dastmalchi F, Karachi A, Mitchell D. The role of CMV in glioblastoma and implications for immunotherapeutic strategies. Oncoimmunology. 2019;**8**(1):e1514921

[64] Vaccine Therapy in Treating Patients With Newly Diagnosed Glioblastoma Multiforme (ATTAC). US National Library of Medicine; 2008 [cited 2021]. Available from: https://clinicaltrials.gov/ct2/show/NCT00639639

[65] Mitchell DA, Batich KA, Gunn MD, Huang MN, Sanchez-Perez L, Nair SK, et al. Tetanus toxoid and CCL3 improve dendritic cell vaccines in mice and glioblastoma patients. Nature. 2015;**519**(7543):366-369

[66] Batich KA, Reap EA, Archer GE, Sanchez-Perez L, Nair SK, Schmittling RJ, et al. Long-term survival in glioblastoma with cytomegalovirus pp65-targeted vaccination. Clinical Cancer Research. 2017;**23**(8):1898-1909

[67] Vaccine Therapy for the Treatment of Newly Diagnosed Glioblastoma Multiforme (ATTAC-II). US National Library of Medicine; 2015 [cited 2021]. Available from: https://clinicaltrials.gov/ct2/show/NCT02465268

[68] DC Migration Study for Newly-Diagnosed GBM (ELEVATE). US National Library of Medicine; 2015 [cited 2021]. Available from: https://clinicaltrials.gov/ct2/show/NCT02366728

[69] Van Brussel I, Berneman ZN, Cools N. Optimizing dendritic cell-based immunotherapy: Tackling the complexity of different arms of the immune system. Mediators of Inflammation. 2012;**2012**:1-14

[70] Mailliard RB, Wankowicz-Kalinska A, Cai Q, Wesa A, Hilkens CM, Kapsenberg ML, et al. alpha-type-1 polarized dendritic cells: A novel immunization tool with optimized CTL-inducing activity. Cancer Research. 2004;**64**(17):5934-5937

[71] Okada H, Kalinski P, Ueda R, Hoji A, Kohanbash G, Donegan TE, et al. Induction of CD8(+) T-cell responses against novel glioma-associated antigen peptides and clinical activity by vaccinations with alpha-type 1 polarized dendritic cells and polyinosinic-polycytidylic acid stabilized by lysine and carboxymethylcellulose in patients with recurrent malignant glioma. Journal of Clinical Oncology. 2011;**29**(3):330-336

[72] Sprent J, Kishimoto H. The thymus and central tolerance. Philosophical Transactions of the Royal Society of London. Series B, Biological Sciences. 2001;**356**(1409):609-616

[73] Buchbinder EI, Desai A. CTLA-4 and PD-1 pathways similarities, differences, and implications of their inhibition. American Journal of Clinical Oncology. 2016;**39**(1):98-106

[74] Fife BT, Bluestone JA. Control of peripheral T-cell tolerance and autoimmunity via the CTLA-4 and PD-1 pathways. Immunological Reviews. 2008;**224**:166-182

[75] Garon EB, Rizvi NA, Hui RN, Leighl N, Balmanoukian AS, Eder JP, et al. Pembrolizumab for the treatment of non-small-cell lung cancer. The New England Journal of Medicine. 2015;**372**(21):2018-2028

[76] Larkin J, Hodi FS, Wolchok JD. Combined nivolumab and ipilimumab or monotherapy in untreated melanoma REPLY. The New England Journal of Medicine. 2015;**373**(13):1270-1271

[77] Motzer RJ, Escudier B, McDermott DF, George S, Hammers HJ, Srinivas S, et al. Nivolumab versus

everolimus in advanced renal-cell carcinoma. The New England Journal of Medicine. 2015;**373**(19):1803-1813

[78] Robert C, Schachter J, Long GV, Arance A, Grob JJ, Mortier L, et al. Pembrolizumab versus ipilimumab in advanced melanoma. The New England Journal of Medicine. 2015;**372**(26): 2521-2532

[79] Yang KL, Li JR, Bai CM, Sun Z, Zhao L. Efficacy of immune checkpoint inhibitors in non-small-cell lung cancer patients with different metastatic sites: A systematic review and meta-analysis. Frontiers in Oncology. 2020;**10**:1

[80] Tawbi HA, Forsyth PA, Algazi A, Hamid O, Hodi FS, Moschos SJ, et al. Combined nivolumab and ipilimumab in melanoma metastatic to the brain. The New England Journal of Medicine. 2018;**379**(8):722-730

[81] Nduom EK, Wei J, Yaghi NK, Huang N, Kong LY, Gabrusiewicz K, et al. PD-L1 expression and prognostic impact in glioblastoma. Neuro-Oncology. 2016;**18**(2):195-205

[82] Mu LY, Long Y, Yang CL, Jin LC, Tao HP, Ge HT, et al. The IDH1 mutation-induced oncometabolite, 2-hydroxyglutarate, may affect dna methylation and expression of PD-L1 in gliomas. Frontiers in Molecular Neuroscience. 2018;**11**

[83] A Study of the Effectiveness and Safety of Nivolumab Compared to Bevacizumab and of Nivolumab With or Without Ipilimumab in Glioblastoma Patients (CheckMate 143). US National Library of Medicine; 2013. Available from: https://clinicaltrials.gov/ct2/show/NCT02017717

[84] Reardon DA, Brandes AA, Omuro A, Mulholland P, Lim M, Wick A, et al. Effect of nivolumab vs bevacizumab in patients with recurrent glioblastoma: The checkmate 143 phase 3 randomized clinical trial. JAMA Oncology. 2020;**6**(7):1003-1010

[85] An Investigational Immuno-therapy Study of Nivolumab Compared to Temozolomide, Each Given With Radiation Therapy, for Newly-diagnosed Patients With Glioblastoma (GBM, a Malignant Brain Cancer) (CheckMate 498). US National Library of Medicine; 2015 [cited 2021]. Available from: https://clinicaltrials.gov/ct2/show/NCT02617589

[86] Bristol-Myers Squibb Announces Phase 3 CheckMate –498 Study Did Not Meet Primary Endpoint of Overall Survival with Opdivo (nivolumab) Plus Radiation in Patients with Newly Diagnosed MGMT-Unmethylated Glioblastoma Multiforme. 2019. Available from: https://news.bms.com/news/corporate-financial/2019/Bristol-Myers-Squibb-Announces-Phase-3-CheckMate--498-Study-Did-Not-Meet-Primary-Endpoint-of-Overall-Survival-with-Opdivo-nivolumab-Plus-Radiatio-n-in-Patients-with-Newly-Diagnosed-MGMT-Unmethylated-Glioblastoma-Multiforme/default.aspx

[87] An Investigational Immuno-therapy Study of Temozolomide Plus Radiation Therapy With Nivolumab or Placebo, for Newly Diagnosed Patients With Glioblastoma (GBM, a Malignant Brain Cancer) (CheckMate548). US National Library of Medicine; 2016 [cited 2021]. Available from: https://clinicaltrials.gov/ct2/show/NCT02667587

[88] Bristol-Myers Squibb Provides Update on Phase 3 Opdivo (nivolumab) CheckMate –548 Trial in Patients with Newly Diagnosed MGMT-Methylated Glioblastoma Multiforme. 2019. Available from: https://news.bms.com/news/corporate-financial/2019/Bristol-Myers-Squibb-Provides-Update-on-Phase-3-Opdivo-nivolumab-CheckMate--548-Trial-in-Patients-with-Newly-Diagnosed-MGMT-Methylated-Glioblastoma-Multiforme/default.aspx

[89] Keenan TE, Burke KP, Van Allen EM. Genomic correlates of response to immune checkpoint blockade. Nature Medicine. 2019;**25**(3):389-402

[90] Chongsathidkiet P, Jackson C, Koyama S, Loebel F, Cui XY, Farber SH, et al. Sequestration of T cells in bone marrow in the setting of glioblastoma and other intracranial tumors. Nature Medicine. 2018;**24**(9):1459-+

[91] Marin-Acevedo JA, Kimbrough EO, Lou YY. Next generation of immune checkpoint inhibitors and beyond. Journal of Hematology & Oncology. 2021;**14**(1):45

[92] Rayner AA, Grimm EA, Lotze MT, Chu EW, Rosenberg SA. Lymphokine-activated killer (LAK) cells. Analysis of factors relevant to the immunotherapy of human cancer. Cancer. 1985;**55**(6): 1327-1333

[93] Hayes RL, Koslow M, Hiesiger EM, Hymes KB, Hochster HS, Moore EJ, et al. Improved long term survival after intracavitary interleukin-2 and lymphokine-activated killer cells for adults with recurrent malignant glioma. Cancer. 1995;**76**(5):840-852

[94] Dillman RO, Duma CM, Schiltz PM, DePriest C, Ellis RA, Okamoto K, et al. Intracavitary placement of autologous lymphokine-activated killer (LAK) cells after resection of recurrent glioblastoma. Journal of Immunotherapy. 2004;**27**(5):398-404

[95] Dillman RO, Duma CM, Ellis RA, Cornforth AN, Schiltz PM, Sharp SL, et al. Intralesional lymphokine-activated killer cells as adjuvant therapy for primary glioblastoma. Journal of Immunotherapy. 2009;**32**(9):914-919

[96] Wang J, Shen F, Yao Y, Wang LL, Zhu Y, Hu J. Adoptive cell therapy: A novel and potential immunotherapy for glioblastoma. Frontiers in Oncology. 2020;**10**:59

[97] Law TM, Motzer RJ, Mazumdar M, Sell KW, Walther PJ, Oconnell M, et al. Phase-III randomized trial of interleukin-2 with or without lymphokine-activated killer-cells in the treatment of patients with advanced renal-cell carcinoma. Cancer. 1995;**76**(5):824-832

[98] Burger MC, Zhang C, Harter PN, Romanski A, Strassheimer F, Senft C, et al. CAR-engineered nk cells for the treatment of glioblastoma: Turning innate effectors into precision tools for cancer immunotherapy. Frontiers in Immunology. 2019;**10**:2683

[99] Chiossone L, Dumas PY, Vienne M, Vivier E. Natural killer cells and other innate lymphoid cells in cancer. Nature Reviews. Immunology. 2018;**18**(11): 671-688

[100] Ishikawa E, Tsuboi K, Saijo K, Harada H, Takano S, Nose T, et al. Autologous natural killer cell therapy for human recurrent malignant glioma. Anticancer Research. 2004;**24**(3b):1861-1871

[101] Campbell KS, Hasegawa J. Natural killer cell biology: An update and future directions. The Journal of Allergy and Clinical Immunology. 2013;**132**(3):536-544

[102] Cornel AM, Mimpen IL, Nierkens S. MHC class i downregulation in cancer: Underlying mechanisms and potential targets for cancer immunotherapy. Cancers (Basel). 2020;**12**(7):536

[103] Dhatchinamoorthy K, Colbert JD, Rock KL. Cancer immune evasion through loss of mhc class i antigen presentation. Frontiers in Immunology. 2021;**12**:1

[104] Zagzag D, Salnikow K, Chiriboga L, Yee H, Lan L, Ali MA, et al. Downregulation of major histocompatibility complex antigens in

invading glioma cells: Stealth invasion of the brain. Laboratory Investigation. 2005;**85**(3):328-341

[105] Intracranial Injection of NK-92/5.28.z Cells in Patients With Recurrent HER2-positive Glioblastoma (CAR2BRAIN). US National Library of Medicine; 2017 [cited 2021]. Available from: https://clinicaltrials.gov/ct2/show/NCT03383978

[106] Natural Killer Cell (CYNK-001) IV Infusion or IT Administration in Adults With Recurrent GBM (CYNK001GBM01). US National Library of Medicine; 2020. Available from: https://clinicaltrials.gov/ct2/show/NCT04489420

[107] Intra-tumoral Injection of Natural Killer Cells in High-Grade Gliomas (NK HGG). 2020 [cited 2021]. Available from: https://clinicaltrials.gov/ct2/show/NCT04254419

[108] Rosenberg SA, Dudley ME. Cancer regression in patients with metastatic melanoma after the transfer of autologous antitumor lymphocytes. Proceedings of the National Academy of Sciences of the United States of America. 2004;**101**:14639-14645

[109] Maxwell R, Luksik AS, Garzon-Muvdi T, Lim M. The potential of cellular- and viral-based immunotherapies for malignant glioma-dendritic cell vaccines, adoptive cell transfer, and oncolytic viruses. Current Neurology and Neuroscience Reports. 2017;**17**(6):50

[110] Berghoff AS, Kiesel B, Widhalm G, Rajky O, Ricken G, Wohrer A, et al. Programmed death ligand 1 (PD-L1) expression and tumor infiltrating lymphocytes in diffuse and anaplastic gliomas. European Journal of Cancer. 2015;**51**:S593-S

[111] Schuessler A, Smith C, Beagley L, Boyle GM, Rehan S, Matthews K, et al. Autologous t-cell therapy for cytomegalovirus as a consolidative treatment for recurrent glioblastoma. Cancer Research. 2014;**74**(13): 3466-3476

[112] Evaluation of Recovery From Drug-Induced Lymphopenia Using Cytomegalovirus-specific T-cell Adoptive Transfer (ERaDICATe). US National Library of Medicine; 2008 [cited 2021]. Available from: https://clinicaltrials.gov/ct2/show/NCT00693095

[113] Reap EA, Suryadevara CM, Batich KA, Sanchez-Perez L, Archer GE, Schmittling RJ, et al. Dendritic cells enhance polyfunctionality of adoptively transferred t cells that target cytomegalovirus in glioblastoma. Cancer Research. 2018;**78**(1):256-264

[114] Maus MV, Grupp SA, Porter DL, June CH. Antibody-modified T cells: CARs take the front seat for hematologic malignancies. Blood. 2014;**123**(17): 2625-2635

[115] Autologous T Cells Redirected to EGFRVIII-With a Chimeric Antigen Receptor in Patients With EGFRVIII+ Glioblastoma. US National Library of Medicine; 2014 [cited 2021]. Available from: https://clinicaltrials.gov/ct2/show/NCT02209376

[116] O'Rourke DM, Nasrallah MP, Desai A, Melenhorst JJ, Mansfield K, Morrissette JJD, et al. A single dose of peripherally infused EGFRvIII-directed CAR T cells mediates antigen loss and induces adaptive resistance in patients with recurrent glioblastoma. Science Translational Medicine. 2017;**9**(399):1-15

[117] Zhang JG, Eguchi J, Kruse CA, Gomez GG, Fakhrai H, Schroter S, et al. Antigenic profiling of glioma cells to generate allogeneic vaccines or dendritic cell-based therapeutics. Clinical Cancer Research. 2007;**13**(2 Pt 1):566-575

[118] Schlegel J, Stumm G, Brandle K, Merdes A, Mechtersheimer G, Hynes NE, et al. Amplification and differential expression of members of the erbB-gene family in human glioblastoma. Journal of Neuro-Oncology. 1994;**22**(3):201-207

[119] Koka V, Potti A, Forseen SE, Pervez H, Fraiman GN, Koch M, et al. Role of Her-2/neu overexpression and clinical determinants of early mortality in glioblastoma multiforme. American Journal of Clinical Oncology. 2003;**26**(4):332-335

[120] Andersson U, Guo D, Malmer B, Bergenheim AT, Brannstrom T, Hedman H, et al. Epidermal growth factor receptor family (EGFR, ErbB2-4) in gliomas and meningiomas. Acta Neuropathologica. 2004;**108**(2): 135-142

[121] CMV-specific Cytotoxic T Lymphocytes Expressing CAR Targeting HER2 in Patients With GBM (HERT-GBM). US National Library of Medicine; 2010 [cited 2021]. Available from: https://clinicaltrials.gov/ct2/show/NCT01109095

[122] Ahmed N, Brawley V, Hegde M, Bielamowicz K, Kalra M, Landi D, et al. HER2-specific chimeric antigen receptor-modified virus-specific t cells for progressive glioblastoma a phase 1 dose-escalation trial. JAMA Oncology. 2017;**3**(8):1094-1101

[123] Taal W, Oosterkamp HM, Walenkamp AM, Dubbink HJ, Beerepoot LV, Hanse MC, et al. Single-agent bevacizumab or lomustine versus a combination of bevacizumab plus lomustine in patients with recurrent glioblastoma (BELOB trial): A randomised controlled phase 2 trial. The Lancet Oncology. 2014;**15**(9):943-953

[124] Debinski W, Gibo DM. Molecular expression analysis of restrictive receptor for interleukin 13, a brain tumor-associated cancer/testis antigen. Molecular Medicine. 2000;**6**(5):440-449

[125] Thaci B, Brown CE, Binello E, Werbaneth K, Sampath P, Sengupta S. Significance of interleukin-13 receptor alpha 2-targeted glioblastoma therapy. Neuro-Oncology. 2014;**16**(10): 1304-1312

[126] Brown CE, Badie B, Barish ME, Weng L, Ostberg JR, Chang WC, et al. Bioactivity and safety of IL13Ralpha2-redirected chimeric antigen receptor CD8+ T cells in patients with recurrent glioblastoma. Clinical Cancer Research. 2015;**21**(18):4062-4072

[127] Cellular Adoptive Immunotherapy Using Genetically Modified T-Lymphocytes in Treating Patients With Recurrent or Refractory High-Grade Malignant Glioma. US National Library of Medicine; 2008 [cited 2021]. Available from: https://clinicaltrials.gov/ct2/show/NCT00730613

[128] Genetically Modified T-cells in Treating Patients With Recurrent or Refractory Malignant Glioma. US National Library of Medicine; 2014 [cited 2021]. Available from: https://clinicaltrials.gov/ct2/show/NCT02208362

[129] Brown CE, Alizadeh D, Starr R, Weng LH, Wagner JR, Naranjo A, et al. Regression of glioblastoma after chimeric antigen receptor t-cell therapy. The New England Journal of Medicine. 2016;**375**(26):2561-2569

[130] Liu GN, Rui W, Zhao XQ, Lin X. Enhancing CAR-T cell efficacy in solid tumors by targeting the tumor microenvironment. Cellular & Molecular Immunology. 2021;**18**(5):1085-1095

[131] Vora P, Venugopal C, Salim SK, Tatari N, Bakhshinyan D, Singh M, et al. The rational development of CD133-targeting immunotherapies for glioblastoma. Cell Stem Cell. 2020;**26**(6):832-844, e6

[132] Shaim H, Shanley M, Basar R, Daher M, Gumin J, Zamler DB, et al. Targeting the alphav integrin/TGF-beta axis improves natural killer cell function against glioblastoma stem cells. The Journal of Clinical Investigation. 2021;**131**(14):1

[133] Majzner RG, Mackall CL. Clinical lessons learned from the first leg of the CAR T cell journey. Nature Medicine. 2019;**25**(9):1341-1355

[134] Sterner RC, Sterner RM. CAR-T cell therapy: Current limitations and potential strategies. Blood Cancer Journal. 2021;**11**(4):69

[135] Bielamowicz K, Fousek K, Byrd TT, Samaha H, Mukherjee M, Aware N, et al. Trivalent CAR T cells overcome interpatient antigenic variability in glioblastoma. Neuro-Oncology. 2018;**20**(4):506-518

[136] Krenciute G, Prinzing BL, Yi Z, Wu MF, Liu H, Dotti G, et al. Transgenic expression of IL15 improves antiglioma activity of IL13Ralpha2-CAR T cells but results in antigen loss variants. Cancer Immunology Research. 2017;**5**(7):571-581

[137] Nazha B, Inal C, Owonikoko TK. Disialoganglioside GD2 expression in solid tumors and role as a target for cancer therapy. Frontiers in Oncology. 2020;**10**:1000

[138] 3rd Generation GD-2 Chimeric Antigen Receptor and iCaspase Suicide Safety Switch, Neuroblastoma, GRAIN (GRAIN). US National Library of Medicine; 2013 [cited 2021]. Available from: https://clinicaltrials.gov/ct2/show/NCT01822652

[139] Heczey A, Louis CU, Savoldo B, Dakhova O, Durett A, Grilley B, et al. CAR T cells administered in combination with lymphodepletion and PD-1 inhibition to patients with neuroblastoma. Molecular Therapy. 2017;**25**(9):2214-2224

[140] Moghimi B, Muthugounder S, Jambon S, Tibbetts R, Hung L, Bassiri H, et al. Preclinical assessment of the efficacy and specificity of GD2-B7H3 SynNotch CAR-T in metastatic neuroblastoma. Nature Communications. 2021;**12**(1):511

[141] Jin L, Ge H, Long Y, Yang C, Chang YE, Mu L, et al. CD70, a novel target of CAR T-cell therapy for gliomas. Neuro-Oncology. 2018;**20**(1):55-65

[142] Jin L, Tao H, Karachi A, Long Y, Hou AY, Na M, et al. CXCR1- or CXCR2-modified CAR T cells co-opt IL-8 for maximal antitumor efficacy in solid tumors. Nature Communications. 2019;**10**(1):4016

[143] Weber EW, Parker KR, Sotillo E, Lynn RC, Anbunathan H, Lattin J, et al. Transient rest restores functionality in exhausted CAR-T cells through epigenetic remodeling. Science. 2021;**372**(6537):49

[144] Raychaudhuri B, Rayman P, Ireland J, Ko J, Rini B, Borden EC, et al. Myeloid-derived suppressor cell accumulation and function in patients with newly diagnosed glioblastoma. Neuro-Oncology. 2011;**13**(6):591-599

[145] Alban TJ, Bayik D, Otvos B, Rabljenovic A, Leng L, Jia-Shiun L, et al. Glioblastoma myeloid-derived suppressor cell subsets express differential macrophage migration inhibitory factor receptor profiles that can be targeted to reduce immune suppression. Frontiers in Immunology. 2020;**11**:1191

[146] Wightman SM, Alban TJ, Chen X, Lathia JD, Wang Y, Stark GR. Bazedoxifene inhibits sustained STAT3 activation and increases survival in GBM. Translational Oncology. 2021;**14**(11):101192

[147] Alghamri MS, McClellan BL, Avvari RP, Thalla R, Carney S, Hartlage MS, et al. G-CSF secreted by

mutant IDH1 glioma stem cells abolishes myeloid cell immunosuppression and enhances the efficacy of immunotherapy. Science Advances. 2021;7(40):eabh3243

[148] Voloshin T, Kaynan N, Davidi S, Porat Y, Shteingauz A, Schneiderman RS, et al. Tumor-treating fields (TTFields) induce immunogenic cell death resulting in enhanced antitumor efficacy when combined with anti-PD-1 therapy. Cancer Immunology, Immunotherapy. 2020;**69**(7):1191-1204

[149] Flores CT, Wildes TJ, Drake JA, Moore GL, Dean BD, Abraham RS, et al. Lin(−)CCR2(+) hematopoietic stem and progenitor cells overcome resistance to PD-1 blockade. Nature Communications. 2018;**9**(1):4313

[150] Flores-Toro JA, Luo D, Gopinath A, Sarkisian MR, Campbell JJ, Charo IF, et al. CCR2 inhibition reduces tumor myeloid cells and unmasks a checkpoint inhibitor effect to slow progression of resistant murine gliomas. Proceedings of the National Academy of Sciences of the United States of America. 2020;**117**(2):1129-1138

[151] Sabbagh A, Beccaria K, Ling X, Marisetty A, Ott M, Caruso H, et al. Opening of the blood-brain barrier using low-intensity pulsed ultrasound enhances responses to immunotherapy in preclinical glioma models. Clinical Cancer Research. 2021;**27**(15):4325-4337

[152] Srivastava S, Riddell SR. Chimeric antigen receptor T cell therapy: Challenges to bench-to-bedside efficacy. Journal of Immunology. 2018;**200**(2):459-468

[153] van der Burg SH, Arens R, Ossendorp F, van Hall T, Melief CJ. Vaccines for established cancer: Overcoming the challenges posed by immune evasion. Nature Reviews. Cancer. 2016;**16**(4):219-233

[154] van der Burg SH, Bijker MS, Welters MJ, Offringa R, Melief CJ. Improved peptide vaccine strategies, creating synthetic artificial infections to maximize immune efficacy. Advanced Drug Delivery Reviews. 2006;**58**(8): 916-930

[155] Zom GG, Khan S, Filippov DV, Ossendorp F. TLR ligand-peptide conjugate vaccines: Toward clinical application. Advances in Immunology. 2012;**114**:177-201

[156] Wen Y, Collier JH. Supramolecular peptide vaccines: Tuning adaptive immunity. Current Opinion in Immunology. 2015;**35**:73-79

[157] Grada Z, Hegde M, Byrd T, Shaffer DR, Ghazi A, Brawley VS, et al. TanCAR: A novel bispecific chimeric antigen receptor for cancer immunotherapy. Molecular Therapy: Nucleic Acids. 2013;**2**:e105

[158] Collins JM, Redman JM, Gulley JL. Combining vaccines and immune checkpoint inhibitors to prime, expand, and facilitate effective tumor immunotherapy. Expert Review of Vaccines. 2018;**17**(8):697-705

[159] Ren J, Liu X, Fang C, Jiang S, June CH, Zhao Y. Multiplex genome editing to generate universal CAR T cells resistant to PD1 inhibition. Clinical Cancer Research. 2017;**23**(9):2255-2266

[160] Rupp LJ, Schumann K, Roybal KT, Gate RE, Ye CJ, Lim WA, et al. CRISPR/Cas9-mediated PD-1 disruption enhances anti-tumor efficacy of human chimeric antigen receptor T cells. Scientific Reports. 2017;**7**(1):737

[161] Suarez ER, de Change K, Sun J, Sui J, Freeman GJ, Signoretti S, et al. Chimeric antigen receptor T cells secreting anti-PD-L1 antibodies more effectively regress renal cell carcinoma in a humanized mouse model. Oncotarget. 2016;7(23):34341-34355

[162] Liu X, Ranganathan R, Jiang S, Fang C, Sun J, Kim S, et al. A chimeric

switch-receptor targeting PD1 augments the efficacy of second-generation CAR T cells in advanced solid tumors. Cancer Research. 2016;**76**(6):1578-1590

[163] Prosser ME, Brown CE, Shami AF, Forman SJ, Jensen MC. Tumor PD-L1 co-stimulates primary human CD8(+) cytotoxic T cells modified to express a PD1:CD28 chimeric receptor. Molecular Immunology. 2012;**51**(3-4):263-272

[164] Salehi A, Paturu MR, Patel B, Cain MD, Mahlokozera T, Yang AB, et al. Therapeutic enhancement of blood-brain and blood-tumor barriers permeability by laser interstitial thermal therapy. Neuro-Oncology Advances. 2020;**2**(1):vdaa071

[165] Leuthardt EC, Duan C, Kim MJ, Campian JL, Kim AH, Miller-Thomas MM, et al. Hyperthermic laser ablation of recurrent glioblastoma leads to temporary disruption of the peritumoral blood brain barrier. PLoS One. 2016;**11**(2):e0148613

Chapter 8

Crossing Blood-Brain Barrier with Nano-drug Carriers for Treatment of Brain Tumors: Advances and Unmet Challenges

Sukanya Bhunia and Arabinda Chaudhuri

Abstract

Blood-brain barrier (BBB), a unique membrane barrier formed by closely stitched brain capillary endothelial cells (BCEC) with tight cellular junctions, separates brain from the circulating blood to protect it from bloodborne pathogens. BBB greatly limits the entry of chemotherapeutics to brain, and in consequence, it is a major obstacle for treating brain tumor. Advances in designing efficient nano-drug carriers are opening new avenues for overcoming this uphill systemic challenge. This book chapter describes current understanding of nanocarriers-mediated noninvasive drug targeting to brain tumor. Design principles behind the construction of the most promising recently designed receptor and transporter selective nano-drug carriers for combating brain tumors have been highlighted.

Keywords: blood-brain barrier, brain tumor, nanocarrier, drug delivery, nanomedicine

1. Introduction

Gliomas are the deadliest primary central nervous system (CNS) neoplasms arising from rapid proliferation of glial cells, the non-neuronal cells present in brain. Based on histopathologic features and progression of the disease, gliomas are classified by WHO into four grades: grade I (pilocytic astrocytoma), grade II (astrocytomas and oligodendrogliomas), grade III (anaplastic astrocytomas and oligodendrogliomas), and grade IV (glioblastoma multiforme). The low-grade (I and II) glial tumors often evolved with time into high-grade (grade IV) glioblastoma multiforme (GBM). However, irrespective of their grading, glial tumors almost invariably exhibit marked infiltrative growth pattern with tumor cells traveling long distances away from their origin into the surrounding healthy brain tissue. Furthermore, they are highly proliferative along with their significant angiogenic potential and resistance to apoptosis. GBM has a median survival of 14–17 months post diagnosis and only 3–5% survivability beyond 5 years. Current standard of care to treat gliomas includes safe surgical resection of the tumor followed by radiotherapy and chemotherapy. Despite significant advances in the cancer treatment, therapeutic success against gliomas remained an unmet challenge mainly because of their diffusive infiltrating growth pattern with rapid proliferation rate and physiological location, which made them difficult to cure completely either by surgical excision or application of radiotherapy/chemotherapy [1, 2]. More often than not rapid recurrence of tumor ensues. Poor drug accumulation in glioblastoma tissue, unfavorable pharmacokinetic behavior, and toxicity to off-target organs are retarding the clinical success of systemic chemotherapy of glioblastoma.

1.1 Physiology and anatomy of human brain

Toward developing an effective therapeutic strategy for combating glioblastoma, a basic understanding of brain physiology is very important. Brain is an integral part of the central nervous system. Primary brain cells include equal number of neuron and glial cells [3]. Where neurons connect different body parts by transmitting information, glial cells provide structural support and protection to the neurons. Both cells together organize into specialized structures, which can be classified as gray matter (dominated by cell bodies) and white matter (dominated by axons). The three major subdivisions of human brain are the cerebrum, cerebellum, and the brain stem (**Figure 1**) [4]. The largest part cerebrum is divided into the right and left hemispheres along the mid-sagittal plane. These hemispheres are made up of an outer layer of gray matter named as the cerebral cortex responsible for language and information processing. Cerebral cortex cells communicate with each other and with the spinal cord via the underlying cerebral white matter. Communication between the two cerebral hemispheres primarily occurs via a major white matter tract called the corpus callosum. The cerebellum contains a similar kind of gray and white matter organization but at a smaller scale. It functions primarily to control balance and coordinated movement. The brain stem, responsible for involuntary functions such as heart rate and breathing, connects the brain to the spinal cord. It also contains both gray and white matter regions. However, unlike in cerebrum and cerebellum, they are not organized into inner and outer layers. Most of the brain tumors occur in the parenchymal space of the cerebrum [5]. However, getting drugs into the brain is much more difficult than that into other body tissues as brain tissue is highly protected both externally and internally. Skull externally protects brain tissue and regulates intracranial tissue pressure by constraining the volume [6], which limits the regional mode of drug delivery to brain. Brain is internally protected by the blood-brain barrier (BBB), which prevents random entry of

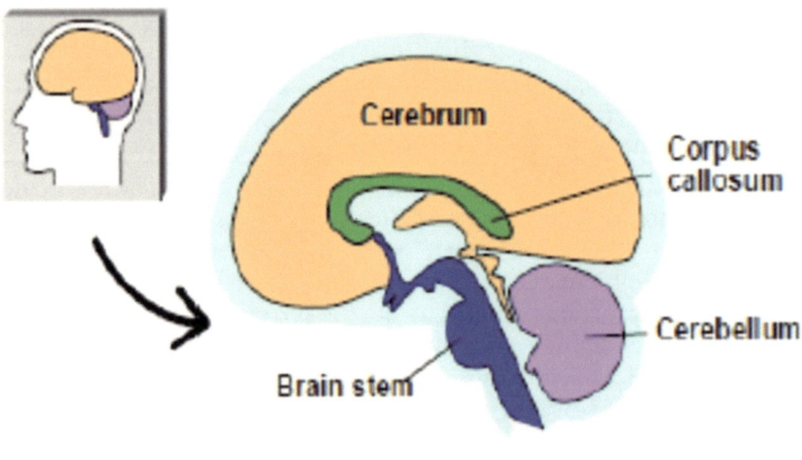

Figure 1.
Basic anatomy of human brain; cerebrum, cerebellum, and brain stem are the three major subdivisions of human brain.

molecules from blood circulation into brain tissue making delivery of systemically administered drugs to brain an arduous task.

1.2 Blood-brain barrier (BBB)

Blood-brain barrier (BBB) is a highly selective and protective membrane barrier that separates the central nervous system (CNS) and prevents entry of random substances from circulating blood to CNS. It protects brain from bloodborne pathogens and maintains the homeostatic regulation of the brain microenvironment [7, 8]. The presence of BBB was first presumed in 1885 when the German bacteriologist Paul Ehrlich found no trace of a water-soluble aniline dye in the brain and cerebrospinal fluid (CSF) after injecting it in the peripheral circulation while it was found in other organ. It was initially assumed that the dye has bonding affinity toward other organ except the brain and CNS [9]. However, in 1913 when E. Goldman, a student of Ehrlich, repeated the same experiment and performed additional experiment by injecting the dye into CSF of dogs, the presence of dye was found in the CNS including brain and the spinal cord only when it is injected in CSF of dogs [10]. Then it strengthened the hypothesis, previously suggested by Bield, Kraus, and Lewandowsky, that there must be a barrier that is preventing the transfer of dyes between blood and brain [7]. In 1937, after the invention of the scanning electron microscopy (SEM), the actual membrane barrier was observed.

The BBB is primarily composed of a continuous layer of brain capillary endothelial cells (BCEC) securely interconnected by tight junctions and adherens junctions, a basement membrane, pericytes, and perivascular astrocyte end-foot processes. The BCEC cells are highly interconnect via tight junction to form a thin wall-like structure (~200 nm), which is from the luminal side (BBB facing blood), covered by heparan sulfate proteoglycans, laminin, collagen type IV, and other extracellular matrix proteins. In comparison with the endothelial cells at the peripheral micro-vessel, BCEC differs in majorly two ways. Firstly, due to the presence of tight junction, the connection between endothelial cells at BBB is ~50–100 times tighter than endothelial cells at the peripheral micro-vessel wall, and there is no fenestration in BBB [11–13]. In addition, BBB endothelial cells have very few pinocytotic vesicles unlike endothelial cells in the rest of the body. As a consequence, transport of nutrients from the blood to the brain requires energy-dependent active transport pathway indicating the presence of ~5–6 times more mitochondria. BBB endothelial cells offer an enzymatic barrier due to the presence of proteolytic enzymes including c-glutamyl transpeptidase, alkaline phosphatase, and aromatic acid decarboxylase [14]. This enzymatic barrier has the capability to break down the neuroactive bloodborne solutes and drugs. The pericytes are covering 20% of the outer surface of endothelial cells. The primary function of pericytes is to form two basal laminas (BL1 and BL2) together with the smooth muscle. The BL1 is the distinct extracellular space between endothelial cells and pericytes, whereas BL2 is the extracellular matrix between pericytes and the glial end feet bounding the brain parenchyma. They are responsible for the regulation of the blood flow in the brain capillary through contraction and relaxation. Astrocytes are a type of glial cells in the CNS with an important role in BBB. The end feet of astrocytes form a complex supporting network surrounding the endothelial cells, which connects endothelial cells with neurons and microglia [15]. This complex network structure of astrocyte end feet is essential for proper function of BBB. Astrocytes can also enhance the level of tight junction proteins, which is crucial for the structural integrity and low permeability of BBB [16]. Moreover, it protects BBB from oxidative stress by inducing anti-oxidative activity in the endothelial cells.

Other than the role in BBB, astrocytes are also essential for maintaining brain homeostasis, injury protection, clearing of synapses. For all the versatile roles, astrocytes are considered as the primary workhorse of the CNS [17].

Other two notable cellular components of BBB are basement membranes and microglia. Basement membranes are composed of extracellular matrix proteins. It provides structural support for endothelial cells and separates themselves from the inner brain tissue [18]. Microglia are a subtype of monocyte cells present throughout the brain and spinal cord [19]. They primarily help in immune defense and maintaining CNS [20]. In addition, current evidence indicates that the activated microglia can enhance the expression of tight junctions, which helps in maintaining the integrity and proper function of BBB [21].

Other than the cellular component in BBB, there exists three types of intercellular junctions, which are responsible for the extremely tight connection between two neighboring endothelial cells: tight junction, adherens junction, and gap junction (**Figure 2**). Tight junctions are formed by many transmembrane proteins and cytoplasmic proteins. Junction adhesion molecules (JAMs), occludins, and claudins are some examples of transmembrane proteins, whereas cytoplasmic proteins include zonula occludins (ZO), cingulin, afadin, calcium/calmodulin-dependent serine protein kinase (CASK), etc. JAM proteins in BBB are expressed by endothelial

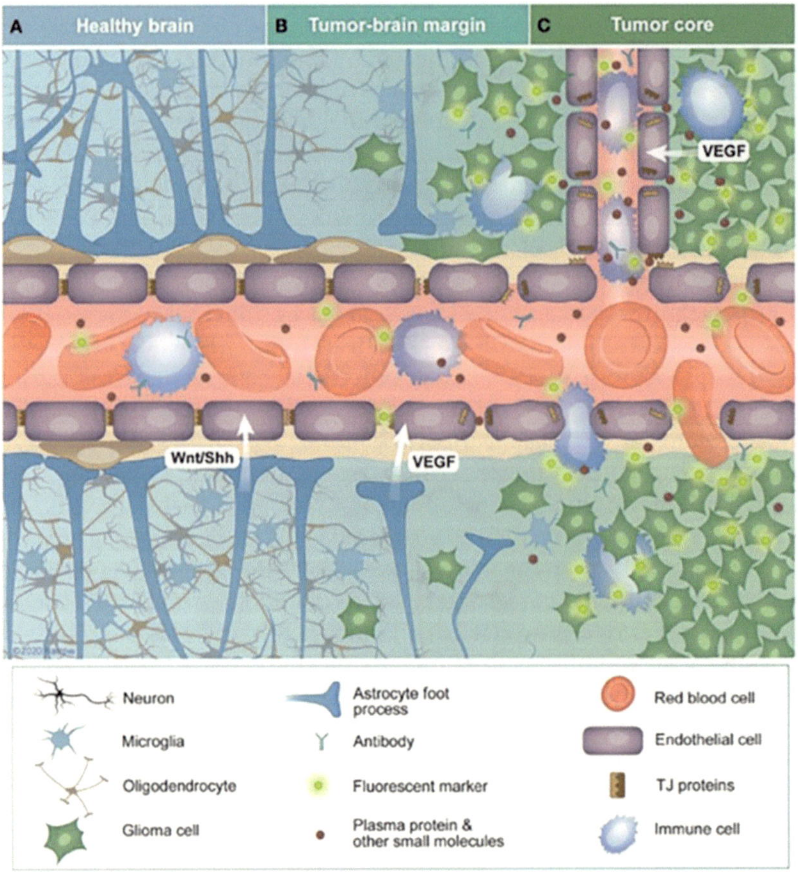

Figure 2.
Characteristics of the blood-brain (BBB) in healthy and glioma bearing brain (blood-brain tumor barriers). (A) Healthy BBB selectively permits entry of solute from blood circulation to brain parenchyma, (B) in tumor margin zone, tight junctions become weak, tumor cells penetrate or rupture BBB, (C) at tumor core, BBB structure is greatly disrupted (adopted from Ref. [22]).

cells and also expressed by leukocytes and platelets. They are highly localized on the tight junctions of BBB [23, 24] and control endothelium permeability, leukocytes migration, and cell polarity [25]. The extracellular domain of JAMs mediates the adhesive interaction between the endothelial cell and platelets as well as interaction with the leukocytes, whereas the cytoplasmic domain of JAMs interacts with various tight junction associated proteins such as ZO-1 and AF-622 [24, 25]. Claudins and occludins are the most crucial transmembrane proteins in the tight junctions of BBB [15, 26]. Claudins are small transmembrane proteins of ~27 kDa at the BBB. The extracellular domains of claudins built the tight junctions among adjacent endothelial cells and seal the paracellular cleft, whereas its intracellular parts connect to the actin filaments. Another type of transmembrane protein is occludin, which is expressed by brain microvascular endothelial cells and exclusively localized at the tight junctions. Occludins have similar function of claudins [27] (**Figure 3**). Besides these abovementioned transmembrane proteins, several other cytoplasmic proteins also contribute to constituting the intact tight junction structures.

Adherens junction is another type of junction that is crucial for the structural integrity of interendothelial cell connections and proper assembly of tight junction proteins. Any alteration of the adherens junction leads to the BBB disruption [29]. Gap junction is newly invented junction located between the tight and the adherens junction. Structurally it is an intercellular channel that connects to endothelial cells. Gap junctions allow the exchange of ions, small metabolites, and metabolic signals between adjacent endothelial cells in BBB and thereby play crucial role of maintaining tissue homeostasis in BBB [30]. In addition, gap junction also regulates permeability of BBB by interacting with scaffolding proteins ZO-1 via afadin-6 protein. Overall, the presence of tight junctions between endothelial cells significantly

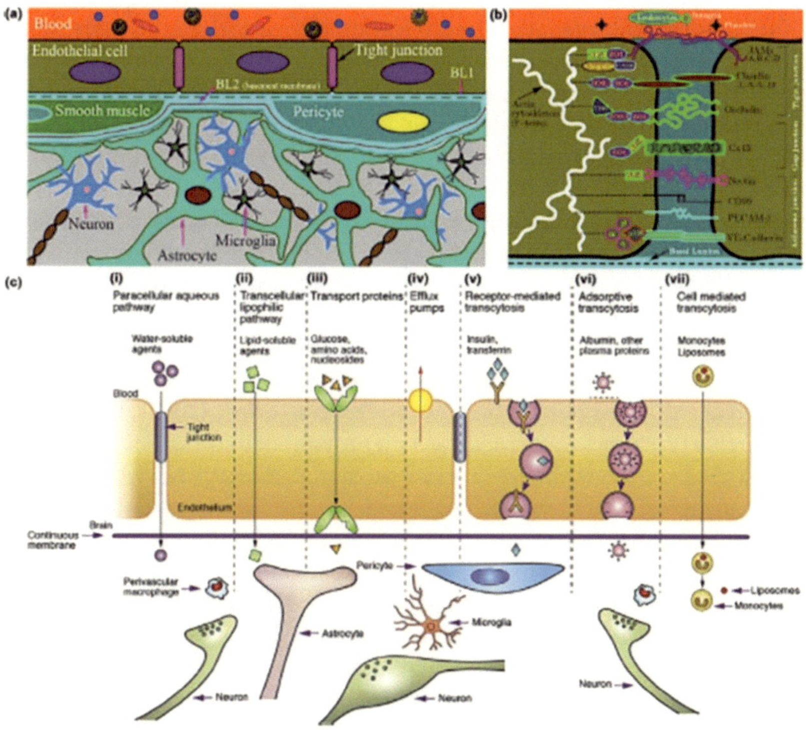

Figure 3.
(a) The cellular components of BBB; (b) structure of junctions at the BBB; (c) transport routes across the BBB (adopted from Ref. [28] with permission).

restricts the random exchange of substances through the BBB. Also, x there exists high electrical resistance (1500–2000 Ω cm^2) between the endothelial cells caused by the encapsulation of capillaries by the astrocytes and pericytes [31].

In the presence of a primary or secondary brain tumor, structural integrity of BBB is disrupted during tumor progression and then the BBB in glioma-bearing brain is named as the blood-tumor barrier (BTB) [32]. BTB is characterized by loss of junctional proteins in endothelial cells, loss of astrocytic end feet and neuronal connections, aberrant distribution of pericytes, and tumor vascularization, which greatly hampered the structural integrity of BBB with progression of glioma [33, 34]. The compromised structural integrity in BTB allows circulating immune cells, e.g., T cell and peripheral monocytes to enter in brain tumor area [35]. Notably, although BBB is disrupted at the tumor core, it may retain its characteristics intact in other area of brain and still act as barrier there. For instance, with an average-size tumor about 10% may have open junction and 30% may have fenestrations, which permits 330 kDa or smaller nanoparticles (NPs) through it [36, 37]. BTB retains the characteristics of expressing efflux transporters in endothelial cells and tumor cells and often exhibits higher expression of some receptors favoring the tumor growth such as GLUT1 and BCRP [38].

1.3 Crossing the bar: transport pathways across the blood-brain barrier

Current approaches of drug delivery to brain include regional and systemic mode of delivery. In regional mode of delivery, therapeutics are directly injected (intracranial injection) into the brain by stereotactic surgery. However, this method results only in localized delivery of drug around the injection site with limited penetration into the brain parenchymal space. Moreover, stereotactic surgery of brain involves drilling of the skull, which is too invasive for human therapy. Systemic mode of delivery via intravenous administration is the ideal noninvasive therapeutic modality to deliver chemotherapeutics into the brain. Rich vascularity of the brain, with blood capillaries spreading virtually throughout all the brain cells, enables efficient assimilation of chemotherapeutic agents into the brain parenchyma provided the therapeutics could cross the BBB [39]. A great deal of effort, therefore, is presently focused on development of BBB-permeable therapeutics. Recent trends to overcome BBB are directed toward exploitation of some active transporter expressed in BBB for supplying nutrients to maintain brain homeostasis. The transports of molecules across BBB can be broadly classified into two ways, passive transport and active transport (**Figure 4**). The passive transport is nonspecific and energy (ATP)-independent process, for example, diffusional transport via paracellular or transcellular transcytosis and passive accumulation of drugs in tumor vasculature via enhanced permeability and retention effect (EPR). On the other hand, the active transport routes such as receptor-mediated transcytosis (RMT), carrier-mediated transcytosis, adsorption-mediated transcytosis (AMT), and cell-mediated transcytosis, all of which require adenosine triphosphate (ATP).

In paracellular diffusion, solute molecules enter the brain through the space between two adjacent endothelial cells. Only aqua-soluble small molecule with molecular weight less than 500 Da can pass through the paracellular space driven by the negative concentration gradient from blood to brain [41]. Modulation in the tight junction can enhance paracellular diffusion rate although it may expose brain parenchyma to unwanted substances [42]. In transcellular diffusion, the solute particles diffuse through the endothelial cells from blood to brain driven by negative concentration gradient similarly. However, for transcellular diffusion, the solutes should be non-ionized, with desirable hydrophilicity and lipid solubility. For instance, steroid and hormones cross BBB via transcellular diffusion.

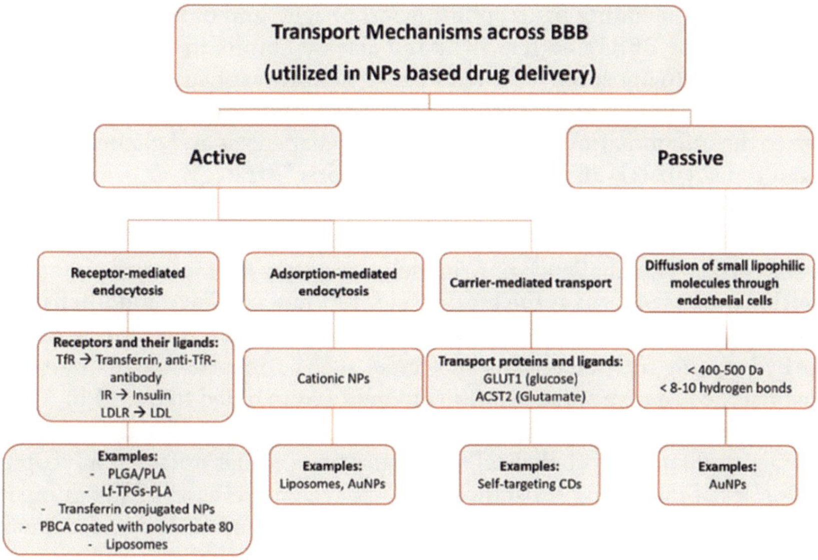

Figure 4.
Different types of transport pathway across BBB (adopted from Ref. [40] with permission).

Among active transport systems, receptor-mediated transcytosis (RMT), where the particles cross BBB by using the receptors expressed on apical surface of the BBB endothelial cells, is an important pathway for transporting drugs to the brain. Currently, it is widely being used for nanocarrier-mediated targeting of drug to the brain. The mechanism of RMT relies on endocytosis where the ligand specifically binds to the receptor followed by formation of an intracellular vesicle via membrane invagination. The membrane invagination occurs either via clathrin or via caveolae-mediated mechanism. In both cases, after vesicle formation, the vesicles are detached from the membrane and trafficked to three different fates. The major portion is directed to the basolateral membrane, fuses, and releases their payload, whereas some vesicles are recycled to the apical side, and some other undergoes lysosomal degradation. Transferrin receptors, low-density lipoprotein receptors, lactoferrin receptors, etc., are some of the most commonly targeted receptors for drug delivery to brain tumor.

Carrier-mediated transcytosis or transporter-mediated transcytosis is another active transport mechanism across BBB. Nutrients such as glucose, amino acids, etc., are transported via specific transporter protein. In this process, nutrient molecule first binds to the specific transporter at the blood side and then the transporter protein undergoes some conformational changes to transfer the nutrients molecules into the brain side. Large amino-acid transporter (LAT) and glucose transporter isoform (GLUT-1) are examples of such transporter. High specificity of the ligand-transporter interaction of this process limits its applicability in transporting large-molecular drugs.

Charged nanoparticles or macromolecules generally cross BBB via adsorption-mediated transcytosis (AMT), which uses the electrostatic interaction between the positively charged nanocarriers and the negatively charged cell surface of endothelial cells facing blood side. In this process, the interactions are nonspecific, and many nanoparticles can be delivered. However, this nonspecific method of nanoparticles transport may also lead to accumulation in other organs under systemic settings.

Besides the transport routes mentioned above, cell-mediated transcytosis can also be used for drug delivery across BBB. This approach depends on exploiting the immune cells including neutrophils, macrophages, and monocytes, which are capable of crossing BBB in both healthy and diseased brain. In this strategy, drugs are first loaded into liposome followed by internalization of such liposome in immune cells circulating in the blood. Then those immune cells cross the BBB and migrate to the inflammation sites in the brain by diapedesis and chemotaxis. Cell-mediated transcytosis is also named as 'Trojan horse" strategy.

Despite the presence of transporters or receptors mentioned above, drug delivery across BBB is still challenging due to the presence of tight junction as discussed earlier. This challenge of drug delivery across BBB is further enhanced by some efflux pumps present at the luminal side of brain capillary endothelial cells. The efflux pumps are protein complex in the endothelial cell surface that expel out the hydrophilic anticancer drug molecules such as doxorubicin, daunorubicin etc., against the negative concentration gradient (from blood to brain) in ATP-dependent pathway. Those pumps also prevent accumulation of hydrophobic drugs in the brain capillary endothelial cells by mitigating cellular uptake. P-glycoprotein (P-gp) is class of multidrug resistance proteins, which acts as an efflux pump in drug-resistant tumor. Therefore, regulation of efflux pump at BBB is also another potential strategy for delivering drug to brain tumor, although the efflux pumps positively impact healthy brain by protecting it from harmful neurotoxin.

1.4 Nanoparticles for drug delivery across BBB for combating glioma

Various approaches have been developed to enhance accumulation of chemotherapeutics across BBB. They include both invasive methods such as post-surgical local delivery into the brain [43, 44], convection enhanced delivery [45, 46], and noninvasive method, e.g., temporary opening of the tight junctions by external energy [47], and nanoparticles-mediated delivery [48]. However, application of external energy such as ultrasound [49], osmotic pressure [50], or microbubbles [51] to open BBB via temporary disruption of tight junctions is risky. They hamper integrity of the BBB making CNS susceptible to unwanted toxins or an uncontrolled influx of medicines [52]. To this end, nanoparticles (NPs) drug delivery through the BBB, although challenging, holds significant promise to achieve a reasonable concentration of chemotherapeutics in brain tumor and to avoid unwanted off-target toxicity in other organs.

Over the past few decades, many types of nanocarriers including polymeric, inorganic, liposomes, etc., have been explored for delivery of chemotherapeutics such as small molecules, nucleotides, peptides, proteins to brain tumor. Such NPs are designed to load drugs efficiently, to selectively deliver the payloads to brain tumor crossing the BBB or BBTB by avoiding opsonization followed by clearance by the reticuloendothelial system (RES). Delivery of the NPs across the BBB is broadly mediated by two ways: passive accumulation of plain nanocarriers and active targeting of the BBB or BBTBs via nanocarrier decorated with targeting ligand on their exo-surface [53].

Among polymeric NPs, poly(butylcyanoacrylate) (PBCA) NPs are the first (in 1995) to be used for drug delivery across the BBB [54]. Surface modification of the PBCA NPs by coating with a surfactant polysorbate 80 was reported to enhance their cellular uptake in human and bovine endothelial cells by 20-fold compared with the conventional NPS [55]. The surface coating of PBCA NPs with polysorbate 80 causes absorption of plasma apolipoprotein E (Apo-E), which further enables recognition of the coated NPs by low-density lipoprotein (LDL) receptor expressed in the brain endothelial cells. Thus, the polysorbate 80 coated PBCA NPs are internalized by the brain endothelial cells through LDL receptor-mediated endocytosis [56]. Since then, polysorbate 80 coated nanoparticles of PBCA or other polymers such as PLA, solid lipid nanoparticles (SLNs), SPION NPs are being used to deliver

Nanoparticles	Chemotherapeutics	In vivo model	Outcome	References
Polysorbate 80 coated PBCA nanoparticles	TMZ	Biodistribution in healthy rats	Enhanced uptake of TMZ in brain	[57]
	DOX	Biodistribution in glioma models	Enhanced DOX accumulation in tumor tissue	[58]
	Gemcitabine	Survival analysis in rat glioma model	Prolonged survival of glioma bearing rat	[59]
PLA NPs coated with polysorbate 80	TMZ	Pharmacokinetic and biodistribution in rats	Enhancement in half-life of TMZ with higher deposition in the brain	[60]
SLN NPs coated with polysorbate 80	CPT	Pharmacokinetic and biodistribution in rats	Increased brain accumulation of CPT	[61]
SPION NPs coated with polysorbate 80	DOX	Biodistribution and efficacy in C6/ Sprague Dawley glioma model	Enhanced brain accumulation of SPION and increased anti-tumor efficacy under magnetic field	[62]

Table 1.
Nanocarrier-mediated passive targeting of drug to brain tumor.

different drugs including temozolomide, doxorubicin, gemcitabine, etc., to brain tumor that are listed in **Table 1**.

Solid lipid nanoparticles (SLNs) have also been explored for drug delivery across BBB into glioma via passive lipophilic interaction. Such NPs are demonstrated to stabilize therapeutics such as temozolomide, or RNA-based therapeutics from non-enzymatic degradation in the blood stream. Such NPs also prevent rapid clearance from blood circulation and enhance therapeutics efficacy [63–65]. Also, the positively charged nanoparticles enhance cellular uptake in BBTB cells or glioma cells [65]. In addition, such SLNs and liposomes increase the circulation time and mediate better accumulation in brain tumor via EPR effect [66]. It is worth mentioning here that such NPs are often nontoxic, and they do not hamper BBB integrity, which is consistent with the observed insignificant changes in expression levels of BBB junction proteins occludin and claudin-1 (analyzed by Western blot) in the BBB cells following SLN administration [67]. Similarly, SLNs coated with surfactants such as polysorbate 80 or Brij 78 also enhance BBB permeability and improve drug accumulation in glioma-bearing rat brain [67, 68].

Cell penetrating peptides (CPPs) are also explored for facilitating drug delivery across BBB. For instance, pegylated liposomes decorated with CPP CB5005 in their exo-surface showed better penetration to glioma cells, delivered DOX, and enhanced the survival of animals xenografted with glioblastoma [69]. Other than polymeric NPs and SLNs, additional nanoparticles that have been used for passive delivery of drugs across BBB are listed in **Table 1**.

The most widely used approaches for drug delivery across the BBB is **active targeting** of some receptor or transporter expressed in BBB or BBTB by nanoparticles exo-surface of which is decorated with targeting ligands of such receptors/ transporters (for achieving RMT or AMT to cross the BBB).

Several receptors including transferrin, LDL, GLUT1, integrin receptors, nicotinic acetylcholine, etc., have been employed during the past decades. Transferrin receptor (TfR) and LDLR are the most widely used receptors to facilitate BBB crossing of NPs due to the high affinity of their ligands transferrin and LDL. For instances, using an *in vitro* BBB model, Chang et al. have demonstrated that the uptake of TfR-coated PLGA NPs is 20 times higher than that of non-coated PLGA NPs, and the uptake is mediated via receptor-mediated endocytosis (RMT) [70]. Many other NPs such as gold nanopartcile (AuNP) [71], SPION [72], etc., have also been explored for drug delivery to glioma. For example, conjugation of carbon dots (CDs) with transferrin increased the efficiency of DOX delivery into brain tumor [73]. Transferrin receptor-mediated drug delivery across BBB is reviewed in detail elsewhere [74]. However, the major limitation of using transferrin as a ligand for TfR is that the endogenous transferrin competes with transferrin-tagged NPs for the receptor binding leading to reduced cellular uptake and compromised efficacy of the NPs. To overcome it, antibodies against TfR (such as OX26, R17-217 and 8D3, etc.) that bind TfR at different location other than transferrin are now being used as ligands to graft exo-surface of the NPs. These antibodies exhibit different level affinity and different organ selectivity for the same receptor. For example, uptake of 8D3 in brain is higher than that of R17-217 while both exhibit selectivity toward TfR expressed on the brain over that on the kidney [75].

1.4.1 Transferrin receptor

Transferrin receptors (TfRs) are attractive target for nanocarrier-mediated drug delivery to the brain. TfRs are of two subtypes, TfR1 and TfR2, with high homology in their extracellular domain. TfRs are associated with controlling the extracellular iron levels by using their natural ligand transferrin, which bind to iron directly. These receptors are highly expressed in luminal membrane of brain endothelium and overexpressed in glioma tissues, which make them attractive target for NPs-mediated glioma therapy. There are many reports demonstrating active targeting of nanocarriers decorated with TfR targeting ligand (such as transferrin (Tf) itself, antibodies, or peptides) for combating glioma. For example, Cui et al. have developed a transferrin-conjugated magnetic silica PLGA nanoparticles (MNP-MSN-PLGA-Tf NPs) and have demonstrated that such NPs when loaded with DOX and PTX can effectively inhibit tumor growth in a intracranial U-87 BALB/c nude mice model [76]. In other studies, Tf-conjugated PEG-PLA polymeric NPs are reported to deliver TMZ, which results in prolonged survival of glioma-bearing C6 rat [77]. Guo et al. have reported enhanced glioma growth inhibition in C6 rat when resveratrol was conjugated with Tf-modified PEG-PLA NPs compared with free resveratrol [78].

Other than polymeric nanoparticles, gold nanopartciles (AuNPs), liposomes, polymersomes have also been used for TfR-mediated drug targeting to brain tumor. For instance, Dixit et al. have reported Tf-conjugated AuNPs to deliver a photodynamic prodrug, Pc 4, to mouse brain, which exhibits a significant brain accumulation after 4 h of administration [71]. To overcome the drug resistance of TMZ, Lam e al. have used combination chemotherapy of TMZ and bromodomain inhibitor. They have reported that transferrin-functionalize pegylated liposomes co-loaded with TMZ and bromodomain inhibitor decreased the tumor burden and prolonged survival of glioma-bearing mice compared with the control groups with no significant systemic drug toxicity observed [79]. Tf is also combined with other targeting ligand for double targeting to achieve a better drug targeting efficacy. For instance, a dual-targeting liposomes containing Tf and RGD (ligand for integrin receptor) at their exo-surface have been developed by Qin et al. This dual-targeting liposome

RGD/Tf-LP has shown significantly higher brain tumor accumulation compared with only Tf-conjugated liposome (Tf-LP), which exhibits further much higher brain tumor accumulation than RGD-tagged liposomes (RGD-LP) in BALB/C mice bearing C6 glioma [80]. Tf is also combined with liposome containing cell penetrating peptide TAT on their exo-surface to develop dual-targeting liposome of TAT/Tf-LP. In vivo biodistribution of coumarin-loaded liposomes reveals that the dual-targeting liposomes TAT/Tf-LP have shown significantly higher brain accumulation in comparison with only Tf-LP (1.5 times) and only TAT-LP (~2 times). The anti-GBM effect of DOX-loaded Tf/TAT-LP has been demonstrated by monitoring the survival of U87 GBM-bearing rats. Treatment of DOX-loaded Tf/TAT-LP enhances the median survival of GBM-bearing rat by 59 days where as it was only 10 days for free-DOX-treated rat [81].

Other than transferrin (80 kD protein), antibodies, antibody fragments, and peptides are also used as ligands for TfR-mediated drug targeting to brain via endocytosis and transcytosis on BBB. For instance, OX26, a monoclonal antibody (mAb) against TfR1, was used for the first time in 1992 to examine BBB-crossing ability of the antibody-drug conjugate (ABC) via TfR-mediated transcytosis. This study resulted in similar rate of brain accumulation for free OX26 and drug-conjugated OX26. Recently, Yue et al. have developed an immunomicelle where micelles are covalently linked with OX26 antibody and have demonstrated much higher BBB-crossing ability of the OX26-micelle compared with the free OX26 antibody [82]. Notably, similar two other monoclonal antibodies Ri7 and 8D3 are also developed that can target TfR expressed on BCEC although not yet used in drug delivery to the brain [83]. It is worth mentioning that antibody-toxin conjugates that target TfR have progressed till clinical trial III for anti-glioma therapy. Initially, human Tf is conjugated to a diphtheria toxin with CRM107 point mutation via thioester bond to develop Tf-CRM107 IT, which exhibits higher tumor growth inhibition in preclinical mouse model (U251 tumor-bearing mice) in a dose-dependent manner than the free toxins [84]. Later, a phase I study following intra-tumoral injection reveals no adverse effect leading to a phase II study in recurrent high-grade brain tumor patient where 35% of the patients exhibit tumor response and improved survival. Unfortunately, Tf-CRM107 fails to exhibit superior activity over the standard of care in an early phase III clinical trial, and CNS toxicity is observed, which lead to termination of this trial [85].

Despite the high targeting ability of mAb, difficulty in their preparation and purification in rigorous laboratory condition introduces hurdle in quality control of the mAbs, which further limit real application of mAb-tagged nanoparticles in drug delivery. Alternatively, short peptide fragment of the antibody with similar affinity toward the receptor has been proposed due to its small size and ease of incorporation in nano-formulation. For instance, a heptapeptide T7 (HAIYPRH) has been reported to specifically bind to TfR with high affinity (Kd = 10 nM) comparable to Tf [86]. Using T7 as TfR-targeting ligand, Jiang's group has co-delivered chemotherapeutic DOX and gene therapy agent pORF-hTRAIL to enhance the survivability of U87 tumor-bearing mice [87]. Similarly, Kuang et al., have used another pegylated nanoparticle decorated with T7 to achieve RNAi mediated in BABLB/c mice bearing U87 glioma [88]. In another interesting study by Kawamoto et al., a hybrid peptide containing a targeting peptide (T7 as TfR-targeting peptide) followed by a lytic peptide (therapeutic part) has been developed. Using this hybrid peptide in nano-formulation, this group has reported significant *in vivo* anti-tumor effect in Gl261 glioblastoma-bearing C57 mice without significant cytotoxicity [89]. All these preclinical studies indicate that targeting TfR for drug delivery across BBB may have future clinical potential.

1.4.2 Apolipoprotein receptors

Apolipoprotein receptors, specifically low-density lipoprotein receptor (LDL-R) and LDL-R-related proteins (LRP), which help lipids transportation into CNS [90] are also widely being explored to facilitate drug delivery to the brain tumor. These receptors are overexpressed on the BBB endothelium as well as glioma cells [91] compared with that in healthy brain tissue and thereby explored as potential molecular target for selective drug delivery to combat glioma. Apolipoprotein E (APOE) is the most studied ligand of such receptors used for delivering NPs to the brain. Mainly two strategies of LDL-R-mediated transcytosis are used in APOE-facilitated transport of NPs, which rely on (i) the high avidity of APOE to the NPs and (ii) the conjugation of NPs with APOE or its derivatives on their exo-surface. In the first strategy, NPs are coated with certain surfactant, i.e., polysorbate 80 (PS80) and poloxamer 188, which recruit APOE in the bloodstream for high-affinity-based association with the NPs facilitating their recognition and subsequent transcytosis by LDL-R in the brain parenchyma. Notably, J. Kreuter and his coworkers have significant contribution to reveal the mechanism of such enhanced accumulation of PS80-coated NPs. In a preliminary study, they have found that the concentration of DOX in rat brain 2–4 h post i.v. administration with DOX-loaded PBCA NPs coated with PS80 is 6 μg/g, which is much higher than that treated with non-coated NPs (non-detectable) [92]. Subsequent *in vitro* study shows that PS80-coated PBCA NPs, when incubated in plasma, adsorb apolipoproteins [93]. They further evaluated anti-glioma efficacy of the DOX-loaded PBCA NPs coated with PS80 in glioma model of Wistar rat and observed enhanced survivability of the animals without any neurotoxicity, which is associated with free DOX treatment [94]. Later on, many other groups have used such PS80-coated PBCA NPs for delivering different anticancer drugs such as DOX [94, 95], temozolomide [96], gemcitabine [97], etc., to glioma tissue. However, concerns are raised regarding use of surfactant PS80 due to the possible disruption of the BBB via modulation of the capillary's tight junctions and emerging adverse immune response [98] in rat, which lead to necessity of modification of the surfactant or directly conjugating LDL-R ligand to the NPs.

In the second strategy, the ligand of LDL-R is directly conjugated with the exo-surface of the NPs to achieve LDL receptor-mediated transcytosis. Initially, native LDL lipoprotein is presumed to be an ideal carrier due to its inherent structural core-shell features (highly hydrophobic core surrounded by a hydrophilic shell), which is capable of drug loading in addition to the targeting LDL-R binding domain. However, its challenging purification and limited drug loading capacity of the whole protein trigger development of alternate short binding sequence (synthetic peptides) as targeting ligand. For example, Grafals-Ruiz et al. reported development of gold-liposome nanoparticles grafted with ApoE peptides to achieve systemic delivery of small-nucleic acids (SNA) to glioma-bearing mouse brain [99]. In another study, Zhang et al. have conjugated peptide-22, a ligand of LDL-R, to PEG-PLA NPs for delivering paclitaxel to mouse brain, which enhances the median survivability of glioma-bearing mice [100]. Liposomes functionalized with synthetic ligand of apoB, another ligand of LDL-R, are also demonstrated to enhance drug accumulation in the brain parenchyma and to exhibit significant apoptotic effect in glioma tissue. The involvement of LDL-R is confirmed by using a LDLR inhibitor, namely suramin, which significantly diminishes the apoptotic effect of the NPs when treated in combination [101, 102].

Another receptor of the same family, namely LDL-R related proteins (LRP), has also attracted significant attention for BBB crossing not only due to its high expression level in glioma and BBB but also for its ability to act as a common receptor for other ligands such as lactoferin and melanotransferrin. Specifically, angiopep-2 peptide has attracted huge attention for its potential in glioma therapy [103, 104]. For instance, PTX-loaded PEG-PCL NPs conjugated to angiopep-2 peptide have been demonstrated to enhance survivability by 15% in U87 brain tumor mouse model [105]. Most importantly, a phase I clinical trial with angiopep-2 peptide conjugated to paclitaxel, namely ANG1005, has resulted a stable disease among eight out of 27 patients with a median of 51 days, which triggered its entry in a phase II clinical trial (NCT01967810) for examining its efficacy in patient with high-grade glioma [106]. Furthermore, ANG1005 is very recently demonstrated to exhibit clinical benefit in a phase II clinical trial for treating patient with recurrent brain metastasis from breast cancer [107]. Thus, angiopep-2 is now being considered as one of the leading ligands among the brain-targeting peptide finding its application in conjugation with different NPs to deliver different chemotherapeutics to glioma.

1.4.3 Targeting of adhesion molecules

Cell adhesion molecules (CAMs), other than mediating adhesion of cells to extracellular matrix (ECM), play important roles in tumor development and progression, tumor vasculature development, cellular migration, etc. There are five main classes of CAMs: integrins, cadherins, selectins, the immunoglobulin (Ig) superfamily, and cluster of differentiation (CD) molecules. The different expression level in healthy brain and tumor-bearing brain indicated a potential role of such CAMs in brain tumor and targeting such CAMs in glioma hold promises for antitumor therapy.

1.4.3.1 Integrin-mediated targeting systems

Integrins are heterodimeric transmembrane glycoprotein (cell surface receptors) mediating adhesion of cells to the extracellular matrix or, in some cases, to adjacent cells. Intracellularly, integrins are connected via associated proteins to the actin cytoskeleton. In the human genome, 18 α and 8 β subunits are encoded from 24 different functional integrins. Integrins are directly involved in tumor progression by facilitating angiogenesis (sprouting of new blood vessels) in tumor area and by mediating invasion and migration of both tumor endothelial cells and tumor cells. Thus, such integrin receptors are overexpressed in brain tumor cells and tumor endothelial cells and are attractive target of drug delivery for cancer therapy. RGD is an exogenous peptide ligand (Arg-Gly-Asp amino acid sequence) that can specifically binds $\alpha v\beta 3$, $\alpha v\beta 5$, $\alpha 5\beta 1$ integrin receptors, which are generally overexpressed in tumor and tumor endothelial cells including for brain tumor. Therefore, RGD ligand is widely used for integrin receptor-mediated drug targeting into brain tumor. Zhan et al. are the first to report RGD-mediated drug targeting for combating brain tumor. They have developed cyclic RGDyK-PEG-PLA micelle for delivering PTX to brain tumor and demonstrated that the PTX-loaded micelles (cRGDyK-PEG-PLA-PTX) significantly enhanced the median survival of mice bearing intracranial U87MG tumor xenografts compared with non-targeting micelle (PEG-PLA-PTX) [108]. Similarly, Jian et al. also delivered PTX to the brain of U87MG glioma-bearing Balb/c mice using a integrin-targeting poly(trimethylene carbonate)-based nanoparticles c(RGDyK)–NP, which enhances the median survival of the glioma-bearing mice by 22 days compared with mice treated with free PTX [109]. In another study, McNerny et al., have functionalized poly(amidoamine) (PAMAM) dendrons with cRGDyK at the surface for multivalent binding and with drug molecule to methotrexate to the focal point for achieving anti-glioma efficacy [110]. A multifunctional dual-targeting liposomal system (c(RGDyK)/pHA-LS) containing integrin receptor-targeting RGD moiety and dopamine receptors targeting p-hydroxybenzoic acid (pHA) has also been reported by Belhadj et al. for delivering DOX to intracranial U87MG glioma-bearing BALB/c nude mice [111]. Peiris et al. have developed a nanochain conjugated to cyclic RGD peptide for delivering CNS-1 tumor-bearing athymic nude mice. A 2.6-fold higher DOX accumulation was observed when mice are treated with targeting NPs compared with that of the non-targeted counterpart [112]. Another chemotherapeutic agent Epirubicin is also loaded to an integrin-targeting micelle via a pH-sensitive hydrazone bond (cRGD-Epi/m) by Quader et al. High concentration of epirubicin is observed in brain tumor when mice are treated with cRGD-Epi/m, which eventually lead to inhibition of intracranial glioblastoma growth [113].

Combination of chemotherapeutics is also delivered using integrin receptor-targeting RGD ligand. For example, DOX and PTX are co-delivered in mouse brain tumor by using RGD functionalized Pluronic micelle, which resulted in significant tumor accumulation following in vivo fluorescence [114]. To this end, recently our lab has reported co-delivery of WP-1066, a small-molecule inhibitor of STAT3 and STAT3 siRNA to mouse brain tumor using $\alpha5\beta1$ integrin receptor-targeting RGDK-liposomes [115]. Cellular uptake study in the presence and absence of integrin receptor-specific antibody shows that liposomes of RGDK enter mouse glioblastoma cells GL261 via $\alpha5\beta1$ integrin receptor. The combination of WP-1066 and STAT3 siRNA delivered by RGDK-liposomes significantly inhibits the glioblastoma growth and prolonged the survival of C57 mice bearing Gl261 orthotopic glioblastoma. Collectively, all the aforementioned reports demonstrate potential of integrin receptor-mediated drug delivery for combating brain tumor.

1.4.3.2 Selectin-targeted nanocarriers

Selectins are single-chain transmembrane proteins including E, L, and P selectins, which are involved in cell adhesion via binding of sugar polymers. Selectin has distinct role in tumor inflammation and progression. Tumor cells exhibit cell tethering and rolling via selectin-dependent recognition of carbohydrates ligands to enhance distance during migration. An overexpression of E-selectin is observed in endothelial cells of high-grade glioma, although their definite role is not well established yet. Recently, Ferber et al. have reported that p-selectin is overexpressed not only in tumor endothelial cells but also in glioblastoma cells [116]. Using a dendritic polyglycerol sulfate (dPGS) nanocarrier, this group has delivered paclitaxel (PTX) in combination with a peptidomimetic of the anti-angiogenic protein thrombospondin-1 (TSP-1 PM) to inhibit the tumor growth *in vivo* using both murine and human orthotopic GB mouse models.

1.4.3.3 Connexin-targeted nanocarriers

Connexins, four-transmembrane glycoproteins, are major constituents of gap junction channels. Six connexin subunits assemble to form a hemi channel in the plasma membrane that docks with another such hemi channels of the adjacent cells to assemble the tight junction and mediate cell-cell interaction. A membrane protein connexin 43 (Cx43) is preferentially expressed in brain tumor and peritumoral area. To achieve Cx43-targeted drug delivery, Nukolova et al. have developed Cx43 mAb-conjugated nanogels loaded with cisplatin and using a C6 glioma model, the authors have shown that these nanogels can effectively inhibit tumor growth and significantly enhance the survival of animals while reducing the systemic toxicity of cisplatin [117]. In addition, the same group also functionalized this Cx43-targeting nanogels with another antibody of brain-specific anion transporter (BSAT1) to achieve additional tumor growth inhibition efficacy via dual targeting [118].

1.4.4 Other receptor and transporter-mediated targeting systems

Beyond these receptors mentioned above, there are many other receptors or transporters protein such as insulin receptor, acetylcholine receptor, glucose transporter (GLUT), large amino acid transporter-1, organic cation transporter OCT3 and OCTN2, etc., are expressed on BBB or on tumor cells that are explored for nanocarrier-mediated drug delivery to brain tumor. For example, Zhang et al. reported PEGylated immunoliposomes (PILs) modified with 83-14 mAb to the human insulin receptor to target gene that EGFR gene (which plays a major role in brain tumor progression) in U87 cancer cells [119], and later the same group modified the nanocarrioers with additional transferrin receptor for achieving RNAi in mice intracranially xenografted with human U87 glioma [120]. Nicotine acetylcholine receptors (nAChRs) expressed on BCEC are also targeted for delivering chemotherapeutics to brain tumor. To this end, Saha et al., from our group, have developed a nicotinylated liposomes to deliver small-molecule STAT-3 inhibitor WP-1066 for combating mouse glioblastoma [121]. The same group has also developed another BBB-crossing liposomes grafted with amphetamine at their exo-surface and using this liposome they deliver combination of paclitaxel (PTX) and PD-L1siRNA (RNAi agent for immune checkpoint inhibitor) to the glioblastoma-bearing mouse brain. This combination therapy is reported to enhance the median survival of mouse till 45 days while the untreated control mice died at 17 days [122]. Among transporters, glucose transporters (GLUTs) and large amino acid transporters (LAT-1) are widely used for nanocarrier-mediated drug delivery to brain tumor. During tumor progression, tumor cells continuously need supply of nutrients such as glucose and amino acids, which leads to overexpression of such transporter in glioma cells as well as BBB [123, 124]. Recently, Anraku et al. have developed a self-assembled supramolecular ~30 nm nanocarrier containing multiple glucose molecules via association of oppositely charged pairs of polyethylene glycol (PEG)-based block ionomers. A remarkable enhancement in brain accumulation of the micelle post ~15 min administration is observed, which is much higher than that for other nanoparticles [125]. Bhunia et al. from our group have reported a LAT-1-targeting liposomes containing L-DOPA on their exo-surface (Amphi-DOPA liposome) for delivering small-molecule STAT-3 inhibitor WP-1066 to glioblastoma-bearing mouse brain. A significant tumor growth inhibition is observed when mice are treated with WP-1066-loaded Amphi-DOPA liposomes compared with the untreated or non-targeting control-treated mice [124].

1.5 Conclusion and future perspectives

During the past decades, significant progressed has been made in developing nanocarriers for glioma therapy. Major focus in this research area has been implementation of different ligands or targeting different receptors and transporters overexpressed on BBB and brain tumor cells for delivering the payload to brain tumor tissue. However, less is known about the key critical design parameters of the nanoparticles facilitating BBB crossing. For example, it has been observed that nanocarriers with size 20–30 nm are most effective in BBB crossing while among the different shapes, nanorod is most efficient in BBB crossing followed by spherical nanocarrier. More detail information is needed in future regarding the role of surface potential, formulation or composition, drug loading method, etc., in facilitating transport across BBB. In addition, the factors influencing pharmacokinetic behaviors of the nanocarriers should be well studied and evaluated, which is very crucial for developing an effective brain-targeting drug carrier. The poor prognosis of GBM has also prompted to develop many new therapeutic strategies exploiting inherent physical properties of the nanomaterials such as photodynamic or photothermal therapies and hyperthermia. However, biodegradability and nanotoxicity of such newly developed materials should be studied in detail. In this regard, liposomal or lipid-based nanocarriers exhibit reasonable safety profiles. Furthermore, as brain tumor cells are highly infiltrating, nanocarriers that only deliver the payload to tumor core via leaky BBB are not sufficient, rather an image-guided delivery of therapeutics has attracted significant attention in recent years indicating the need of developing theragnostic nanoparticles. Significant attention should also be paid in enhancing targeting efficiency of the nanocarrier, which is far away from satisfactory yet, either by increasing number of targeting ligand or using high-affinity ligands with optimum ratio.

In conclusion, the following aspects should be considered on designing efficient brain tumor targeting nanocarrier in future:

1. The small nanocarriers with multiple functionalities on the surface and with high fluorescence. The multiple anchoring site can facilitate conjugation with a greater number of same ligands or different ligands specific to multiple receptors and loading of more drug molecules. The fluorescence can facilitate the bioimaging. 2. Biocompatibility of the nanocarriers to eliminate scope of nanotoxicity. 3. Optimum circulation stability and biodegradability of the nanocarriers. 4. Accessibility by noninvasive advanced imaging technique such as magnetic resonance imaging and real-time in vivo microscopy to avoid unnecessary sacrifice of the animal. 5. Application of multiple approaches to develop multimodal nanocarriers for effective BBB penetration followed by chemotherapy and bioimaging.

Author details

Sukanya Bhunia[1]* and Arabinda Chaudhuri[2]

1 Department of Immunology and Nanomedicine, Florida International University, Miami, Florida, USA

2 Department of Chemical Sciences, Indian Institute of Science Education and Research (IISER) Kolkata, Mohanpur, West Bengal, India

*Address all correspondence to: sbhunia@fiu.edu

References

[1] Giese A, Bjerkvig R, Berens ME, Westphal M. Cost of migration: Invasion of malignant gliomas and implications for treatment. Journal of Clinical Oncology. 2003;**21**(8):1624-1636

[2] Rao JS. Molecular mechanisms of glioma invasiveness: The role of proteases. Nature Reviews. Cancer. 2003;**3**(7):489-501

[3] Azevedo FA, Carvalho LR, Grinberg LT, Farfel JM, Ferretti RE, Leite RE, et al. Equal numbers of neuronal and nonneuronal cells make the human brain an isometrically scaled-up primate brain. The Journal of Comparative Neurology. 2009;**513**(5): 532-541

[4] Huynh GH, Deen DF, Szoka FC Jr. Barriers to carrier mediated drug and gene delivery to brain tumors. Journal of Controlled Release. 2006;**110**(2):236-259

[5] Berger MS, Bernstein M. Neuro-Oncology: The Essentials. New York, NY: Thieme Medical Publishers; 2000

[6] Mokri B. The Monro-Kellie hypothesis: Applications in CSF volume depletion. Neurology. 2001;**56**(12): 1746-1748

[7] Ribatti D, Nico B, Crivellato E, Artico M. Development of the blood-brain barrier: A historical point of view. Anatomical Record. Part B, New Anatomist. 2006;**289**(1):3-8

[8] Keaney J, Walsh Dominic M, O'Malley T, Hudson N, Crosbie Darragh E, Loftus T, et al. Autoregulated paracellular clearance of amyloid-β across the blood-brain barrier. Science Advances. 2015;**1**(8):e1500472

[9] Béduneau A, Saulnier P, Benoit JP. Active targeting of brain tumors using nanocarriers. Biomaterials. 2007;**28**(33): 4947-4967

[10] Goldmann EE. Neue untersuchungen über die äussere und innere sekretion des gesunden und kranken organismus im lichte der "vitalen färbung". Deutsche Zeitschrift für Nervenheilkunde. 1912;**117**:403-404

[11] Sohet F, Lin C, Munji RN, Lee SY, Ruderisch N, Soung A, et al. LSR/ angulin-1 is a tricellular tight junction protein involved in blood–brain barrier formation. Journal of Cell Biology. 2015;**208**(6):703-711

[12] Sweeney MD, Sagare AP, Zlokovic BV. Blood-brain barrier breakdown in Alzheimer disease and other neurodegenerative disorders. Nature Reviews. Neurology. 2018;**14**(3): 133-150

[13] Abbott NJ. Astrocyte-endothelial interactions and blood-brain barrier permeability. Journal of Anatomy. 2002;**200**(6):629-638

[14] Persidsky Y, Ramirez SH, Haorah J, Kanmogne GD. Blood-brain barrier: Structural components and function under physiologic and pathologic conditions. Journal of Neuroimmune Pharmacology. 2006;**1**(3):223-236

[15] Abbott NJ, Patabendige AA, Dolman DE, Yusof SR, Begley DJ. Structure and function of the blood-brain barrier. Neurobiology of Disease. 2010;**37**(1):13-25

[16] Yao Y, Chen Z-L, Norris EH, Strickland S. Astrocytic laminin regulates pericyte differentiation and maintains blood brain barrier integrity. Nature Communications. 2014;**5**(1):3413

[17] Schroeter ML, Mertsch K, Giese H, Müller S, Sporbert A, Hickel B, et al. Astrocytes enhance radical defence in capillary endothelial cells constituting the blood-brain barrier. FEBS Letters. 1999;**449**(2-3):241-244

[18] Oddo A, Peng B, Tong Z, Wei Y, Tong WY, Thissen H, et al. Advances in microfluidic blood-brain barrier (BBB) models. Trends in Biotechnology. 2019;**37**(12):1295-1314

[19] Ginhoux F, Lim S, Hoeffel G, Low D, Huber T. Origin and differentiation of microglia. Frontiers in Cellular Neuroscience. 2013;**7**(45)

[20] Daneman R. The blood-brain barrier in health and disease. Annals of Neurology. 2012;**72**(5):648-672

[21] da Fonseca AC, Matias D, Garcia C, Amaral R, Geraldo LH, Freitas C, et al. The impact of microglial activation on blood-brain barrier in brain diseases. Frontiers in Cellular Neuroscience. 2014;**8**:362

[22] Belykh E, Shaffer KV, Lin C, Byvaltsev VA, Preul MC, Chen L. Blood-brain barrier, blood-brain tumor barrier, and fluorescence-guided neurosurgical oncology: Delivering optical labels to brain tumors. 2020;**10**(739)

[23] Weber C, Fraemohs L, Dejana E. The role of junctional adhesion molecules in vascular inflammation. Nature Reviews. Immunology. 2007;**7**(6):467-477

[24] Ebnet K, Suzuki A, Ohno S, Vestweber D. Junctional adhesion molecules (JAMs): More molecules with dual functions? Journal of Cell Science. 2004;**117**(Pt 1):19-29

[25] Garrido-Urbani S, Bradfield PF, Imhof BA. Tight junction dynamics: The role of junctional adhesion molecules (JAMs). Cell and Tissue Research. 2014;**355**(3):701-715

[26] Kniesel U, Wolburg H. Tight junctions of the blood-brain barrier. Cellular and Molecular Neurobiology. 2000;**20**(1):57-76

[27] Furuse M, Hirase T, Itoh M, Nagafuchi A, Yonemura S, Tsukita S, et al. Occludin: A novel integral membrane protein localizing at tight junctions. The Journal of Cell Biology. 1993;**123** (6 Pt 2):1777-1788

[28] Ding S, Khan AI, Cai X, Song Y, Lyu Z, Du D, et al. Overcoming blood–brain barrier transport: Advances in nanoparticle-based drug delivery strategies. Materials Today. 2020;**37**: 112-125

[29] Rustenhoven J, Jansson D, Smyth LC, Dragunow M. Brain pericytes as mediators of neuroinflammation. Trends in Pharmacological Sciences. 2017;**38**(3):291-304

[30] Spéder P, Brand AH. Gap junction proteins in the blood-brain barrier control nutrient-dependent reactivation of Drosophila neural stem cells. Developmental Cell. 2014;**30**(3): 309-321

[31] Zhang T-T, Li W, Meng G, Wang P, Liao W. Strategies for transporting nanoparticles across the blood–brain barrier. Biomaterials Science. 2016;**4**(2):219-229

[32] Watkins S, Robel S, Kimbrough IF, Robert SM, Ellis-Davies G, Sontheimer H. Disruption of astrocyte-vascular coupling and the blood-brain barrier by invading glioma cells. Nature Communications. 2014;**5**:4196

[33] Dubois LG, Campanati L, Righy C, D'Andrea-Meira I, Spohr TC, Porto-Carreiro I, et al. Gliomas and the vascular fragility of the blood brain barrier. Frontiers in Cellular Neuroscience. 2014;**8**:418

[34] Achrol AS, Rennert RC, Anders C, Soffietti R, Ahluwalia MS, Nayak L, et al. Brain metastases. Nature Reviews. Disease Primers. 2019;**5**(1):5

[35] Ratnam NM, Gilbert MR, Giles AJ. Immunotherapy in CNS cancers: The role of immune cell trafficking. Neuro-Oncology. 2019;**21**(1):37-46

[36] Hobbs SK, Monsky WL, Yuan F, Roberts WG, Griffith L, Torchilin VP, et al. Regulation of transport pathways in tumor vessels: Role of tumor type and microenvironment. Proceedings of the National Academy of Sciences of the United States of America. 1998;**95**(8): 4607-4612

[37] Sarin H, Kanevsky AS, Wu H, Brimacombe KR, Fung SH, Sousa AA, et al. Effective transvascular delivery of nanoparticles across the blood-brain tumor barrier into malignant glioma cells. Journal of Translational Medicine. 2008;**6**:80

[38] van Tellingen O, Yetkin-Arik B, de Gooijer MC, Wesseling P, Wurdinger T, de Vries HE. Overcoming the blood-brain tumor barrier for effective glioblastoma treatment. Drug Resistance Updates. 2015;**19**:1-12

[39] Schlachetzki F, Zhang Y, Boado RJ, Pardridge WM. Gene therapy of the brain: The trans-vascular approach. Neurology. 2004;**62**(8):1275-1281

[40] Zhou Y, Peng Z, Seven ES, Leblanc RM. Crossing the blood-brain barrier with nanoparticles. Journal of Controlled Release. 2018;**270**:290-303

[41] Burek M, Förster CY. Culturing of rodent brain microvascular endothelial cells for in vitro modeling of the blood-brain barrier. In: Barichello T, editor. Blood-Brain Barrier. New York, NY: Springer New York; 2019. pp. 45-54

[42] Nitta T, Hata M, Gotoh S, Seo Y, Sasaki H, Hashimoto N, et al. Size-selective loosening of the blood-brain barrier in claudin-5-deficient mice. The Journal of Cell Biology. 2003;**161**(3): 653-660

[43] Bastiancich C, Vanvarenberg K, Ucakar B, Pitorre M, Bastiat G, Lagarce F, et al. Lauroyl-gemcitabine-loaded lipid nanocapsule hydrogel for the treatment of glioblastoma. Journal of Controlled Release. 2016;**225**:283-293

[44] Bastiancich C, Lemaire L, Bianco J, Franconi F, Danhier F, Préat V, et al. Evaluation of lauroyl-gemcitabine-loaded hydrogel efficacy in glioblastoma rat models. Nanomedicine (London, England). 2018;**13**(16):1999-2013

[45] Lollo G, Vincent M, Ullio-Gamboa G, Lemaire L, Franconi F, Couez D, et al. Development of multifunctional lipid nanocapsules for the co-delivery of paclitaxel and CpG-ODN in the treatment of glioblastoma. International Journal of Pharmaceutics. 2015;**495**(2):972-980

[46] Lopez-Bertoni H, Kozielski KL, Rui Y, Lal B, Vaughan H, Wilson DR, et al. Bioreducible polymeric nanoparticles containing multiplexed cancer stem cell regulating miRNAs inhibit glioblastoma growth and prolong survival. Nano Letters. 2018;**18**(7):4086-4094

[47] Landhuis E. Ultrasound for the brain. Nature. 2017;**551**(7679):257-259

[48] Koo YE, Reddy GR, Bhojani M, Schneider R, Philbert MA, Rehemtulla A, et al. Brain cancer diagnosis and therapy with nanoplatforms. Advanced Drug Delivery Reviews. 2006;**58**(14):1556-1577

[49] Chu P-C, Chai W-Y, Tsai C-H, Kang S-T, Yeh C-K, Liu H-L. Focused ultrasound-induced blood-brain barrier opening: Association with mechanical index and cavitation index analyzed by dynamic contrast-enhanced magnetic-resonance imaging. Scientific Reports. 2016;**6**:33264-33264

[50] Gumerlock MK, Belshe BD, Madsen R, Watts C. Osmotic blood-brain barrier disruption and chemotherapy in the treatment of high grade malignant glioma: Patient series and literature review. Journal of Neuro-Oncology. 1992;**12**(1):33-46

[51] Wu SK, Chu PC, Chai WY, Kang ST, Tsai CH, Fan CH, et al. Characterization

of different microbubbles in assisting focused ultrasound-induced blood-brain barrier opening. Scientific Reports. 2017;7:46689

[52] Upadhyay RK. Drug delivery systems, CNS protection, and the blood brain barrier. BioMed Research International. 2014;**2014**:869269

[53] Gastaldi L, Battaglia L, Peira E, Chirio D, Muntoni E, Solazzi I, et al. Solid lipid nanoparticles as vehicles of drugs to the brain: Current state of the art. European Journal of Pharmaceutics and Biopharmaceutics. 2014;**87**(3):433-444

[54] Kreuter J, Alyautdin RN, Kharkevich DA, Ivanov AA. Passage of peptides through the blood-brain barrier with colloidal polymer particles (nanoparticles). Brain Research. 1995;**674**(1):171-174

[55] Ramge P, Unger RE, Oltrogge JB, Zenker D, Begley D, Kreuter J, et al. Polysorbate-80 coating enhances uptake of polybutylcyanoacrylate (PBCA)-nanoparticles by human and bovine primary brain capillary endothelial cells. The European Journal of Neuroscience. 2000;**12**(6):1931-1940

[56] Kulkarni PV, Roney CA, Antich PP, Bonte FJ, Raghu AV, Aminabhavi TM. Quinoline-n-butylcyanoacrylate-based nanoparticles for brain targeting for the diagnosis of Alzheimer's disease. Wiley Interdisciplinary Reviews. Nanomedicine and Nanobiotechnology. 2010;**2**(1):35-47

[57] Tian XH, Lin XN, Wei F, Feng W, Huang ZC, Wang P, et al. Enhanced brain targeting of temozolomide in polysorbate-80 coated polybutylcyanoacrylate nanoparticles. International Journal of Nanomedicine. 2011;**6**:445-452

[58] Ambruosi A, Khalansky AS, Yamamoto H, Gelperina SE, Begley DJ, Kreuter J. Biodistribution of polysorbate 80-coated doxorubicin-loaded [14C]-poly(butyl cyanoacrylate) nanoparticles after intravenous administration to glioblastoma-bearing rats. Journal of Drug Targeting. 2006;**14**(2):97-105

[59] Wang CX, Huang LS, Hou LB, Jiang L, Yan ZT, Wang YL, et al. Antitumor effects of polysorbate-80 coated gemcitabine polybutylcyanoacry late nanoparticles in vitro and its pharmacodynamics in vivo on C6 glioma cells of a brain tumor model. Brain Research. 2009;**1261**:91-99

[60] Jain D, Bajaj A, Athawale R, Shrikhande S, Goel PN, Nikam Y, et al. Surface-coated PLA nanoparticles loaded with temozolomide for improved brain deposition and potential treatment of gliomas: development, characterization and in vivo studies. Drug Delivery. 2016;**23**(3):999-1016

[61] Martins SM, Sarmento B, Nunes C, Lúcio M, Reis S, Ferreira DC. Brain targeting effect of camptothecin-loaded solid lipid nanoparticles in rat after intravenous administration. European Journal of Pharmaceutics and Biopharmaceutics: Official Journal of Arbeitsgemeinschaft fur Pharmazeutische Verfahrenstechnik e. V. 2013;**85**(3 Pt A):488-502

[62] Xu H-L, Mao K-L, Huang Y-P, Yang J-J, Xu J, Chen P-P, et al. Glioma-targeted superparamagnetic iron oxide nanoparticles as drug-carrying vehicles for theranostic effects. Nanoscale. 2016;**8**(29):14222-14236

[63] Chen Z, Lai X, Song S, Zhu X, Zhu J. Nanostructured lipid carriers based temozolomide and gene co-encapsulated nanomedicine for gliomatosis cerebri combination therapy. Drug Delivery. 2016;**23**(4):1369-1373

[64] Wu M, Fan Y, Lv S, Xiao B, Ye M, Zhu X. Vincristine and temozolomide combined chemotherapy for the

treatment of glioma: A comparison of solid lipid nanoparticles and nanostructured lipid carriers for dual drugs delivery. Drug Delivery. 2016;**23**(8):2720-2725

[65] Jin J, Bae KH, Yang H, Lee SJ, Kim H, Kim Y, et al. In vivo specific delivery of c-Met siRNA to glioblastoma using cationic solid lipid nanoparticles. Bioconjugate Chemistry. 2011;**22**(12): 2568-2572

[66] Tapeinos C, Battaglini M, Ciofani G. Advances in the design of solid lipid nanoparticles and nanostructured lipid carriers for targeting brain diseases. Journal of Controlled Release. 2017;**264**:306-332

[67] de Mendoza E-HA, Préat V, Mollinedo F, Blanco-Prieto MJ. In vitro and in vivo efficacy of edelfosine-loaded lipid nanoparticles against glioma. Journal of Controlled Release. 2011;**156**(3):421-426

[68] Koziara JM, Lockman PR, Allen DD, Mumper RJ. Paclitaxel nanoparticles for the potential treatment of brain tumors. Journal of Controlled Release. 2004;**99**(2):259-269

[69] Zhang Y, Zhang L, Hu Y, Jiang K, Li Z, Lin YZ, et al. Cell-permeable NF-κB inhibitor-conjugated liposomes for treatment of glioma. Journal of Controlled Release. 2018;**289**:102-113

[70] Chang J, Jallouli Y, Kroubi M, Yuan XB, Feng W, Kang CS, et al. Characterization of endocytosis of transferrin-coated PLGA nanoparticles by the blood-brain barrier. International Journal of Pharmaceutics. 2009;**379**(2):285-292

[71] Dixit S, Novak T, Miller K, Zhu Y, Kenney ME, Broome A-M. Transferrin receptor-targeted theranostic gold nanoparticles for photosensitizer delivery in brain tumors. Nanoscale. 2015;**7**(5):1782-1790

[72] Jiang W, Xie H, Ghoorah D, Shang Y, Shi H, Liu F, et al. Conjugation of Functionalized SPIONs with Transferrin for Targeting and Imaging Brain Glial Tumors in Rat Model. PLoS One. 2012;**7**(5):e37376

[73] Li S, Amat D, Peng Z, Vanni S, Raskin S, De Angulo G, et al. Transferrin conjugated nontoxic carbon dots for doxorubicin delivery to target pediatric brain tumor cells. Nanoscale. 2016;**8**(37):16662-16669

[74] Choudhury H, Pandey M, Chin PX, Phang YL, Cheah JY, Ooi SC, et al. Transferrin receptors-targeting nanocarriers for efficient targeted delivery and transcytosis of drugs into the brain tumors: A review of recent advancements and emerging trends. Drug Delivery and Translational Research. 2018;**8**(5):1545-1563

[75] Lee HJ, Engelhardt B, Lesley J, Bickel U, Pardridge WM. Targeting rat anti-mouse transferrin receptor monoclonal antibodies through blood-brain barrier in mouse. The Journal of Pharmacology and Experimental Therapeutics. 2000;**292**(3): 1048-1052

[76] Cui Y, Xu Q, Chow PK, Wang D, Wang CH. Transferrin-conjugated magnetic silica PLGA nanoparticles loaded with doxorubicin and paclitaxel for brain glioma treatment. Biomaterials. 2013;**34**(33): 8511-8520

[77] Sun T, Wu H, Li Y, Huang Y, Yao L, Chen X, et al. Targeting transferrin receptor delivery of temozolomide for a potential glioma stem cell-mediated therapy. Oncotarget. 2017;**8**(43): 74451-74465

[78] Guo W, Li A, Jia Z, Yuan Y, Dai H, Li H. Transferrin modified PEG-PLA-resveratrol conjugates: in vitro and in vivo studies for glioma. European Journal of Pharmacology. 2013;**718**(1-3):41-47

[79] Lam FC, Morton SW, Wyckoff J, Vu Han TL, Hwang MK, Maffa A, et al. Enhanced efficacy of combined temozolomide and bromodomain inhibitor therapy for gliomas using targeted nanoparticles. Nature Communications. 2018;**9**(1):1991

[80] Qin L, Wang CZ, Fan HJ, Zhang CJ, Zhang HW, Lv MH, et al. A dual-targeting liposome conjugated with transferrin and arginine-glycine-aspartic acid peptide for glioma-targeting therapy. Oncology Letters. 2014;**8**(5):2000-2006

[81] Zheng C, Ma C, Bai E, Yang K, Xu R. Transferrin and cell-penetrating peptide dual-functioned liposome for targeted drug delivery to glioma. International Journal of Clinical and Experimental Medicine. 2015;**8**(2):1658-1668

[82] Yue J, Liu S, Wang R, Hu X, Xie Z, Huang Y, et al. Fluorescence-labeled immunomicelles: Preparation, in vivo biodistribution, and ability to cross the blood-brain barrier. Macromolecular Bioscience. 2012;**12**(9):1209-1219

[83] Paris-Robidas S, Emond V, Tremblay C, Soulet D, Calon F. In vivo labeling of brain capillary endothelial cells after intravenous injection of monoclonal antibodies targeting the transferrin receptor. Molecular Pharmacology. 2011;**80**(1):32-39

[84] Laske DW, Ilercil O, Akbasak A, Youle RJ, Oldfield EH. Efficacy of direct intratumoral therapy with targeted protein toxins for solid human gliomas in nude mice. Journal of Neurosurgery. 1994;**80**(3):520-526

[85] Weaver M, Laske DW. Transferrin receptor ligand-targeted toxin conjugate (Tf-CRM107) for therapy of malignant gliomas. Journal of Neuro-Oncology. 2003;**65**(1):3-13

[86] Du W, Fan Y, Zheng N, He B, Yuan L, Zhang H, et al. Transferrin receptor specific nanocarriers conjugated with functional 7peptide for oral drug delivery. Biomaterials. 2013;**34**(3):794-806

[87] Liu S, Guo Y, Huang R, Li J, Huang S, Kuang Y, et al. Gene and doxorubicin co-delivery system for targeting therapy of glioma. Biomaterials. 2012;**33**(19):4907-4916

[88] Kuang Y, An S, Guo Y, Huang S, Shao K, Liu Y, et al. T7 peptide-functionalized nanoparticles utilizing RNA interference for glioma dual targeting. International Journal of Pharmaceutics. 2013;**454**(1):11-20

[89] Kawamoto M, Horibe T, Kohno M, Kawakami K. A novel transferrin receptor-targeted hybrid peptide disintegrates cancer cell membrane to induce rapid killing of cancer cells. BMC Cancer. 2011;**11**:359

[90] Mahley RW. Central nervous system lipoproteins: Apoe and regulation of cholesterol metabolism. Arteriosclerosis, Thrombosis, and Vascular Biology. 2016;**36**(7):1305-1315

[91] Maletínská L, Blakely EA, Bjornstad KA, Deen DF, Knoff LJ, Forte TM. Human glioblastoma cell lines: Levels of low-density lipoprotein receptor and low-density lipoprotein receptor-related protein. Cancer Research. 2000;**60**(8):2300-2303

[92] Gulyaev AE, Gelperina SE, Skidan IN, Antropov AS, Kivman GY, Kreuter J. Significant transport of doxorubicin into the brain with polysorbate 80-coated nanoparticles. Pharmaceutical Research. 1999;**16**(10): 1564-1569

[93] Nuisin R, Krongsin J, Noppakundilograt S, Kiatkamjornwong S. Microencapsulation of menthol by crosslinked chitosan via porous glass membrane emulsification technique and their controlled release properties. Journal of Microencapsulation. 2013;**30**(5):498-509

[94] Steiniger SC, Kreuter J, Khalansky AS, Skidan IN, Bobruskin AI, Smirnova ZS, et al. Chemotherapy of glioblastoma in rats using doxorubicin-loaded nanoparticles. International Journal of Cancer. 2004;**109**(5):759-767

[95] Kreuter J. Nanoparticulate systems for brain delivery of drugs. Advanced Drug Delivery Reviews. 2001;**47**(1):65-81

[96] Nam L, Coll C, Erthal LCS, de la Torre C, Serrano D, Martínez-Máñez R, et al. Drug delivery nanosystems for the localized treatment of glioblastoma multiforme. Materials (Basel). 2018;**11**(5)

[97] Alyaudtin RN, Reichel A, Löbenberg R, Ramge P, Kreuter J, Begley DJ. Interaction of poly(butylcyanoacrylate) nanoparticles with the blood-brain barrier in vivo and in vitro. Journal of Drug Targeting. 2001;**9**(3):209-221

[98] Kim HR, Andrieux K, Gil S, Taverna M, Chacun H, Desmaële D, et al. Translocation of poly(ethylene glycol-co-hexadecyl)cyanoacrylate nanoparticles into rat brain endothelial cells: Role of apolipoproteins in receptor-mediated endocytosis. Biomacromolecules. 2007;**8**(3):793-799

[99] Grafals-Ruiz N, Rios-Vicil CI, Lozada-Delgado EL, Quiñones-Díaz BI, Noriega-Rivera RA, Martínez-Zayas G, et al. Brain targeted gold liposomes improve RNAi delivery for glioblastoma. International Journal of Nanomedicine. 2020;**15**:2809-2828

[100] Zhang B, Sun X, Mei H, Wang Y, Liao Z, Chen J, et al. LDLR-mediated peptide-22-conjugated nanoparticles for dual-targeting therapy of brain glioma. Biomaterials. 2013;**34**(36):9171-9182

[101] Nikanjam M, Gibbs AR, Hunt CA, Budinger TF, Forte TM. Synthetic nano-LDL with paclitaxel oleate as a targeted drug delivery vehicle for glioblastoma multiforme. Journal of Controlled Release. 2007;**124**(3):163-171

[102] Nikanjam M, Blakely EA, Bjornstad KA, Shu X, Budinger TF, Forte TM. Synthetic nano-low density lipoprotein as targeted drug delivery vehicle for glioblastoma multiforme. International Journal of Pharmaceutics. 2007;**328**(1):86-94

[103] Ruan S, Yuan M, Zhang L, Hu G, Chen J, Cun X, et al. Tumor microenvironment sensitive doxorubicin delivery and release to glioma using angiopep-2 decorated gold nanoparticles. Biomaterials. 2015;**37**:425-435

[104] Li Y, Zheng X, Gong M, Zhang J. Delivery of a peptide-drug conjugate targeting the blood brain barrier improved the efficacy of paclitaxel against glioma. Oncotarget. 2016;7(48):79401-79407

[105] Xin H, Sha X, Jiang X, Zhang W, Chen L, Fang X. Anti-glioblastoma efficacy and safety of paclitaxel-loading Angiopep-conjugated dual targeting PEG-PCL nanoparticles. Biomaterials. 2012;**33**(32):8167-8176

[106] Kurzrock R, Gabrail N, Chandhasin C, Moulder S, Smith C, Brenner A, et al. Safety, pharmacokinetics, and activity of GRN1005, a novel conjugate of angiopep-2, a peptide facilitating brain penetration, and paclitaxel, in patients with advanced solid tumors. Molecular Cancer Therapeutics. 2012;**11**(2):308-316

[107] Kumthekar P, Tang SC, Brenner AJ, Kesari S, Piccioni DE, Anders C, et al. ANG1005, a brain-penetrating peptide-drug conjugate, shows activity in patients with breast cancer with leptomeningeal carcinomatosis and recurrent brain metastases. Clinical Cancer Research. 2020;**26**(12):2789-2799

[108] Zhan C, Gu B, Xie C, Li J, Liu Y, Lu W. Cyclic RGD conjugated

poly(ethylene glycol)-co-poly(lactic acid) micelle enhances paclitaxel anti-glioblastoma effect. Journal of Controlled Release. 2010;**143**(1):136-142

[109] Jiang X, Sha X, Xin H, Xu X, Gu J, Xia W, et al. Integrin-facilitated transcytosis for enhanced penetration of advanced gliomas by poly(trimethylene carbonate)-based nanoparticles encapsulating paclitaxel. Biomaterials. 2013;**34**(12):2969-2979

[110] McNerny DQ, Kukowska-Latallo JF, Mullen DG, Wallace JM, Desai AM, Shukla R, et al. RGD dendron bodies; synthetic avidity agents with defined and potentially interchangeable effector sites that can substitute for antibodies. Bioconjugate Chemistry. 2009;**20**(10): 1853-1859

[111] Belhadj Z, Zhan C, Ying M, Wei X, Xie C, Yan Z, et al. Multifunctional targeted liposomal drug delivery for efficient glioblastoma treatment. Oncotarget. 2017;**8**(40):66889-66900

[112] Peiris PM, Abramowski A, McGinnity J, Doolittle E, Toy R, Gopalakrishnan R, et al. Treatment of invasive brain tumors using a chain-like nanoparticle. Cancer Research. 2015;**75**(7):1356-1365

[113] Quader S, Liu X, Chen Y, Mi P, Chida T, Ishii T, et al. cRGD peptide-installed epirubicin-loaded polymeric micelles for effective targeted therapy against brain tumors. Journal of Controlled Release. 2017;**258**:56-66

[114] Huang Y, Liu W, Gao F, Fang X, Chen Y. c(RGDyK)-decorated Pluronic micelles for enhanced doxorubicin and paclitaxel delivery to brain glioma. International Journal of Nanomedicine. 2016;**11**:1629-1641

[115] Vangala V, Nimmu NV, Khalid S, Kuncha M, Sistla R, Banerjee R, et al. Combating glioblastoma by codelivering the small-molecule inhibitor of STAT3 and STAT3siRNA with α5β1 integrin receptor-selective liposomes. Molecular Pharmaceutics. 2020;**17**(6):1859-1874

[116] Ferber S, Tiram G, Sousa-Herves A, Eldar-Boock A, Krivitsky A, Scomparin A, et al. Co-targeting the tumor endothelium and P-selectin-expressing glioblastoma cells leads to a remarkable therapeutic outcome. eLife. 2017;**6**

[117] Nukolova NV, Baklaushev VP, Abakumova TO, Mel'nikov PA, Abakumov MA, Yusubalieva GM, et al. Targeted delivery of cisplatin by connexin 43 vector nanogels to the focus of experimental glioma C6. Bulletin of Experimental Biology and Medicine. 2014;**157**(4):524-529

[118] Baklaushev VP, Nukolova NN, Khalansky AS, Gurina OI, Yusubalieva GM, Grinenko NP, et al. Treatment of glioma by cisplatin-loaded nanogels conjugated with monoclonal antibodies against Cx43 and BSAT1. Drug Delivery. 2015;**22**(3):276-285

[119] Zhang Y, Jeong Lee H, Boado RJ, Pardridge WM. Receptor-mediated delivery of an antisense gene to human brain cancer cells. The Journal of Gene Medicine. 2002;**4**(2):183-194

[120] Zhang Y, Zhang YF, Bryant J, Charles A, Boado RJ, Pardridge WM. Intravenous RNA interference gene therapy targeting the human epidermal growth factor receptor prolongs survival in intracranial brain cancer. Clinical Cancer Research. 2004;**10**(11): 3667-3677

[121] Saha S, Venu Y, Bhattacharya D, Kompella SD, Madhusudana K, Chakravarty S, et al. Combating established mouse glioblastoma through nicotinylated-liposomes-mediated targeted chemotherapy in combination with dendritic-cell-based genetic immunization. Advanced Biosystems. 2017;**1**(1-2):1600009

[122] Saha S, Yakati V, Shankar G, Jaggarapu MMCS, Moku G, Madhusudana K, et al. Amphetamine decorated cationic lipid nanoparticles cross the blood–brain barrier: Therapeutic promise for combating glioblastoma. Journal of Materials Chemistry B. 2020;**8**(19):4318-4330

[123] Patching SG. Glucose transporters at the blood-brain barrier: Function, regulation and gateways for drug delivery. Molecular Neurobiology. 2017;**54**(2):1046-1077

[124] Bhunia S, Vangala V, Bhattacharya D, Ravuri HG, Kuncha M, Chakravarty S, et al. Large amino acid transporter 1 Selective liposomes of l-DOPA functionalized amphiphile for combating glioblastoma. Molecular Pharmaceutics. 2017;**14**(11):3834-3847

[125] Anraku Y, Kuwahara H, Fukusato Y, Mizoguchi A, Ishii T, Nitta K, et al. Glycaemic control boosts glucosylated nanocarrier crossing the BBB into the brain. Nature Communications. 2017;**8**(1):1001